REVISED
AND UPDATED

MAYO CLINIC GUIDE TO ARTHRITIS

MANAGING JOINT PAIN FOR AN ACTIVE LIFE

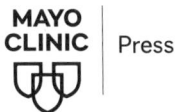

MAYO CLINIC | Press

COURTNEY A. ARMENT, M.D.

Medical Editor

Courtney A. Arment, M.D.

Contributors

Brent A. Bauer, M.D.

Joshua S. Bingham, M.D.

Jen M. Davison, M.D., M.P.H.

Kostas J. Economopoulos, M.D.

Floranne C. Ernste, M.D.

Ali A. Duarte Garcia, M.D.

Alicia M. Hinze, M.D., M.H.S.

Anushka Irani, B.M.B.Ch., Ph.D.

Stephanie N. Kannas, C.H.T., O.T.

Edward R. Laskowski, M.D.

Elena Myasoedova, M.D., Ph.D.

Amir B. Orandi, M.D.

Ashley O. Otto, Pharm.D., R.Ph.

Cassie L. Ramel, Pharm.D., R.Ph.

David Raslau, M.D., M.P.H.

Griffin J. Reed, M.D.

Christopher D. Sletten, Ph.D., L.P.

Can M. Sungur, M.D., Ph.D.

Kenneth J. Warrington, M.D.

Kerry Wright, M.B.B.S.

Katherine A. Zeratsky, R.D.N., L.D.

The medical information in this book is true and complete to the best of our knowledge. This book is intended only as an informative guide for those wishing to learn more about health issues. It is not intended to replace, countermand or conflict with advice given to you by your own physician. The ultimate decision concerning your care should be made between you and your healthcare team. Information in this book is offered with no guarantees. The author and publisher disclaim all liability in connection with the use of this book. Any references to specific products, processes or services by trade name, trademark, manufacturer or otherwise do not constitute or imply endorsement, recommendation or favoring by Mayo Clinic.

Proceeds from the sale of every book benefit important medical research and education at Mayo Clinic.

To stay informed about Mayo Clinic Press, subscribe to our free e-newsletter at MCPress.MayoClinic.org or follow us on social media. For bulk sales contact Mayo Clinic at SpecialSalesMayoBooks@mayo.edu.

Image Credits All photographs and illustrations are copyright of Mayo Foundation for Medical Education and Research (MFMER) except for the following: Cover image credits: vejaa/iStock/Getty Images Plus

MAYO CLINIC PRESS

200 First St. SW

Rochester, MN 55905

MCPress.MayoClinic.org

ISBN 9798887702858 (hardcover) |
ISBN 9798887702865 (ebook)

Library of Congress Control Number: 2025017265

Library of Congress Cataloging-in-Publication Data is available upon request.

Printed in China

First printing: 2026

Contents

From the editor

Every day at Mayo Clinic, I try to help patients to live full and comfortable lives. In updating this new edition of *Mayo Clinic Guide to Arthritis*, I also had my own family in mind. My middle name was given in honor of my great-aunt Alice, and growing up, I was curious about this person who left a lasting impression. Through stories, I heard about Alice's genuine love and interest in her niece, my mom. I also learned of her crippling rheumatoid arthritis, the impact it had on her daily life and that it caused her to die too young. Those stories reflected the love and invaluable support of Alice's family. Alice's brother Ted also passed away early in life due to systemic lupus erythematosus, another rheumatologic disease. While I was not fortunate enough to get to meet my great aunt and uncle, their legacy and that of their loving family lives on.

Thankfully, with advances in medical care, the impact of these diseases on functioning and longevity has dramatically improved over the years. Doctors have more tools than ever to help people with joint pain — effectively treating pain symptoms, caring for mental health and putting the disease into remission. What has not changed over time is the importance of connection and of continuing the activities and relationships you value.

In that sentiment, I give a hearty thank you to the medical editor of the prior edition, Dr. Lynne Peterson. Her fingerprint remains throughout this book, and her legacy in rheumatology care continues to inspire. I also thank many colleagues who contributed to this update, bringing Mayo Clinic's expertise and person-centered care to every page. I hope this book can help empower anyone affected by arthritis to get the care and support they need.

In these pages you'll find the latest information regarding different types of arthritis, available treatments and ways to manage your symptoms so you can keep — or get back to — doing what you love. Part 1 introduces the different types of arthritis and the difference between inflammatory and noninflammatory arthritis. Also covered are common musculoskeletal and spine disorders, childhood arthritis, and pain conditions. In addition, Chapter 9 describes tests and medical specialists that may be helpful in diagnosing and treating arthritis.

In Part 2, you'll find information on different treatment options. Simple, clear explanations cover a wide range of medications, surgeries, injections and holistic therapies to help with joint pain.

Part 3 is a guide to living as normally as possible while managing arthritis. Chapters highlight expert tips for being active, eating well, managing your mental health, protecting your joints, boosting your immune system and managing the disease in daily life.

Sometimes arthritis can make every day a struggle. But this book aims to give you hope. When you understand the disease and how to manage it, you can be an active partner in improving your symptoms so you can focus on the activities, people and life you love.

Courtney Alice Arment, M.D.

Courtney A. Arment, M.D., is a rheumatologist at Mayo Clinic in Rochester, Minnesota, and an assistant professor at Mayo Clinic College of Medicine and Science. Her clinical focus includes inflammatory arthritis, such as rheumatoid arthritis, psoriatic arthritis, ankylosing spondylitis, spondyloarthropathy, gout and other crystalline arthritis. She enjoys helping patients understand their disease and empowering patients to become partners in managing their health. Dr. Arment is also active in research and education, providing mentorship to residents and fellows.

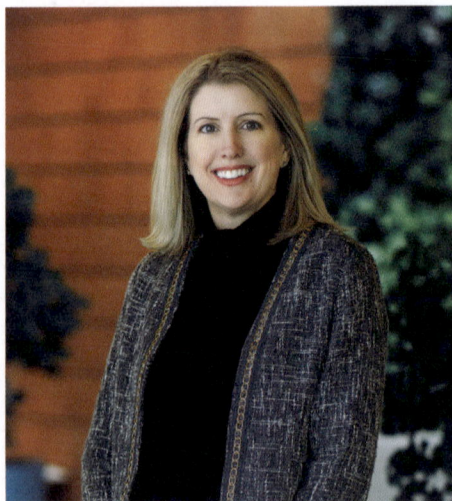

1

Arthritis — Common and complex

When your joints are working smoothly, it's easy to take them for granted. But when they begin to ache, you take notice. If you've ever experienced pain, stiffness, swelling and difficulty moving because of arthritis, you're not alone.

Arthritis is a common condition, affecting about 1 in 5 adults in the United States. About 54 million Americans, including around 220,000 children, have been diagnosed with some form of the disease. And research suggests that the number of people affected by arthritis may be much higher if you include those who have symptoms but haven't been officially diagnosed.

Arthritis is one of the leading causes of disability in the United States. The costs for medical care and lost productivity due to arthritis amount to hundreds of billions of dollars annually. And as the population ages, the number of people with arthritis is expected to increase.

Although people often think of arthritis as one disease, it's not. The term refers to many diseases that can cause joint pain or stiffness, damage to the structure of a joint, or loss of joint function. The word *arthritis* is a blend of the Greek *arthron* + *-itis*, which literally means "joint inflammation." However, the term is commonly used to refer to any disease of the joints.

A WORD ON INFLAMMATION

Inflammation is the body's normal response to infection or injury. To fight infection, the immune system releases chemicals that stimulate a reaction, causing warmth, swelling and pain. But some diseases trigger an abnormal response creating ongoing (chronic) inflammation.

Arthritis occurs in more than 100 different forms. Some forms develop gradually due to the natural wear of joints, while others appear suddenly and then disappear, recurring later. Other forms of arthritis are chronic and progressive, getting worse over time. Signs and symptoms can vary a great deal from one person to another, even if both individuals have the same form of the disease.

The most common symptoms of arthritis are pain while using the affected joints and joint stiffness after periods of rest or inactivity. But many arthritic disorders affect more than your joints. They can also affect the muscles, tendons and ligaments surrounding and supporting the joints, as well as your skin and other organs, such as the lungs, heart, bowel, brain, liver and kidneys.

Although there's no cure for arthritis, treatment options are far ahead of what was available just a decade or two ago, and new research offers hope of even better therapies. Getting the right treatment early on can help prevent joint damage and mobility problems. You can also take steps at home to prevent arthritis or minimize its effects. By actively

WHAT IS RHEUMATISM?

If your grandparents had achy joints, they might have talked about the "rheumatism" in their bones. Rheumatism is an older term used to describe the pain and stiffness of arthritis. Both words — *rheumatism* and *arthritis* — are often used in a general way to describe joint problems.

In fact, arthritis is an umbrella term for more than 100 diseases that cause joint pain, swelling and stiffness. The term *rheumatic disease* has broader significance for any disease of the bones, muscles and joints.

Rheumatology is the branch of medicine devoted to arthritis and other diseases of the musculoskeletal system. This system includes the bones, joints, muscles, tendons, ligaments and other connective tissues that provide a framework and support for your body. Rheumatologists are healthcare professionals who have specialized training in rheumatology and internal medicine.

In addition to treating arthritis, rheumatologists treat autoimmune diseases — illnesses in which your immune system attacks your own body tissues. They also treat musculoskeletal disorders including back pain and bursitis, as well as bone diseases such as osteoporosis.

managing your arthritis, you can enjoy a more active, fulfilling life.

WHO GETS ARTHRITIS?

Arthritis affects people of all ages — around half of people with arthritis are under age 65, and symptoms often begin after age 40. Nevertheless, the risk of getting arthritis increases as you get older. By conservative estimates, nearly half of all adults age 65 and older have some form of arthritis.

Women are at higher risk than men of getting many forms of arthritis, especially after age 40. Researchers believe that female hormones may play a role in how — and when — arthritis develops. Hormones may also affect the severity of arthritis symptoms in women.

The likelihood of having arthritis also varies by race and ethnicity, as well as other factors. White and Black Americans, American Indians, and Alaska Natives are diagnosed with arthritis at higher rates than people of Hispanic or Asian heritage.

People who are overweight have a higher risk of developing arthritis, especially in the knees and hips. In addition, arthritis is more common in military veterans than nonveterans. And a past joint injury can also increase the risk of arthritis.

WHAT CAUSES ARTHRITIS?

The pain associated with arthritis is caused by joint damage, but the damage can occur in different ways. Osteoarthritis, the most common form of arthritis, involves a wearing away of the tough, lubricated cartilage that normally cushions the ends of the bones in your joints. Rheumatoid arthritis develops from an uncontrolled response of your immune system, which causes chronic inflammation in the lining of your joints.

Most of the underlying causes of arthritis are unclear, but researchers believe that the condition may result from a complex interplay of multiple factors, including genetics and environment.

It's true that wear and tear on joints over time can contribute to osteoarthritis. But arthritis isn't just a normal consequence of aging. Some people never develop it.

Family history can influence whether you get arthritis. Scientists have identified specific genes linked to an increased risk of rheumatoid arthritis. Genetic factors that contribute to osteoarthritis have also been identified. But even people who are genetically predisposed to having arthritis don't necessarily develop it.

Physical trauma, such as an ankle sprain or knee injury, can set the stage for osteoarthritis and other forms of the disease. Lack of physical activity and excess weight also can lead to arthritis. The shape of the joint and issues of body alignment play a role too. Stress or other forms of emotional trauma can worsen symptoms.

Other possible factors that could trigger the onset of arthritis may include

ANATOMY OF A JOINT

Joints are points of connection between two or more bones. The joints are designed to hold the bones together and allow your skeleton to move. The parts of a bone within your joints are covered with shock-absorbing cartilage. Cartilage is a tough, smooth, slippery material that prevents bone-against-bone contact, allowing for easy movement with little friction.

Synovial joints, found in the neck, shoulders, elbows, wrists, fingers, hips, knees, ankles and toes, are the most mobile form of a joint. These joints are surrounded by a tough fibrous capsule that attaches to the bone on each side of the joint. The joint capsule helps stabilize and protect the joint. The capsule is lined with tissue called the synovium. This thin membrane produces synovial fluid, a clear substance that nourishes the cartilage and "oils" the joint so that it can move smoothly.

Ligaments are tough cords of fibrous tissue that attach bone to bone. They help support the joint and keep it properly aligned. Muscles and tendons also hold the joint together. Tendons — which connect muscle and bone — attach to bone just outside the capsule above or below the joint.

Bursae are small, fluid-filled sacs tucked between muscles, tendons and bone. Synovial membrane lines the inside of each bursa, releasing a lubricating fluid to cushion the joint and reduce friction as tendons and muscles glide over bones.

The diagram at right shows how all these parts fit together in a typical knee joint.

cigarette smoking, infectious agents such as viruses, bacteria, fungi or parasites, toxic materials, or substances in food, water or air. An imbalance of certain hormones or enzymes in the body could possibly play a role as well.

TYPES OF ARTHRITIS

Different forms of arthritis can generally be divided into two categories. One involves inflammatory joint symptoms, with joint damage caused by inflammation. The other involves noninflammatory joint symptoms. Dividing arthritis into

TYPICAL JOINT

Joint capsule
This tough, fibrous material encapsulates and helps stabilize your joints.

Synovial membrane and fluid
The synovium is a thin membrane lining the inside of the joint capsule. It releases synovial fluid into the joint cavity to aid in lubrication.

Cartilage
Bones in your joints are capped with shock-absorbing cartilage, a tough, slippery material that reduces friction during movement.

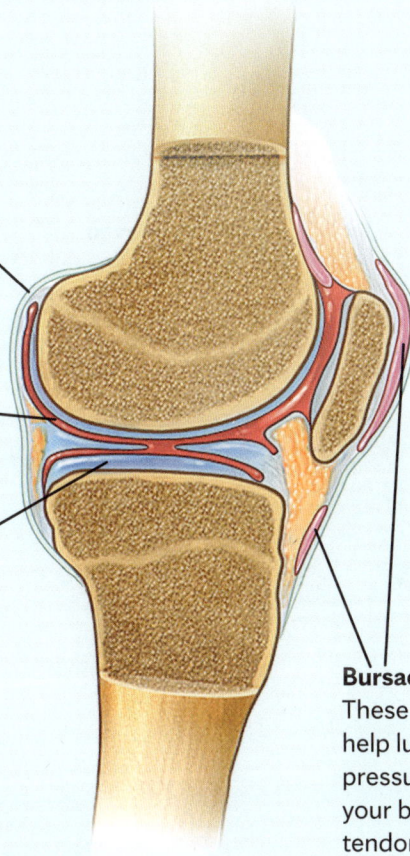

Bursae
These tiny fluid-filled sacs help lubricate and cushion pressure points between your bones, muscles and tendons.

these two categories is important, as the symptoms and treatment options are different.

The vast majority of people who have arthritis have one of two forms — osteoarthritis or rheumatoid arthritis. Osteoarthritis is the most common type of noninflammatory arthritis and is by far the most common form of arthritis overall (see Chapter 2). Rheumatoid arthritis, the most common inflammatory type, affects fewer people, but its symptoms can be much more debilitating (see Chapter 4).

HOW ARTHRITIS CHANGES A JOINT

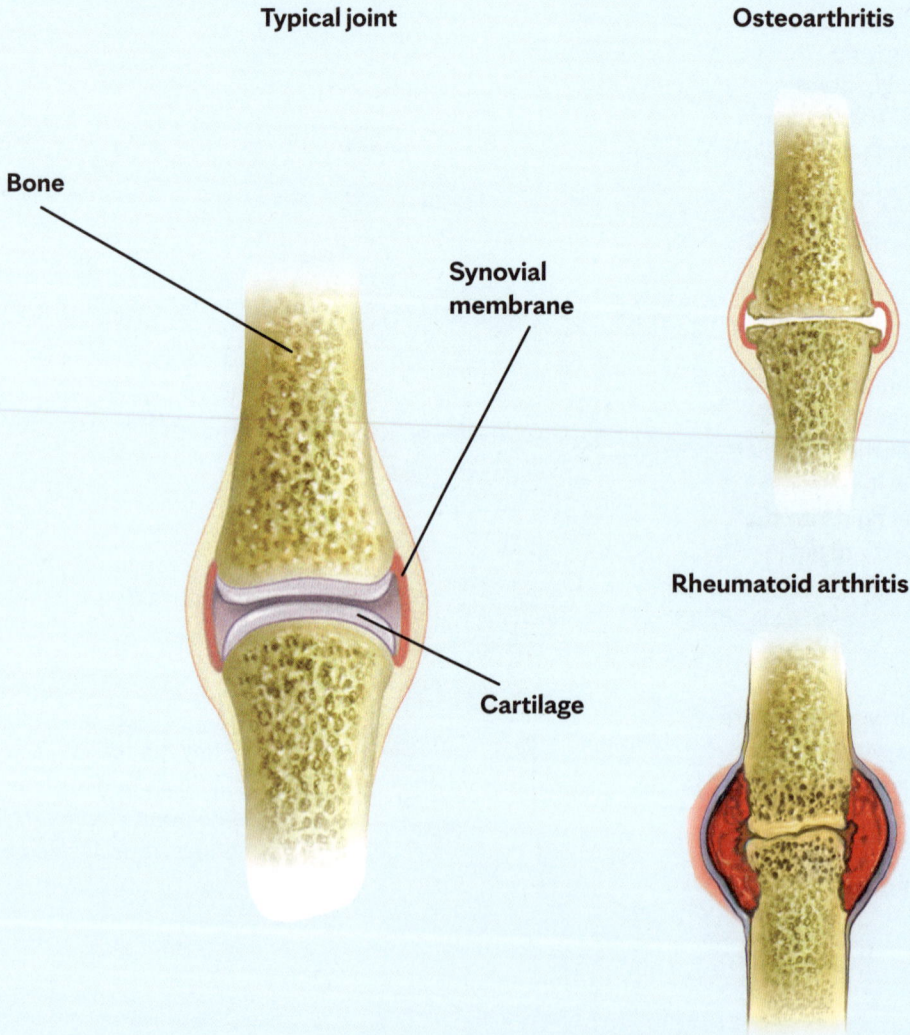

Typical joint

Osteoarthritis

Bone

Synovial
membrane

Rheumatoid arthritis

Cartilage

Osteoarthritis, the most common form of arthritis, involves the wearing away of the cartilage that caps the bones in your joints. With rheumatoid arthritis, the synovial membrane that protects and lubricates joints becomes inflamed, causing pain and swelling. Joint erosion may follow.

CAN ARTHRITIS BE PREVENTED?

Many risk factors for arthritis, such as your heredity, age and sex, aren't under your control. But there are things you can do to help lower your risk of arthritis. Even if you're beginning to experience pain and stiffness, you can influence how the disease affects you.

One of the best ways to prevent pain and joint damage is to see a medical professional as soon as you have signs and symptoms such as joint pain, stiffness or swelling. Early diagnosis and proper treatment can limit much of the damage.

To help prevent arthritis or minimize its effects, follow these guidelines:
- *Stay physically active.* Exercise keeps your joints flexible and strong. Aerobic exercise can help you maintain that flexibility. Strength training strengthens the muscles that stabilize and support joints.
- *Protect your joints from injuries.* Injuries to joints can lead to arthritis. Make sure to warm up before exercise, and stretch appropriately afterward.
- *Treat injuries properly and promptly.* This will help the injury heal correctly and limit possible joint damage.
- *Use good body mechanics to avoid joint stress.* During exercise and daily movements, use your large joints and largest muscles for tasks such as lifting. Don't lift or move things that are too heavy for you.
- *Manage your weight.* Being overweight or obese increases your chance of getting osteoarthritis. If you do have arthritis, the pressure on your joints from extra body weight may make your symptoms a little worse.
- *Avoid cigarette smoke.* Studies suggest that smoking increases the risk of rheumatoid arthritis, and quitting smoking may help prevent it.
- *Pay attention to what you eat.* Although there's no magic diet that can prevent arthritis, foods containing healthy fats, such as olive oil, nuts and certain types of fish, may have anti-inflammatory effects. Antioxidants and other compounds in vegetables and fruits also may help fight inflammation. Calcium and vitamin D help keep bones strong, which helps protect against arthritis damage.

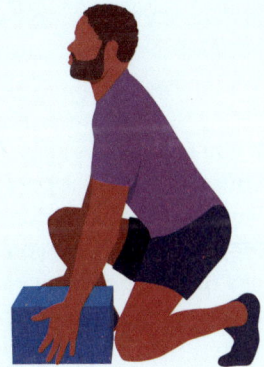

All forms of arthritis have certain signs and symptoms in common, such as joint pain or tenderness, stiffness, difficulty moving, and joint swelling.

However, other musculoskeletal conditions may cause similar symptoms. New technology and tests have made it easier to diagnose arthritis. But there still aren't definitive tests that can pinpoint the specific condition.

For these reasons, diagnosing arthritis can sometimes be a challenge. Healthcare professionals will rely on your description of the symptoms and your risk factors, as well as a physical exam and possibly lab tests. Your honest input is important.

You may have several visits before your healthcare team can confirm a diagnosis and find a treatment that works best for you. Regardless, the earlier you can start treatment, the better it is for your long-term health.

WHEN TO BE SEEN

Most often, arthritis isn't an emergency. But treatment is usually more effective when symptoms are caught in the early stages of the disease. In addition, some symptoms require immediate attention.

If you experience joint pain and stiffness that disappear within a few days, you probably don't need medical care. But if you experience any of the signs and symptoms listed below, call your healthcare team:
- New pain or persistent symptoms lasting several days or more.
- Joint pain with a fever, rash, headache or weight loss.
- Severe or worsening pain in one or more joints.
- Numbness or pain in your hands or legs or pain that radiates from your neck or lower back.
- Joint injury or trauma.

LIVING IN MOTION

Despite the aches and pains and joint problems that arthritis causes, most people with arthritis get on with their lives and control their symptoms successfully. The two most common forms of arthritis, osteoarthritis and rheumatoid arthritis, aren't ordinarily life-threatening, and they respond well to medical treatments and self-care.

Start by learning as much as you can about your form of arthritis, your treatment options and, most importantly, the steps you can take to control the condition. This book will give you information as well as tools and strategies for living with a chronic disease.

Armed with information and a positive attitude, you can move forward, adjusting your lifestyle to manage arthritis without compromising your happiness.

2 Osteoarthritis

Osteoarthritis (OA), also called degenerative joint disease or wear-and-tear arthritis, affects more than 30 million adults in the United States. It is the most common form of arthritis.

OA can affect any joint in your body. It most often occurs in joints that bear weight or are used the most, including the knees, hips, back and hands. Less commonly, it affects the shoulders, elbows, wrists and ankles. It tends to start in only one joint, but it can spread to others.

UNDERSTANDING THE CONDITION

Osteoarthritis occurs when the protective cartilage that cushions the ends of bones in your joints deteriorates. With use, the soft, pliable layer of cartilage may start to wear down, and its smooth surface may become rough. At this point, many people feel intermittent pain in the joint, especially after strenuous use.

If the cartilage wears away completely, you may be left with bone rubbing on bone, which damages the ends of your bones. This is usually painful.

Your body tries to repair the damage, but lost cartilage typically can't be regenerated. When this protective layer wears away, new bone growth forms spurs along the sides of existing bones. Prominent lumps can form around the joint as a result. These occur most often with osteoarthritis of the hands and feet. Pain and tenderness over the bony lumps may be most noticeable early in the disease and less noticeable later on.

OA is typically considered a noninflammatory joint disease. That means it isn't associated with systemic inflammation in the body that causes swelling, redness or warmth in the joints. Still, changes from

JOINT CHANGES IN OSTEOARTHRITIS

Inflammation   **Cartilage wearing away**

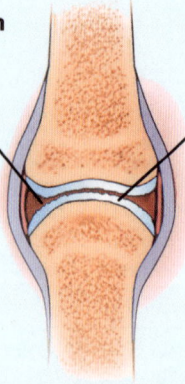 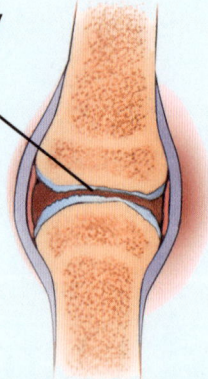

The first signs of osteoarthritis in a joint are microscopic pits and fissures on the surface of cartilage, which are usually accompanied by mild inflammation.

As the cartilage is worn completely through, the contours of the joint are changed and patches of exposed bone appear.

Exposed bone   **Bone spurs**

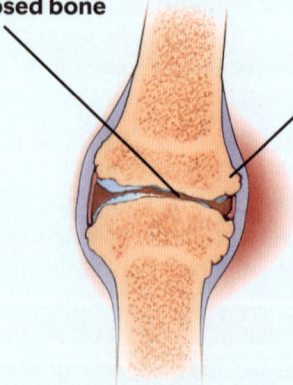 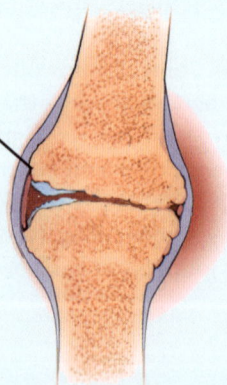

The exposed bone thickens and bone spurs (osteophytes) develop. It becomes painful to use the joint.

In advanced stages, the space between bones may disappear and ligaments loosen, causing further joint instability. The irregular surface of bones can significantly limit the motion of the joint.

OA in a joint can cause inflammation of the joint lining. This can lead to swelling.

Many scientists believe cartilage damage may be due to an enzyme imbalance in the cartilage cells or lining of the joint. When balanced, these enzymes allow for the natural breakdown and regeneration of cartilage. But too many enzymes can cause the cartilage to break down faster than it's being rebuilt. The exact cause of this enzyme imbalance is unclear.

Early changes to the cartilage and bone don't always result in pain or other symptoms. Many older adults have OA but are unaware of it until it's seen on a routine X-ray.

The risk of OA increases with age, with the disease most often developing in people over age 40. It's more common in women than men overall, although before the age of 45 it's more prevalent in men. It's relatively rare among younger adults unless they've had a joint injury, or they have an underlying secondary cause of OA, as discussed on page 23. Those affected often have a family history of the disease.

An active lifestyle may slow the development of osteoarthritis, although almost everyone older than age 65 will experience some joint damage and have mild signs of arthritis that are visible in imaging tests such as X-rays. Still, these mild signs and symptoms may or may not cause pain or affect your activity.

A severe injury to one or more joints at an early age may lead to OA years later. Also, excessively stressful use of joints over many years — such as working at a job that requires repeated knee bending — may cause OA later on. If certain activities are causing joint pain, try to avoid those activities until you can have the joint examined by a medical professional.

Being overweight also increases your risk of developing OA, especially in the knees. The more you weigh, the greater your risk. Increased weight adds stress to weight-bearing joints, such as your hips and knees. Also, fat tissue produces proteins that can cause harmful inflammation in and around your joints. Losing excess weight can help you reduce the risk of OA or relieve some joint pain. (For information on weight management, see Chapter 16.)

SIGNS AND SYMPTOMS

Osteoarthritis symptoms usually develop slowly and worsen over time. At first, many people notice pain and stiffness when getting out of bed in the morning. This feeling of stiff or creaky joints after a period of inactivity, a phenomenon called "gelling," usually passes within 30 minutes. Others often notice OA pain after strenuous activity. Typically, resting the joint helps relieve the pain.

With osteoarthritis you may experience:
- Joint pain or tenderness during or after use, or following a period of inactivity
- Joint discomfort before or during a change in the weather

- Joint swelling and stiffness, particularly after use
- Formation of bony lumps on the middle or end finger joints or at the base of the thumb
- Loss of joint flexibility
- Grating sensation in the joint

For example, you may first feel pain and stiffness in the index finger of one hand, but eventually multiple finger joints in both hands may be affected. Your fingers may be stiff and deformed, making it hard to hold a pen or open a jar. Your knees may start to ache after a game of tennis or a jog in the park.

Be aware that the normal wear and tear on your joints doesn't necessarily result in osteoarthritis. OA is not an inevitable part of aging. But if you develop the condition, the symptoms won't go away without treatment. In the early stages, OA pain often fades within a year, but it can return if you overuse an affected joint. Pain tends to increase over the years and can progressively limit your activity. OA often affects joints on one side of the body at first. Gradually, joints on the opposite side may become involved as well.

Osteoarthritis may affect only one joint, which is called localized OA. If it occurs in many joints, it is known as generalized OA. It often affects the hands and the weight-bearing joints of the hips, knees and feet. You may have pain whenever you stand, walk, get up from a chair or climb stairs. Unless multiple joints are involved, the effects of osteoarthritis are likely to be mild. Keeping active helps prevent problems.

Hand osteoarthritis

In the hands, osteoarthritis is most common in the distal and proximal joints. Those are the joints near the tip and middle of the fingers. The joint at the base of the thumb, the carpometacarpal joint, also is often affected. These joints in the hand may be painful or tender and show some redness or swelling, especially in early stages. This discomfort usually lessens over time.

Bone spurs may form in finger joints with OA. If these growths develop in the joints closer to your fingertips, they are called Heberden's nodes, while growths in the middle joints of the fingers are known as

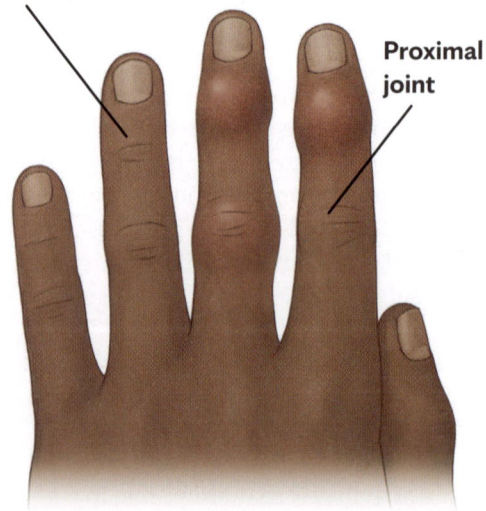

Distal joint

Proximal joint

Some people with hand osteoarthritis have bony lumps in the joints near the tips of the fingers (Heberden's nodes). The nodes may be painful at first but are mostly a cosmetic concern once the pain subsides.

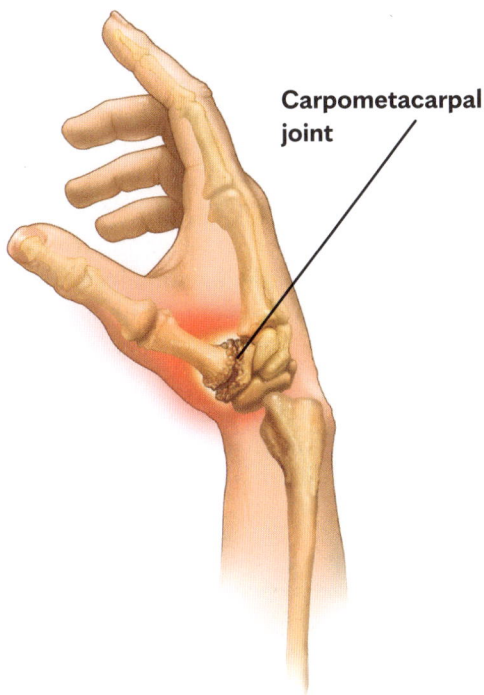

Carpometacarpal joint

typically seen in rheumatoid arthritis, helping differentiate the two.

Knee osteoarthritis

When OA affects the knees, both knees are usually involved, although the condition may be more severe on one side. People who have knee OA often describe a feeling of giving way and may be prone to falls. The knee may be stiff and swollen, and you may feel a grating or catching sensation when you move it. The joint sometimes makes a sound with use.

Bouchard's nodes. This pattern of arthritis is known as nodal osteoarthritis and tends to run in the family. It often is passed down from the mother or maternal grandmother.

Erosive osteoarthritis, also called inflammatory osteoarthritis, is a more severe type of OA that can affect the hands. It is usually more aggressive than typical hand OA, causing joint damage quickly. It affects the distal finger joints, like nodal OA, but is often associated with swelling and warmth. Because of this, it can be confused with an underlying inflammatory arthritis such as rheumatoid arthritis. X-rays will show erosions or "bites" out of the bone, in the center. Erosions on the sides of the bones are

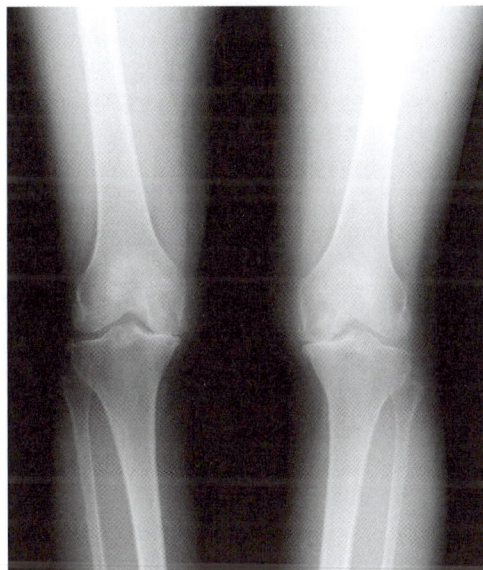

This X-ray image of knees affected by OA shows the uneven spaces and the points of contact between the thigh bone and shinbone — the femur and the tibia, respectively — on the inside of the joints.

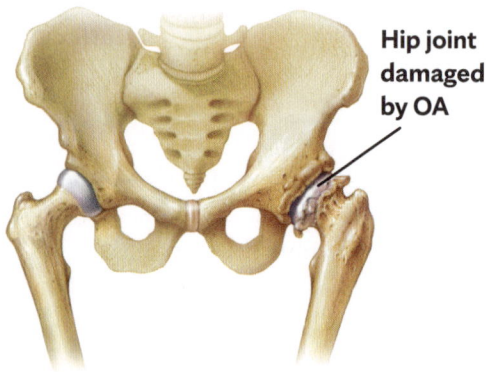

Hip joint damaged by OA

Hip osteoarthritis

Pain from hip OA usually occurs deep in the groin area and not in the sides of the hips or back. Pain is worse with activities such as standing from a seated position and starting to walk after being seated for a while. Unlike knee OA, hip OA frequently affects only one side.

Big toe osteoarthritis

Osteoarthritis in the foot develops most often where the big toe attaches to the foot. This joint gets less flexible and larger with bony swelling. You may find it uncomfortable to wear shoes and painful to walk or stand. When this joint bulges out to the side of your foot, it is called a bunion deformity. Usually both big toes are affected.

Spine osteoarthritis

Osteoarthritis commonly occurs in the neck or back when the cartilage in your spine wears down. Disks of cartilage normally cushion the bones of your spine, called vertebrae. But they can wear down over time, making the spaces between the bones narrower. Bony outgrowths called spurs may form.

When bone surfaces rub together, those areas of the vertebrae become inflamed, causing stiffness and pain. Gradually your spine stiffens and loses flexibility.

If several disks are involved, you may notice a loss of height. Specific spine conditions are discussed in more detail in Chapter 6.

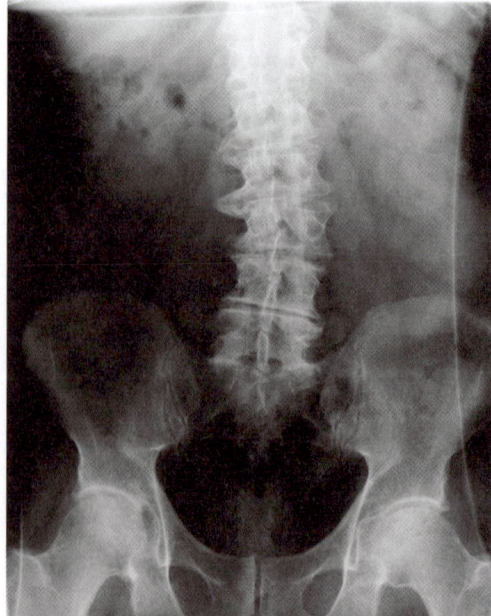

This X-ray image of advanced osteoarthritis of the spine shows vertebrae that have become misaligned and unevenly spaced.

Generalized osteoarthritis

When multiple joints are affected with osteoarthritis, it's called generalized osteoarthritis. It's also known as polyarticular arthritis. Usually the distal joints in the hands, the joints at the base of the thumbs, and the big toes, neck, lower back, knees and hips are involved. The symptoms usually first appear in one or two joints and gradually appear in others.

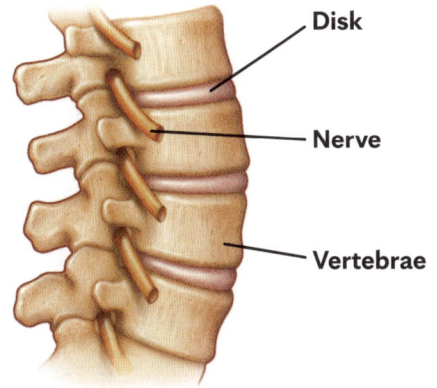

Secondary osteoarthritis

The term *secondary osteoarthritis* refers to arthritis that develops after a known cause, such as a previous joint injury. Other physical factors that can lead to osteoarthritis include obesity, legs of unequal length, previous joint diseases, surgery or fracture. Certain bone disorders, metabolic conditions and hypermobile joints also can predispose someone to developing OA.

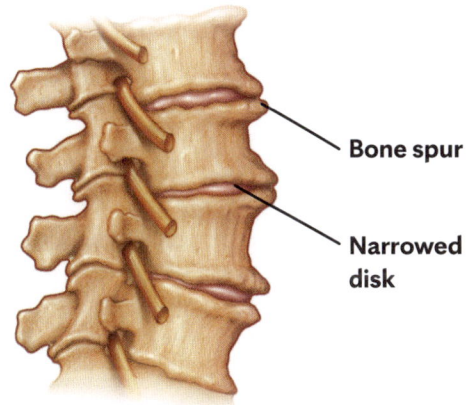

DIAGNOSIS AND TREATMENT

If you have joint pain and stiffness that may be from osteoarthritis, schedule an appointment with your healthcare professional.

A diagnosis of osteoarthritis is usually based on a careful physical examination and your medical history. You may be asked for details about your symptoms, such as pain, swelling or stiffness. The nature of the joint pain and the specific joints that are affected can help distinguish different forms of arthritis.

Disk

Nerve

Vertebrae

Bone spur

Narrowed disk

Elastic structures called disks cushion the vertebrae in the spine, keeping it flexible. In OA, disks may narrow and bone spurs can form. Where bone surfaces rub together, you may have pain and stiffness, and the spine may become less flexible.

You also may be asked whether the symptoms started gradually or suddenly, how they have changed over time, and how they are affected by certain types of activity. For example, mild morning stiffness is common in osteoarthritis and usually gets better after a few minutes of activity. In contrast, morning stiffness that lasts for hours is more likely to be a symptom of rheumatoid arthritis or another type of inflammatory disorder. In addition, you may be asked whether you have other symptoms, such as fever, fatigue or skin problems. It's important to alert your healthcare team to any events or changes that occurred just before your symptoms began and whether you have a family history of arthritis.

QUESTIONS YOUR HEALTHCARE TEAM MAY ASK

Diagnosing any form of arthritis relies heavily on your description of signs and symptoms and other relevant information. It's a good idea to make a list of your signs and symptoms and when and where they occur. Keeping a pain record or diary for two weeks to share with your healthcare team can help in making a diagnosis. Keep track of the intensity of your pain, how long it lasts, what it feels like, and whether anything makes it better or worse.

Here are some questions you may be asked about your arthritis signs and symptoms:
- Which joints are painful?
- Do the same joints on both sides of your body hurt at the same time, or is the pain just on one side?
- Has the pain moved from one joint to another?
- Did the pain start in just one joint and then progress to include others? How quickly did this happen?
- Did your symptoms start gradually or all at once? Have they gotten worse over time or stayed about the same?
- Do you have stiffness in the morning or after a period of inactivity, such as when watching TV? How long does the morning stiffness last?
- What time of day is the pain most severe?
- If you have pain in your hands, which joints hurt the most?
- Have you had times of feeling weak and uncomfortable all over? Have you been unusually tired?
- Does anything make your pain better or worse?
- Does pain or difficulty moving interfere with your work, sleep or daily activities?
- Do you have any other symptoms besides joint problems? Have you had fever, loss of appetite, changes in vision or any other physical changes?
- Does arthritis or rheumatic disease run in your family?
- Did you have any injuries or trauma before your symptoms first appeared?

During a physical exam, your joints will be checked for tenderness, swelling and redness. Your healthcare team will look for bone spurs along the sides of existing bones and listen for a crunching or grating sound. Called crepitation, this sound indicates that the joint cartilage surface has become rough. Your joints may also be moved through their range of motion to check for pain in certain positions and see if you have limited motion.

You may have an X-ray to confirm the diagnosis, rule out other causes of pain and determine the extent of joint damage. Although soft tissue such as bone carti-lage doesn't show up on X-ray images, a narrowing of the space between bones can indicate cartilage loss. X-rays may also show bone spurs developing on the affected joint.

Magnetic resonance imaging (MRI) provides detailed images of bone and soft tissue, which can help determine exactly what's causing the pain. The MRI can pro-vide more insight into the muscles and tendons to see if they are the cause of your symptoms.

There are no blood tests for osteoarthri-tis, but a blood sample may be taken to help rule out rheumatoid arthritis and other forms of arthritis or inflammation.

Keep in mind that many people have no symptoms or disability from osteoarthri-tis. They may not even realize that they have it.

While there are no known cures for osteoarthritis, you and your healthcare team can develop a treatment program that helps you reduce pain, preserve joint movement and maintain a high quality of life. An all-around approach may be recommended, including medications, physical exercise and splints. In addition, physical therapy and occupational therapy may help you learn how to change certain behaviors, such as grip-ping objects, to protect your joints. In some cases, surgery may be necessary. Specific treatments are described more in Part 2: Treating Arthritis. These treat-ments have long-lasting benefits that can help you control the disease and live an active, independent life.

JOINT PAIN: MANY POSSIBILITIES TO CONSIDER

A number of musculoskeletal dis-eases — disorders affecting the bones, muscles and joints — are associated with arthritis. These might cause joint pain and stiffness or occur alongside arthritis, or they may be a result of arthritis. The pain may stem from problems in the joint itself or from problems in nearby bones, ligaments, tendons, muscles, nerves and other tissues. The symptoms often overlap with arthritis symp-toms, which can make diagnosis a challenge. Some of the more common musculoskeletal diseases are discussed in more detail in Chapter 3.

3 Other noninflammatory musculoskeletal disorders

Musculoskeletal disorders are problems with the body's muscles, bones, tendons or ligaments. Osteoarthritis and other forms of arthritis are types of musculoskeletal disorders. But muscle and joint pain can result from many other conditions. This chapter reviews some of the most common causes.

While the conditions discussed here often cause pain and inflammation, they are considered noninflammatory. That's because inflammation is typically the result of these injuries and conditions, not the cause.

See a medical professional if you have any significant joint or muscle pain. Ignoring pain or injury may lead to more serious problems. A careful diagnosis can help you know how to treat the condition, reduce your pain and prevent joint damage.

ANKLE SPRAINS

Ankle sprains are a common injury. They're usually due to the ankle joint rolling in too far. The ligaments that hold the ankle bones together stretch or tear, causing pain and swelling. A sprain often makes it difficult to bear weight on the ankle because of pain and unsteadiness.

Initial treatment of an ankle sprain involves rest, ice, compression and elevation (R.I.C.E.). Rest the ankle and stay off your feet. You may need crutches or a cane to get around and take pressure off the ankle. Ice the ankle every 1 to 2 hours, for 15 minutes each time, to help ease pain and inflammation. Wrapping the ankle in an elastic bandage provides compression, which reduces swelling and gives the joint support. Elevating the foot above the level of your heart also helps keep swelling down. Anti-inflammatory medications may help as well.

Most ankle sprains heal with these conservative therapies. Rarely, surgery is needed to repair a torn ligament, and it is most often performed for multiple sprains. People who have had an ankle sprain are typically at higher risk of future sprains, so it's important to perform ankle strength and stability exercises to help prevent injuries in the future.

AVASCULAR NECROSIS

Avascular necrosis (AVN) is the death of bone tissue due to a lack of blood supply. It can occur when the blood vessels to a joint are disrupted, for example, from a broken bone or a dislocated joint.

AVN can affect any joint, but it's usually most severe when the hip or knee is involved. People who have avascular necrosis of the hip or knee typically develop pain in the joint, especially when walking, and may limp.

Factors that may raise your risk of AVN include alcoholism, steroid use, trauma such as a major bone or joint injury, and smoking. Your risk may also be higher after radiation therapy for cancer.

To diagnose AVN, a healthcare professional will examine the joint and look at imaging tests such as an X-ray, computerized tomography (CT) scan or magnetic resonance imaging (MRI), which can show changes to the bone. Treatment typically includes bed rest, crutches, physical therapy and anti-inflammatory medications. For advanced AVN, surgery might be recommended.

BAKER'S CYST (POPLITEAL CYST)

A Baker's cyst, also called a popliteal cyst, is a fluid-filled sac behind the knee. It usually results from an abnormality or injury in the knee such as arthritis or a cartilage tear. This may cause your knee to produce fluid, which can pool and form a cyst. The cyst can lead to pain or stiffness, or it may not cause any symptoms. You may notice swelling or a bulge at the back of the knee, especially when the leg is straight. The pain and stiffness might feel worse if you stand for a long time. Occasionally, the cyst may tear open, causing the calf to swell and become red. Sometimes a bruise will form in the ankle.

Usually, treating a painful Baker's cyst involves draining (aspirating) the synovial fluid in the knee joint, injecting a steroid into the joint and treating any related arthritis. Rarely, surgery is necessary to

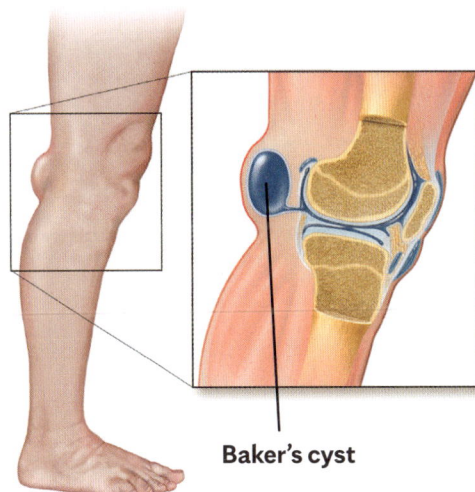

Baker's cyst

remove or repair a cartilage tear that's causing the cyst.

BUNION

A bunion is a bump that may form along the joint at the base of the big toe. The bump develops when the big toe angles toward the toe next to it. The joint begins to stick out, which can lead to swelling, redness and soreness. Bunions occur in women more often than in men, and they tend to run in the family. They also can be associated with wearing tight shoes, such as dress shoes that crunch the toes. A foot deformity from birth also may lead to a bunion.

Most bunions are treatable without surgery. To treat or prevent bunions, it's important to wear properly fitting shoes that don't constrict the toes. A toe spacer placed between the big toe and the second toe can help reduce a bunion deformity. Medial bunion pads — worn on the outside of the big toe joint — may

Bunion

First metatarsal

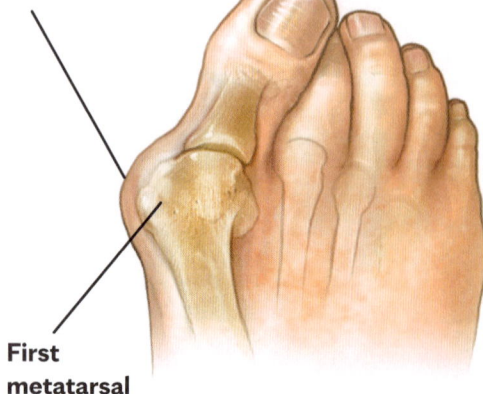

help lessen the pain and other symptoms. When discomfort isn't getting better with conservative management, surgery may be an option.

A similar bump that forms on the outside of the fifth toe is called a bunionette or tailor's bunion. This can lead to a hard corn and, occasionally, painful bursitis. A bunionette is typically caused by tight, poorly fitting shoes. You may need to wear shoes that allow plenty of toe space to decrease pressure on the area and relieve symptoms. As with a bunion, surgery is needed only in rare cases if pain persists.

BURSITIS

Your body has more than 150 bursae — small, fluid-filled sacs that cushion pressure points between the bones, tendons and muscles near your joints. Overuse of a joint or repeated stress on the joint can lead to painful inflammation of a bursa, called bursitis. Bursitis most often affects your shoulders, elbows and hips. But bursitis can also affect your knee, heel or the base of your big toe.

If you have bursitis, you may feel an ache or tenderness around a joint. The joint may be stiff and difficult to move, and it may hurt especially when you move the joint or put pressure on it. If the inflamed bursa is near the skin's surface, the area may be red, swollen and warm to the touch.

The most common causes of bursitis are repetitive motions or positions that irritate the bursae around a joint. For example, if you spend a lot of time kneeling, the pressure on the knee could cause inflammation in a bursa at the front of your kneecap. Swinging a golf club or throwing a ball repeatedly can affect a bursa in your elbow or shoulder. Bursitis may also result from joint stress, infection, gout, or injury to a joint, tendon or ligament. Often the cause is unknown. Some forms of arthritis also can lead to bursitis.

Bursitis may be diagnosed from a physical exam if a healthcare professional can identify specific areas of tenderness. To help rule out other possible causes of the discomfort, you may have an imaging test such as an X-ray, MRI or ultrasound. Treatment includes resting the affected area and applying ice and compression to reduce swelling. Bursitis pain usually goes away within about a week of home treatment. Taking anti-inflammatory drugs such as ibuprofen (Advil, Motrin IB, others) or naproxen sodium (Aleve) can help relieve pain and reduce inflammation.

To avoid having bursitis become a chronic problem, it's important to prevent flare-ups. This includes protecting the joint and avoiding repetitive activities and positions that put pressure on the bursa. Specific types of bursitis are discussed below.

Olecranon bursitis

The bursa that sits at the tip of your elbow is called the olecranon bursa. If it becomes inflamed it can cause swelling, often resembling a golf ball on the elbow. Olecranon bursitis is most commonly caused by trauma or irritation to the elbow — for example, leaning on a table or chair or using an elbow to get out of bed. People with certain jobs, such as carpet laying, are prone to developing the condition.

When the cause is repetitive trauma, the olecranon bursitis usually comes on slowly and the surrounding tissues are not affected. The elbow can still fully extend despite the bursa swelling. Conservative treatments such as elbow pads may be recommended to prevent ongoing irritation to the joint. Typically, for swelling caused by trauma, the first approach will not be to drain the fluid. This is because most swelling resolves with time, compression and protection of the area, and the risk of infection is a bit higher with needle drainage. If swelling

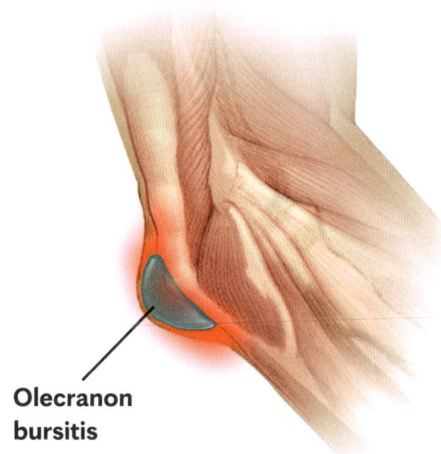

Olecranon bursitis

continues, draining the fluid can be considered.

Inflammatory conditions such as gout, rheumatoid arthritis or infection also can lead to olecranon bursitis. When inflammation is the cause, the elbow becomes swollen, red, warm and very painful. Often, inserting a needle into the bursa to analyze the fluid is necessary to find the cause of the swelling. In rare instances, such as in the context of infection, surgery is needed to remove the bursa.

Trochanteric bursitis

Bursitis around the greater trochanter — a portion of the thigh bone located just below the hip — is a common cause of hip pain. It may occur from irritation, overuse, early hip arthritis, weak hip muscles or obesity. This type of bursitis usually causes a dull, burning pain. It

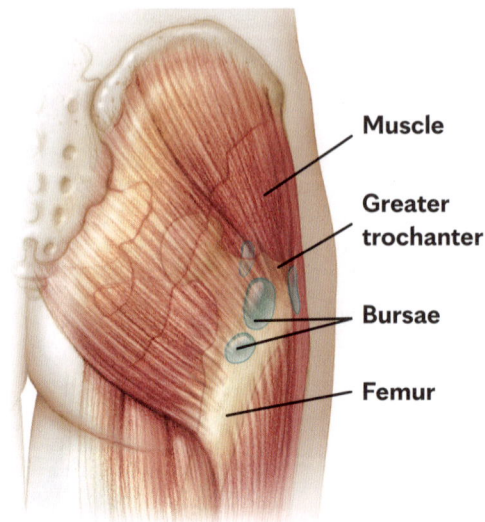

Muscle

Greater trochanter

Bursae

Femur

typically doesn't cause visible swelling or skin redness because the bursae are located beneath bulky muscles.

Rest and physical therapy, especially strengthening of the gluteal muscles, are the first therapies for treating bursitis around the hip. If the problem remains painful, steroid injections may help relieve the inflammation. But these injections are used less frequently, since gluteal weakness is usually the main contributing factor.

DUPUYTREN'S CONTRACTURE

Dupuytren's contracture is a thickening of the connective tissue in the palm of your hand. It most often affects the two fingers farthest from the thumb. Over a period of years, it can pull the fingers into a bent position. Initially, you might notice thickening or a hard lump in the palm of your hand. This lump may feel painful or painless. In later stages, some people have difficulty straightening one or more fingers.

This condition occurs more frequently in men than in women. You may be at higher risk if a family member has the condition, if you have diabetes, or if you use tobacco or alcohol.

There is no treatment to stop Dupuytren's contracture from getting worse, but certain treatments may improve symptoms. Sometimes, a medical professional can break up the thick tissue using either a needle inserted through the skin or a type of enzyme injection. If symptoms are severe, surgery may be needed to break up or remove the tissue.

With mild symptoms, using a cushioned tool handle or padded gloves can reduce pain when gripping or grasping objects.

MERALGIA PARESTHETICA

A numbness or tingling along the outer thigh may be due to meralgia paresthetica. This condition results when the large nerve in your outer thigh, known as the lateral femoral cutaneous nerve, gets pinched, often by a nearby ligament. You might feel tingling in the side of your thigh or burning pain on the surface. However, the condition doesn't cause any weakness to the muscle.

Meralgia paresthetica often occurs in people who are overweight, have diabetes, are older or are pregnant. Trauma to the area, rapid weight gain and wearing clothing that is tight at the waist also can lead to symptoms.

Most of the time, no specific treatment is needed, but you can learn ways to reduce pressure on the nerve. Avoiding tight clothing or belts or other measures may help the problem resolve on its own. Occasionally, medications may be used to help reduce persistent symptoms. Surgery is rarely necessary.

MORTON'S NEUROMA

Morton's neuroma is a thickening of the tissue around one of the nerves that lead

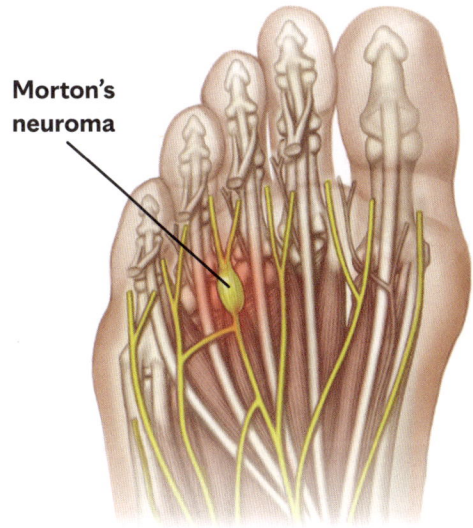

Morton's neuroma

to the toes. The condition most frequently develops between the third and fourth toes. It's more common in women and usually occurs in response to irritation, trauma or excessive pressure on the toes.

Symptoms include a feeling of walking on a marble or burning pain in the ball of the foot that may radiate into the toes. Tingling or numbness in the toes also is common. An exam and imaging tests such as an X-ray or ultrasound can confirm the diagnosis.

High-heeled and tight or narrow shoes tend to aggravate Morton's neuroma. You may need to switch to low-heeled or flat shoes with wider toe boxes and use orthotics to relieve pressure on the area. Taking anti-inflammatory medications also can help. If a neuroma doesn't respond to these types of conservative treatments, a medical professional may recommend steroid injections or, eventually, surgery.

OSGOOD-SCHLATTER DISEASE

Osgood-Schlatter disease causes pain just below the kneecap on the tibia, the large lower leg bone. It usually occurs with swelling or a bump on the front of the knee. Typically, this condition affects children ages 9 to 14. It often occurs in children going through a growth spurt and those who are active in sports that involve running, jumping and fast changes of direction, like basketball and soccer. The repeated stress and activity pull on the tendon connecting the kneecap and the tibia, which in turn pulls on the growth plate of the tibia bone, causing inflammation.

Knee pain from Osgood-Schlatter disease is usually worse with running, jumping or kneeling activities, and it improves with rest. The condition normally goes away after a child's bones stop growing. Icing the area and stretching the quadriceps muscles on the front of the thigh may help the pain. Children with Osgood-Schlatter disease can continue sports and other activities if the pain is manageable.

OSTEOPOROSIS

Osteoporosis is a bone-weakening disease caused by the gradual loss of calcium and other minerals from the bones. Over many years, this makes the bones thinner, weaker and more prone to breaking.

Unlike osteoarthritis, which leads to stiffness and pain, osteoporosis causes no symptoms at first. Painful fractures in the spine, hips, wrists or other bones may be the earliest signs of the disease.

Your bones are living tissue that's continuously changing. Over time, old or worn-out bone is broken down and absorbed, and new bone is made to replace it. By the time you reach your mid-30s, more bone tissue is being lost than replaced, so you gradually begin to lose bone strength. Osteoporosis develops if enough bone is lost that portions of your skeleton become porous, brittle and weak. People over age 50 are most likely to develop the disease, and the risk increases with age.

Osteoporosis is common. Among people over age 65, it affects more than 1 in 4 women and 1 in 20 men in the United States. Your risk depends in part on your bone mass — how much bone tissue you've developed by the time it peaks during young adulthood. How rapidly you lose it later also affects your risk.

Some risk factors are out of your control. The disease is generally more common among women, people with a parent or sibling with osteoporosis, and men and women who are white or of Asian descent. Those with a small frame also are more likely to get osteoporosis, as they have less bone mass to draw from as they age.

In addition, hormone levels, medications, your diet and other lifestyle choices affect your risk. In women, a sudden drop

Typical bone

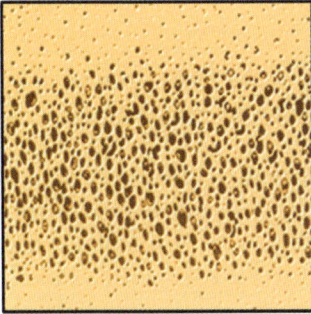

Osteoporotic bone

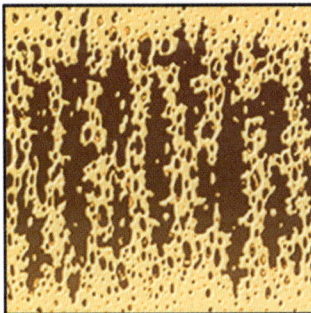

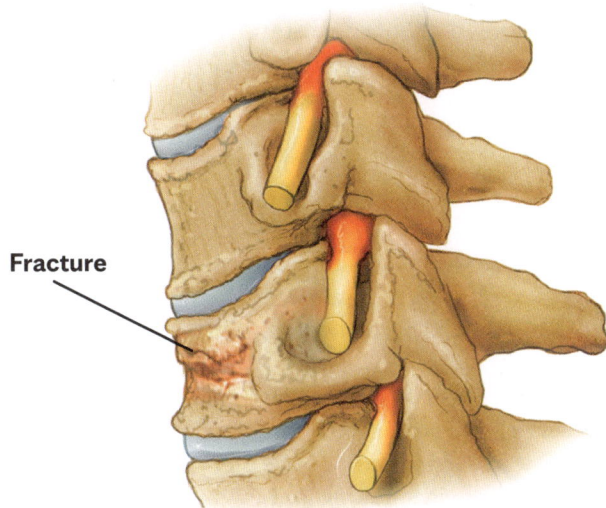

Fracture

in estrogen at menopause can speed up bone loss. Lower testosterone levels in older men can do the same. Not getting enough calcium and vitamin D in your diet also can speed up bone loss. Other factors that raise your risk of osteoporosis include an eating disorder such as anorexia, certain diseases, long-term use of some medications, an inactive lifestyle, and use of alcohol and tobacco.

With osteoporosis, bone breaks may happen more easily than expected. In the spine, vertebrae can become compressed and fracture or collapse. You may have back pain, lose height over time and develop a stooped posture. Hip and wrist fractures also are common.

If you have risk factors for osteoporosis, your healthcare team may recommend diagnostic tests. You'll likely have a bone density scan and a physical exam.

Diagnostic tests are done to:
• Confirm that you have osteoporosis
• Determine the severity of your low bone density
• Establish your baseline values for bone density
• Identify chemical abnormalities that may predispose you to osteoporosis

A bone density test can help your care team determine if you have osteoporosis and predict your risk of a fracture. Bone density scans are generally simple, fast and painless. They use special X-rays or ultrasound technology to measure how much calcium and other minerals — collectively known as bone mineral content — are packed into your bones. The higher your mineral content, the denser the bone. The denser the bone, the stronger it is and the less likely it is to break.

Medications such as bisphosphonates are often prescribed to treat osteoporosis. These drugs slow the breakdown of bone.

Making healthy lifestyle choices also can help preserve bone strength. To maintain bone density, it's important to eat a diet rich in calcium, avoid smoking and drinking in excess, and stay active, especially with weight-bearing exercise and strength training.

PATELLOFEMORAL PAIN SYNDROME

Patellofemoral pain syndrome causes pain in the front of the knee, around the kneecap, also known as the patella.

It's common in runners and others who are active in sports that involve running and jumping. The pain is typically worse with activities that put pressure on the knees, such as squatting, running, going up or down stairs, and sitting for long periods of time. In addition, the knee may make a popping noise while climbing stairs or squatting and standing.

This type of knee pain is more common in women and adolescents or young adults. Studies have linked it with weak or imbalanced muscles around the hip, which don't permit proper movement of

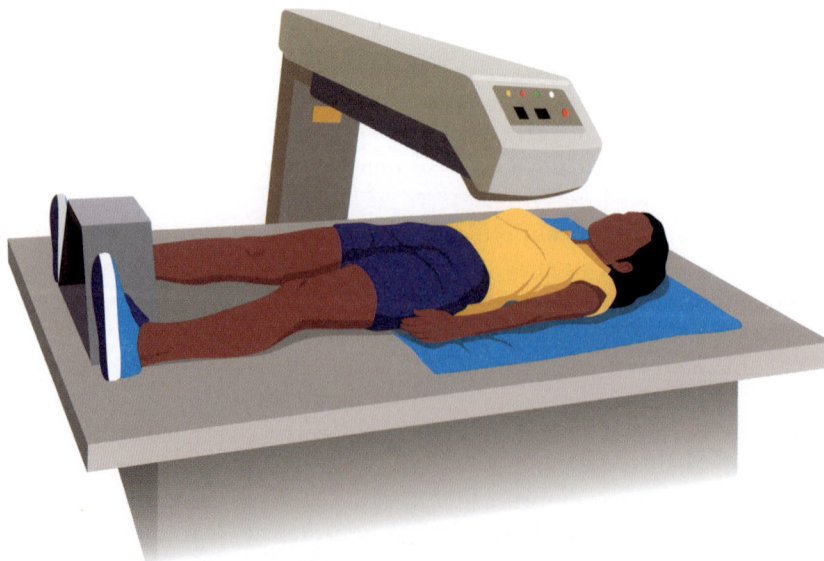

A bone density scan can help identify areas where your bones are growing weaker. The spine, forearm and wrist, fingers, hip, and heel are common areas to have checked.

WHO SHOULD BE TESTED FOR OSTEOPOROSIS?

Ideally, adults at risk of osteoporosis will have a bone mineral density (BMD) test. Other tools that estimate risk, such as the Fracture Risk Assessment Tool (FRAX), can help determine who should have BMD testing. Early testing gives more time to take steps to prevent bone loss. It's also the first and best step toward receiving a diagnosis and starting treatment. A bone density test is recommended for:

- Women age 65 and older.
- Women over age 50 who are at higher risk of osteoporosis. Risk factors include a family history of fractures, a slender frame, a decrease in height and a drop in hormone levels. Your risk is also higher if you've had an organ transplant.
- Men who've had an X-ray showing possible low bone density or who've lost height.
- Adults who've had a fragility fracture — when bone becomes so fragile that it breaks much more easily than expected.
- Adults who have a medical condition associated with lower bone mass, such as rheumatoid arthritis, diabetes and hyperparathyroidism.
- Adults who are taking or will soon take a medication associated with lower bone mass, such as corticosteroid drugs and thyroid hormones.
- Anyone being treated for osteoporosis.

Bone density testing is usually not a one-time thing. The frequency of retesting depends on your age and your risk factors. One year is the minimum amount of time for bones affected by osteoporosis to show a noticeable increase or decrease in density. Even if your bone density is normal at the initial test, talk with your healthcare team about when to repeat the test. Bone density tests over several years can reveal the rate at which you may be losing bone. This rate helps predict your risk of a fracture.

the lower leg during activities. That often causes the knee to turn inward. It's also associated with overuse of the knee or a previous injury or surgery.

A key part of treatment involves strengthening the core and hip muscles. This helps with proper leg alignment when you're active, permits the kneecap to glide easier and reduces the pressure under the kneecap. Avoiding activities that make the pain worse should also help. Icing the knee, taping around the kneecap and wearing a brace for the kneecap may provide additional relief.

PLANTAR FASCIITIS

One of the most common causes of heel pain is plantar fasciitis, an inflammation of the connective tissue that runs from the heel to the base of the toes, called the plantar fascia. This tough layer of fascia supports the arch of the foot. Plantar fasciitis typically causes a sharp pain in the heel when you put weight on it, especially with the first few steps in the morning or after being at rest for a while. The pain usually recedes as you keep moving.

Plantar fasciitis is often caused by repetitive stress on the connective tissue, which can lead to small tears known as microtraumas. The condition is a common injury in runners. Your risk is also higher if you're on your feet for hours at work, if you're overweight or if you don't wear proper foot support.

You can usually manage the pain with rest, acetaminophen (Tylenol, others) and anti-inflammatory medications such as ibuprofen or naproxen sodium, orthotics, and physical therapy focused on stretching the tissue. Wearing a splint at night also may help. Plantar fasciitis tends to run its course, but it can take months to resolve. If

your pain doesn't go away, steroid injections or ultrasound-guided procedures may be recommended to stimulate blood flow or remove damaged tissue.

SHIN SPLINTS

Shin splints cause pain in the front of the legs along the lower part of the shinbone, called the tibia. Usually, this pain starts during or after intense exercise such as running or after a rapid increase in activity. The new duration or intensity can stress the muscles, tendons and bone tissue.

Shin splints typically go away with self-care, including resting, elevating the leg, icing the area and using anti-inflammatory medications. Core and hip strengthening also can help promote proper body mechanics during running. However, sometimes shin splints can lead to a stress fracture (see below). You can reduce your chances of getting shin splints by increasing your activity gradually. Wearing cushioned, supportive shoes also may help.

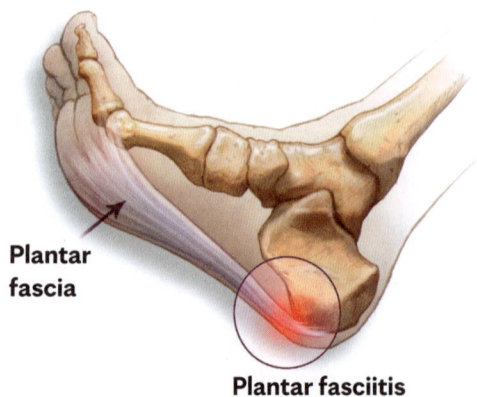

Plantar
fascia

Plantar fasciitis

STRESS FRACTURE

A stress fracture is a tiny fracture of a bone due to repeated force. These fractures are most common in the weight-bearing leg and foot bones. They tend to occur after a sudden increase in activity — doing too much, too hard, too soon — and are often caused by distance running, sports that involve jumping or military training.

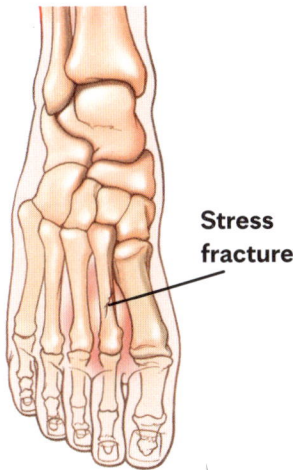

Stress fracture

The pain of a stress fracture develops gradually, becoming more intense with continued activity. At first, rest can relieve the pain. But as the condition worsens, it may be painful even while resting and at night. You may have a specific area of tenderness and swelling, but usually no bruising or discoloration.

To help a stress fracture heal, you'll need to avoid high-impact activities and wear a walking boot or use crutches to decrease stress on the area. With these measures, a stress fracture can generally heal over a period of six to eight weeks.

TENDINITIS

Tendons are thick, fibrous cords that attach muscles to bones and other structures in the body. Tendinitis is traditionally defined as inflammation of the tendons, though in many cases the degree of inflammation may actually be small. With aging and stressful use, the tendons may become worn, frayed and sometimes torn.

Tendinitis causes pain and tenderness just outside a joint — and over the involved tendon — most often around your shoulders, elbows and knees. Tennis elbow, golfer's elbow, pitcher's shoulder, swimmer's shoulder and jumper's knee are common names for different forms of tendinitis. Pain may also occur in the groin area or above your heel, in the Achilles tendon. Pain is usually worse when you use the muscles attached to the tendon. The location depends on which tendon is affected.

The most common causes of tendinitis are injury and overuse from work or play. Professional athletes and weekend warriors alike may be affected by the condition. It can develop along with rheumatoid arthritis and other inflammatory rheumatic diseases. And because of their similar locations in the body, bursitis and tendinitis may occur together. The risk of developing tendinitis increases with age, as your muscles and tendons lose their elasticity. Using proper form and technique while active can help prevent overloading the tendons.

Tendinitis may not require care in a clinic. Treatment usually focuses on resting the tendon, applying ice to reduce swelling, taking pain relievers as needed, and progressive stretching and strengthening of the tendon. Using proper movement technique also is important. If an elbow or knee is involved, wrapping it with an elastic band may be helpful.

Discomfort from tendinitis may disappear within a few weeks. But if pain interferes with your normal activities or doesn't improve after two weeks, see a medical professional. To help rule out other possible problems, you may have an X-ray, MRI or ultrasound.

Tendinitis often heals more slowly if you're older or if you continue to use the affected joint. It may become chronic, and the tendon may even tear or rupture.

Several specific tendinitis conditions are discussed below.

Achilles tendinitis

Achilles tendinitis is an irritation of the Achilles tendon, which connects the calf muscles to the heel bone in the back of the leg. This tendon is used when you walk, run and jump. Achilles tendinitis most often affects people who are physically active, especially in high-impact exercises such as running and jumping, but it can occur in anyone.

Your risk of developing this tendinitis is greater if you suddenly increase your exercise or activity, do the same activities over and over, or exercise without warming up the calf muscles. Your risk is also higher if you exercise in shoes that are worn out or do not have the right support. Arthritis or a bone growth on the back of the heel bone can irritate the tendon too.

Typically, the pain that Achilles tendinitis causes gets worse with exercise and better with rest. Occasionally, the tendon becomes swollen and makes noise with motion. Conservative treatment is usually recommended — resting, avoiding painful activities, icing the area, and using an elastic bandage or a heel lift in your shoe for support. Stretches and strengthening exercises also may be recommended. Specific strength exercises have been found to be especially beneficial for chronic Achilles tendon problems. Meanwhile, acetaminophen and anti-inflammatory medications can help relieve symptoms.

Sudden, severe pain in the back of the leg and difficulty putting weight on your foot can be signs of an Achilles tendon rupture. With this injury, you may hear a pop or experience a sudden feeling of being kicked in the back of the ankle. You might be referred to an orthopedic surgeon to repair the tear. These tears can also be treated without surgery.

If you've had Achilles tendinitis, it's important to warm up your muscles before exercise to keep it from recurring. You'll want to avoid sudden increases in exercise and make sure to ease into a new sport or activity. It also may help to avoid exercising outside in cold weather or on hard surfaces. In addition, keep up strengthening exercises to help the tendons absorb load and wear supportive shoes.

De Quervain's tenosynovitis

This form of tendinitis leads to pain in the base of the thumb and wrist, trouble gripping objects and possibly mild wrist

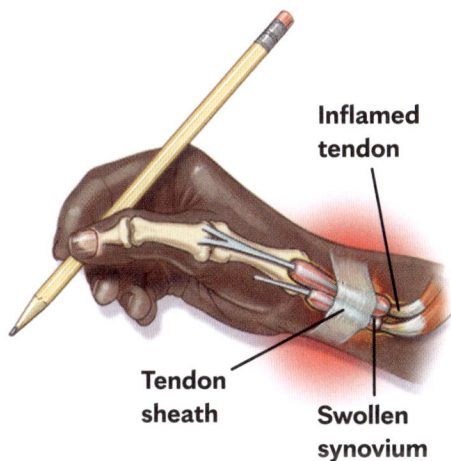

Inflamed tendon

Tendon sheath

Swollen synovium

your forearm or grip an object. The pain of golfer's elbow occurs more on the inside of your elbow, affecting different tendons. The pain typically spreads into the upper arm or down to the forearm. It can cause forearm weakness and difficulty with activities such as throwing a ball.

Sports other than tennis and golf also can cause these conditions. So can work-related activities that involve heavy use of the wrist and forearm muscles. And as people age, tendons can break down, leading to tendon irritation even with normal use.

swelling. De Quervain's tenosynovitis is caused by irritation of the tendons that connect the forearm muscles to the thumb. It also affects the tendons' protective sheaths, a condition called tenosynovitis. It's typically associated with overuse and is more common in manual laborers and during pregnancy.

Treatment includes rest, ice, wearing a splint, and using acetaminophen or anti-inflammatory medications. Sometimes you may need a steroid injection around the inflamed tendon or surgery for relief. After your symptoms improve, exercises to strengthen the muscles in the wrist, hand and arm will help prevent the condition from coming back.

Elbow tendinitis

Tendinitis is one of the most common causes of elbow pain. Tennis elbow, one form of elbow tendinitis, causes pain on the outside of your elbow as you rotate

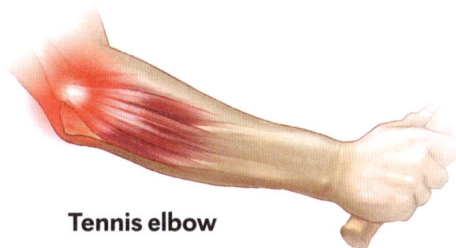

Tennis elbow

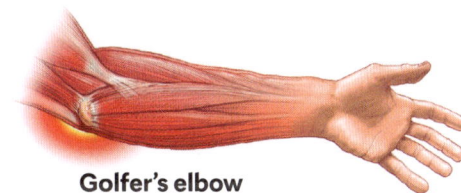

Golfer's elbow

Tennis elbow, a type of tendinitis, causes pain due to tiny tears in a tendon on the outside of the elbow that becomes inflamed.

Golfer's elbow affects tendons on the inside of the elbow.

Symptoms can often be treated with anti-inflammatory medications. Wearing a forearm brace and icing the area can also help bring relief. Specific exercises for the forearm muscles can help to strengthen the muscles and tendons and have been shown to help resolve these conditions. To avoid repeated injury, make sure to use proper technique, whether you're swinging a racket or a golf club.

Rotator cuff tendinitis and subacromial bursitis

Pain in the shoulder may occur when the tendons or bursa of the shoulder joint is irritated. The rotator cuff tendons help hold the arm in place in the shoulder. They may become inflamed with trauma or overuse, such as repeated throwing motion, or as you age.

If a rotator cuff tendon becomes inflamed, it may also irritate the subacromial bursa, which provides a smooth cushion for the tendons to glide along.

Rotator cuff tendinitis generally causes shoulder pain that's worse when you move the arm overhead. It may also limit the range of motion of the shoulder. With continued irritation, the tendon may tear.

If a healthcare professional suspects tendinitis without a tear, you'll likely be referred to physical therapy for treatment. Balanced strength in the shoulder muscles is important to protect the rotator cuff. Sometimes a steroid injection may be helpful. If the pain persists despite conservative therapy, you may need imaging tests such as an MRI scan to be evaluated for a possible rotator cuff tear.

TRIGGER FINGER

Trigger finger occurs when a tendon in your hand becomes inflamed or irritated, leading to a finger that's stuck in the bent (flexed) position. The tendon can't glide easily through its inflamed protective sheath, and it becomes "locked" where it connects to the finger in the palm. You may feel a catching or "triggering" upon waking up in the morning or after rest. At times you may have to use the other hand

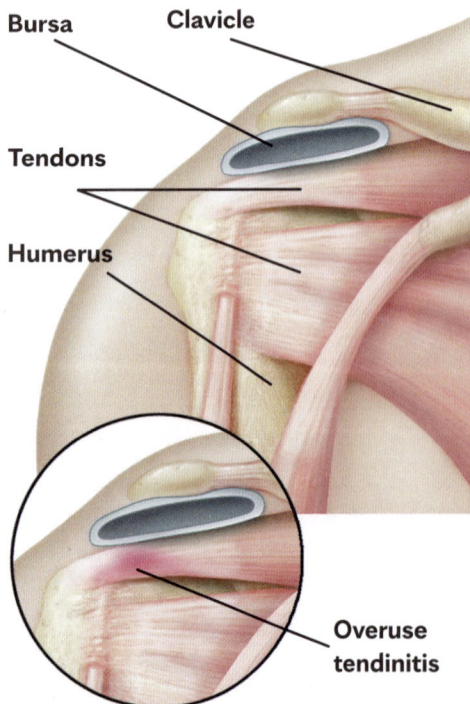

Bursa
Clavicle
Tendons
Humerus
Overuse tendinitis

to straighten out the finger. Trigger finger occurs most often in the ring finger, thumb and second finger.

Healthcare professionals can diagnose trigger finger by examining your hand. They will check for pain, swelling and smooth movement of the tendons as you open and close your hand. To treat the condition, you may try conservative therapies first, including rest, a splint and gentle exercises. Meanwhile, acetaminophen or anti-inflammatory medications can help temporarily relieve pain. If the triggering continues, a steroid injection may be helpful. In some cases, a needling technique or surgery may be needed to relieve the constriction around the tendon.

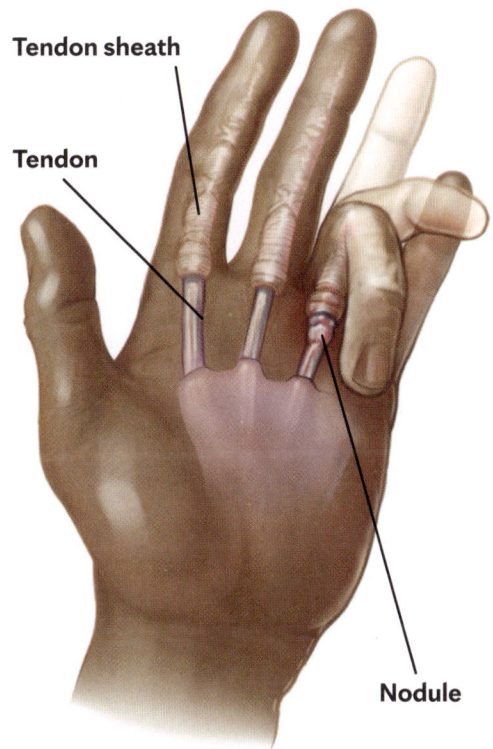

Tendon sheath

Tendon

Nodule

4 Rheumatoid arthritis

Rheumatoid arthritis (RA) causes painful aching and swelling in your joints and leaves you feeling tired and ill. It's the most common form of inflammatory arthritis — caused by inflammation in the body — and it often occurs at a younger age than osteoarthritis typically does. While its exact cause isn't known, the disease appears to be triggered by an abnormal response from your immune system.

The immune system is your body's primary defense against germs, such as bacteria or viruses, that make you sick. When the immune system identifies a threat, it activates special cells, proteins and chemicals that attempt to seek out and destroy the germs. This battle with foreign invaders often results in inflammation — redness, swelling, warmth and pain at the point of infection.

In rheumatoid arthritis and other forms of inflammatory arthritis, something

goes awry with your body's normal immune response. The immune system mistakenly identifies some of your body's own cells as foreign invaders. This triggers an uncontrolled attack on your tissues and organs. Long-term (chronic) inflammation from these misplaced attacks may result in severe damage to parts of your body, including your joints.

Diseases in which the immune system turns against its own body are known as autoimmune disorders. There are more than 80 different autoimmune disorders. Research indicates that some people may be genetically predisposed to develop these diseases. You can find out more about other forms of inflammatory arthritis in Chapter 5.

UNDERSTANDING THE CONDITION

An estimated 1.5 million Americans have rheumatoid arthritis. The disease is more common among women, affecting two to three times more women than men. It occurs more frequently in older people, often beginning in middle age. But it can also affect children and young adults.

Overall, rheumatoid arthritis occurs in about 0.5% to 1% of people, but it's more common in some geographic regions and ethnic groups than in others.

In rheumatoid arthritis, an immune reaction leads to inflammation, causing the body's joints to swell, ache and throb. Pain, swelling and stiffness can make even simple activities, such as opening a jar or taking a walk, difficult to manage. If the inflammation continues over a long period of time, damage may occur to the joint structure, causing it to become deformed.

The primary target of the immune system is a protective layer lining the joints called the synovial membrane or synovium. White blood cells — whose job it is to attack unwanted invaders — move from the bloodstream into the membrane. The blood cells release potent chemicals that cause the membrane to become inflamed.

As inflammation develops, the body recruits more immune cells to enter the synovial tissues. These cells, along with proteins and other substances they release, cause the normally thin synovium to thicken. As a result, the body's joints become painful, tender and swollen.

If joint inflammation persists, the result is often destruction of cartilage, bone and

soft tissues in the joint. Ligaments, muscle and bone also are weakened. This weakening may lead to looseness in the joint and to its eventual destruction. Over time, the involved joints may gradually lose their alignment and shape.

Researchers believe that rheumatoid arthritis begins damaging bones during the first year or two of onset. Because of this, early diagnosis and treatment of the disease are extremely critical.

In contrast to osteoarthritis, which affects primarily bones and cartilage, rheumatoid arthritis can target your whole body. It can affect organs you might not expect to be involved, such as your heart, blood vessels, lungs and eyes. However, the disease most commonly affects your joints.

Rheumatoid arthritis increases your risk of osteoporosis, a bone-thinning disease (see page 32). Taking steroid medications to treat arthritis especially increases the risk.

Some research suggests that people with rheumatoid arthritis also have an increased risk of infections, heart disease and forms of cancer, such as lymphomas. The higher risk of these problems may be due to immune system activity and the effects of inflammation. Medications for rheumatoid arthritis also may play a role.

CAUSES

Scientists still don't know exactly what causes an immune system to turn against

JOINT CHANGES IN RHEUMATOID ARTHRITIS

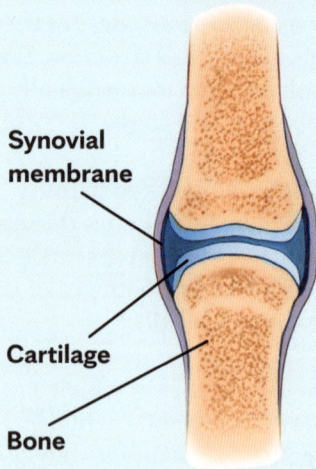

Synovial membrane

Cartilage

Bone

In a typical joint, the synovial membrane forms a protective capsule around a joint. Synovial fluid lubricates the joint.

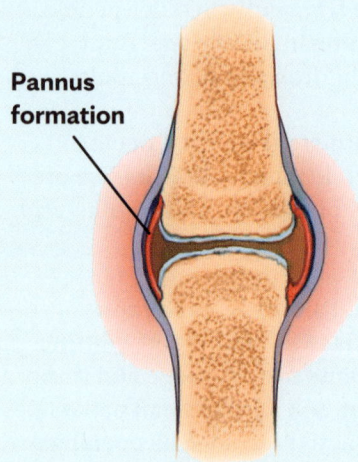

Pannus formation

Inflammation causes the synovial fluid to thicken, forming a layer called the pannus. The joint becomes swollen and warm.

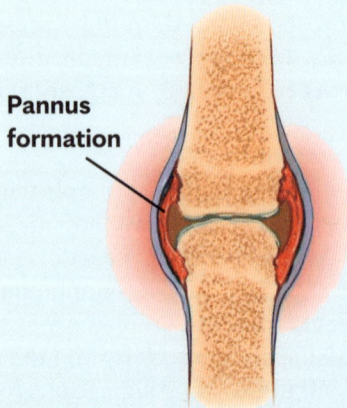

Pannus formation

Cells in the pannus release enzymes that destroy cartilage and bone. Space narrows between the bones of the joint as cartilage is eroded.

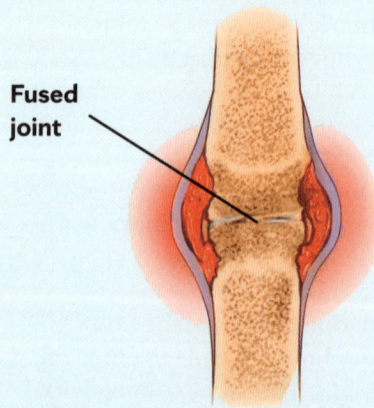

Fused joint

Tendons and the joint capsule may become inflamed. The tendons shorten as the joint becomes too painful to move. This results in fusion of the bones of the joint.

DIFFERENCES BETWEEN OSTEOARTHRITIS AND RHEUMATOID ARTHRITIS

Osteoarthritis	Rheumatoid arthritis
Affects nearly 31 million U.S. adults	Affects 1.5 million U.S. adults
Usually begins after age 40 and symptoms develop slowly	Usually begins in middle age and symptoms may develop suddenly, within weeks or months
May occur in a few joints on one or both sides of the body	Usually affects many joints on both sides of the body
Typically affects only certain joints, most commonly those of the hips, hands, knees and lower back	Affects many joints, especially small joints of the hands and feet as well as the wrists, elbows and shoulders
Usually causes minimal warmth and swelling as well as brief morning stiffness; joints may be hard and bony	Causes warmth, swelling and prolonged morning stiffness, often lasting for hours
Can cause Heberden's nodes — bony growths in the end joints of the fingers	Can cause rheumatoid nodules — soft nodules under the skin, most commonly over elbows or over finger joints
Doesn't cause an overall feeling of sickness and fatigue	Often causes an overall feeling of sickness and fatigue and may lead to weight loss
Blood tests negative for rheumatoid factor and anti-CCP antibodies; normal sed rate and CRP level (see pages 49-50)	Blood tests often positive for rheumatoid factor and anti-CCP antibodies; sed rate and CRP level sometimes elevated (see pages 49-50)

itself in rheumatoid arthritis. But research has identified several factors that seem to increase the risk or trigger the disease.

Certain genes appear to make you more susceptible to rheumatoid arthritis. How severe your symptoms are also may depend on genetics. If you have these specific genes, you're not guaranteed to get rheumatoid arthritis. It's just more likely to develop. People who don't have these genes also can develop RA.

Many researchers suspect that an infection may trigger rheumatoid arthritis, particularly in people whose genes make them more susceptible to the disease.

However, many studies have looked for a connection between specific bacteria or viruses and RA. None have been able to prove that an infection causes this form of arthritis. Recent studies have suggested that infection and inflammation of the mucosal surfaces (such as the lining of your nose, lungs, oral cavity or bowels) may trigger an autoimmune response. This would increase the risk for developing RA, particularly in people with certain genes.

Smoking causes irritation of the airways and increases the risk of rheumatoid arthritis, especially if your genes make you more susceptible to the disease. Smoking may also cause forms of RA that are more severe. For example, smokers may be more likely to develop nodules or have joint erosion seen on X-rays.

Some studies suggest that gum disease may be another trigger for developing rheumatoid arthritis. As with smoking, a type of gum disease may lead to RA in people who are genetically at higher risk. Researchers are also exploring whether an imbalance of bacteria in the gut microbiome — the organisms that live in your gut — may play a role in triggering RA.

Because women are more likely to get rheumatoid arthritis, researchers believe that reproductive hormones such as estrogen also may play a role. The disease often improves during pregnancy but flares up postpartum. In addition, breast-feeding appears to lower women's risk of RA. However, researchers have a limited understanding of how hormones influence the disease.

Experts believe that rheumatoid arthritis develops when several of these genetic, biological and environmental factors combine. The result is an autoimmune disease in which your immune system attacks tissue in the joints of your body.

SIGNS AND SYMPTOMS

Rheumatoid arthritis can affect you in different ways. One common pattern is to have periods when your signs and symptoms are worse, called flares or flare-ups, alternating with periods when you feel better, called remissions.

Some people develop a severe form of the disease that's almost continuously active and lasts for many years. For a few people, the signs and symptoms persist for a certain amount of time — from a few months to a couple of years — and then go away.

The signs and symptoms of rheumatoid arthritis can be more or less severe, and they may be persistent or come and go. Signs and symptoms include:
- Pain in joints, especially the smaller joints of the hands and feet
- Aching or stiffness in joints and muscles, especially in the morning or after periods of rest
- Warmth and swelling in the affected joints
- Loss of motion in the affected joints
- Weakness in the muscles attached to the affected joints
- Fatigue, which can be severe during a flare
- Low-grade fever

- General sense of not feeling well
- Weight loss
- Deformity of the joints
- Anxiety or depression

Morning stiffness is common in both osteoarthritis and rheumatoid arthritis. But with osteoarthritis, it usually goes away quickly — within about 30 minutes. In contrast, morning stiffness associated with rheumatoid arthritis generally lasts more than an hour and may even extend for several hours. Stiffness can recur after periods of rest or inactivity.

Rheumatoid arthritis usually causes problems in several joints at the same time.

While any joint can be affected, most people experience symptoms of inflammation first in their wrists, hands and feet. As the disease spreads to other parts of the body, it may also affect the knees, shoulders, elbows, hips, jaw and neck. Usually both sides of the body experience symptoms at the same time, such as the knuckles of both hands.

Rheumatoid arthritis often is more disabling than osteoarthritis. The affected joints are swollen, painful, tender and warm during the initial attack and during the flares that may follow. Swelling or damage to a joint may limit your range of motion in some joints.

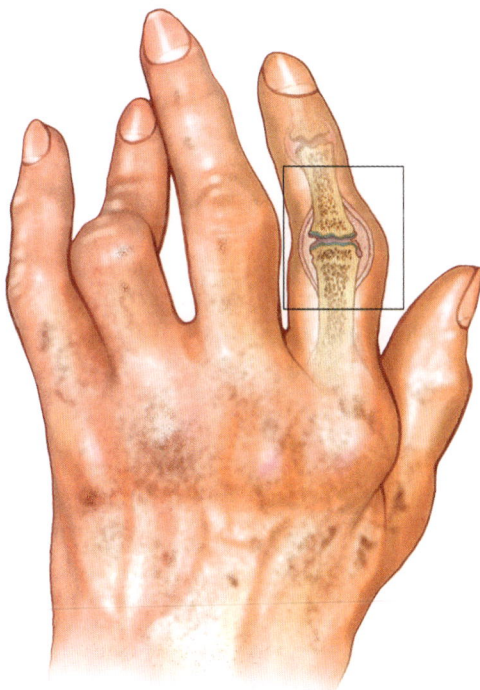

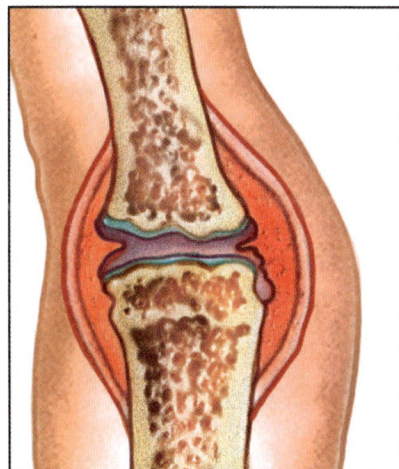

Rheumatoid arthritis often leads to deformity — a change from the usual shape — in the fingers. During flares, your hand may be painful and weak.

Rheumatoid arthritis can affect more than just the joints, too. It may affect all organ systems. This is more common in people who have positive lab tests for rheumatoid arthritis, including rheumatoid factor and CCP antibody tests (see page 50). The disease might involve various organs in the following ways:

Skin

Small lumps called rheumatoid nodules may form under the skin over bony areas, such as your elbows, hands, knees and toes and the back of your scalp. These nodules are usually painless. They may range in size from smaller than a pea to as large as a walnut.

Eyes

Many people with RA develop a condition called Sjögren's syndrome, which causes dryness in the eyes and mouth. In addition, some may have inflammation of the eye. An ophthalmologist should evaluate new pain or redness of the eye in people with rheumatoid arthritis.

Blood vessels

Very rarely, the disease may result in inflammation of the blood vessels, called vasculitis. This can cause red dots to appear on the skin. Another possibility that happens only rarely is that RA affects the vessels supplying the nerves and can cause neuropathy — nerve damage.

Nerves

Carpal tunnel syndrome is common in people with active rheumatoid arthritis. This condition causes numbness and tingling in the hand, especially at night. It occurs when inflammation presses on the nerve that runs through the wrist to the fingers. Usually, once the inflammation is controlled, these symptoms improve. However, surgery is sometimes necessary in severe cases.

Long-standing RA may start to affect the bones of the neck. These bones make up the cervical spine. Sometimes, joint damage from RA causes the vertebrae in your neck to shift partly out of place — known as subluxation — but this is rare. Subluxation can compress the spinal cord and the nerves connecting to the head and arms. If you need surgery for any reason, your healthcare team may check X-rays of your cervical spine before the procedure to make sure the vertebrae are not affected. If there is evidence of inflammation, the anesthesiologist also will take special measures so as not to make any nerve damage worse.

Lungs

The lining around your lungs may become inflamed and cause pain when you take deep breaths, a condition called pleurisy. In some cases, scar tissue in the lungs may lead to problems with the lung tissue — known as interstitial lung disease. Your healthcare professional will refer you to a pulmonologist if these complications develop.

Heart

In a few people with RA, the lining around the heart — the pericardium — may become inflamed. This condition, called pericarditis, typically causes chest pain or shortness of breath. Inflammation in RA can also lead to blocking or narrowing of the vessels in the heart, resulting in a higher risk of heart attacks.

Liver

The liver is rarely involved in rheumatoid arthritis. However, many of the medications used to treat RA can affect the liver, so you'll likely have liver function tests done regularly while being treated.

DIAGNOSIS

It's challenging to diagnose rheumatoid arthritis in its early stages, especially in older people. No single test can confirm the diagnosis, and the signs and symptoms vary from one person to another. Even an experienced rheumatologist may find it hard to tell whether a person has rheumatoid arthritis or another disease that causes similar signs and symptoms.

Healthcare professionals use a variety of tools to diagnose rheumatoid arthritis and to rule out other conditions. An important starting point is your medical history, including a description of your signs and symptoms and when and how they began. For example, your healthcare team may want to know about the morning stiffness you experience and how long it lasts.

A physical exam also can give helpful information. Your healthcare team will look at your joints, skin, reflexes and muscle strength. They will check for typical features of rheumatoid arthritis, such as joint swelling and tenderness, and limited motion of joints or joints out of alignment. You may also be tested on physical functions to check on factors such as your grip strength and walking time.

Blood tests

If you have signs and symptoms of rheumatoid arthritis, you will likely have certain lab tests done. No test offers proof that you have RA, but several different blood tests can provide useful clues to your healthcare team. Along with the physical exam, these tests usually provide enough information to make a diagnosis.

Complete blood count

A complete blood count (CBC) measures different components of your blood to evaluate your overall health and assess a variety of symptoms. For example, a low red blood cell count, a condition known as anemia, often is associated with rheumatoid arthritis. The white blood cell count is usually normal in people with rheumatoid arthritis.

Erythrocyte sedimentation rate

Sometimes referred to as the sed rate, this test can reveal inflammation in your body. In the test, a sample of your blood is placed in a tall, thin tube. Then the rate at which red blood cells, also called erythrocytes, fall to the bottom of the tube is measured.

Cells that settle quickly may indicate the presence of inflammation, which is typical of active rheumatoid arthritis. In contrast, the sed rate in someone with osteoarthritis tends to be normal.

This test is easy and inexpensive. However, it may be less useful for older people. Everyone's sed rate increases with age, making it harder to determine a "typical" level.

C-reactive protein

When you have inflammation, your liver quickly manufactures higher amounts of C-reactive protein (CRP), which is released into your blood. A C-reactive protein test measures the level of this protein in your system. In people with rheumatoid arthritis, the CRP level is usually high.

The CRP test is very sensitive, and it generally measures small degrees of inflammation better than the sed rate does. But sometimes, even during a flare-up of rheumatoid arthritis, the CRP level isn't high. Researchers don't know why this is.

The sed rate and CRP tests are often used to help monitor the degree of inflammation at any given point.

Rheumatoid factor

This test identifies an antibody in your blood called rheumatoid factor.

Antibodies are proteins made by your immune system that normally attach to foreign substances, such as germs, as they enter the body. Antibodies are supposed to deactivate and eliminate these foreign substances, but the rheumatoid factor antibody acts abnormally. Instead of targeting an outside agent, it targets your body's own proteins.

Around 80% of people with rheumatoid arthritis develop this abnormal antibody in their bloodstream at some point. But rheumatoid factor doesn't appear to be a cause of arthritis symptoms, and it isn't specific to RA. While the antibody typically isn't found in people with osteoarthritis, it can be present in some people with other inflammatory diseases or infections.

Anti-cyclic citrullinated peptide (anti-CCP) antibody

The anti-CCP test identifies anti-citrulline antibodies in your blood. Like rheumatoid factor, these antibodies are proteins made by the immune system in response to a perceived threat from your own body. In this case, the perceived threat is from a protein component called citrulline.

This test can help in diagnosing RA early on. That's because anti-CCP antibodies are in the blood of half or more of people with early rheumatoid arthritis, that is, those who have had the disease for less than two years. And someone who tests negative for rheumatoid factor may have an elevated anti-CCP test, which is a more certain sign of RA. Eventually, 60% to 70% of people with rheumatoid arthritis will have anti-CCP antibodies.

Synovial fluid testing

If the cause of the joint swelling isn't clear, some of the synovial fluid from one of the swollen joints may be drawn and analyzed in a lab. In someone with RA, the fluid should have a high white blood cell count — a sign of inflammation.

If the result is noninflammatory, the joint swelling may be due to causes such as osteoarthritis or a joint injury. The lab will also look for markers of other conditions, such as gout, pseudogout or infection, to rule out those diseases.

Studies are ongoing to investigate if sampling of the synovial lining (synovial biopsy) can be helpful for the diagnosis and treatment of RA. So far, this is in the research phase and is not widely used in clinic.

Imaging tests

In addition to lab tests, your care team may order X-rays to examine damage to affected joints. X-rays taken from multiple visits over time can show the progression of rheumatoid arthritis. As the disease progresses, many people develop small holes called erosions near the ends of the bones and a narrowing of the space around the joint from cartilage loss.

It often takes several months of active inflammation before damage appears on an X-ray. So this imaging may not be helpful if your symptoms have just developed.

Magnetic resonance imaging (MRI) may be more useful in detecting rheumatoid arthritis because it can show early inflammation and cartilage damage that isn't seen on an X-ray. Ultrasound imaging also can help your healthcare team detect

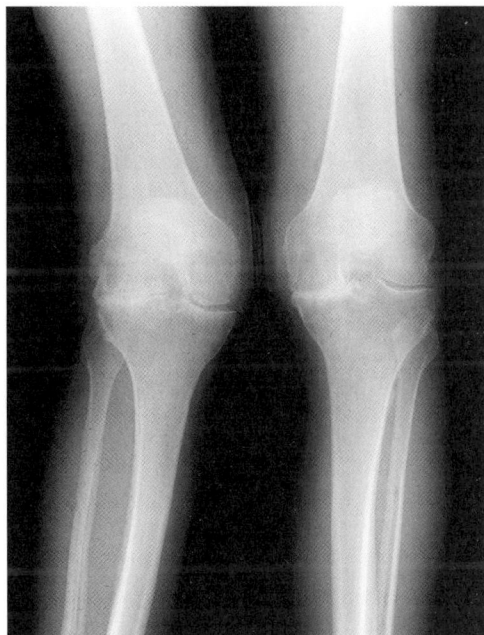

This X-ray image shows two knees affected by rheumatoid arthritis. The cartilage covering the joint surfaces has been eroded, but more severely on one side of each joint.

early joint damage and assess the degree of inflammation.

TREATMENT

Although there's no cure for rheumatoid arthritis, it's best to start treating the condition as early as possible in its course. The goal is to reduce or stop inflammation during the window of opportunity at the disease's onset before irreparable damage occurs to the joints. To this end, treatment strategies now include earlier use of powerful prescription medications that can modify the disease rather than simply treat its symptoms. The medications inhibit an overactive immune system, giving you better control of the disease.

Specific drugs used for treatment of rheumatoid arthritis are discussed in more detail in Chapter 10. Medications can be divided into four main categories:

Nonsteroidal anti-inflammatory drugs (NSAIDs)

These medications help with day-to-day pain and swelling, and they work quickly. Examples include ibuprofen (Advil, Motrin IB, others) and naproxen sodium (Aleve). However, these do not help to slow or stop RA disease activity.

Steroids

Steroids such as prednisone can be very effective in controlling inflammation quickly to treat pain and prevent joint damage, but they have a significant risk of side effects. Often they are used to help control RA symptoms temporarily until slower-acting agents, such as DMARDs or biologics, can take effect. Steroids may be taken in pill form or may be given by injections into the joint.

Disease-modifying antirheumatic drugs (DMARDs)

These medications broadly suppress the immune system to halt the inflammation of RA and stop further progression of the disease. They can take three to six months to kick in, which is why low-dose steroids may be used to control symptoms until these medications have had time to work. In addition, these drugs carry the risk of side effects, including liver damage and lung infections. However, by controlling inflammation, these medications can help reduce the risk of heart disease. Common conventional DMARDs include methotrexate (Trexall, Rasuvo, others), leflunomide (Arava), hydroxychloroquine (Plaquenil) and sulfasalazine (Azulfidine).

Biologics

In the last few decades, many new options for treating rheumatoid arthritis have become available. Biologics, also known as biologic response modifiers, target the specific parts of the immune system that cause inflammation. These medications include tumor necrosis factor inhibitors, such as adalimumab (Humira); interleukin inhibitors, such as tocilizumab (Actemra); the B-cell blocker rituximab (Rituxan); and the T-cell blocker abatacept (Orencia). Most of these drugs are given by self-injection or infusion through an IV. A biologic may be prescribed along with a conventional DMARD to be most effective. Because of the way they work, biologics can increase the risk of infection.

Also available are targeted DMARDs, medications that block specific inflammatory pathways in immune cells. These drugs include Janus kinase (JAK) inhibitors, such as baricitinib (Olumiant) and tofacitinib (Xeljanz).

Biosimilars

In recent years, more biosimilar medications have become available as alternatives to biologics. A biosimilar medicine is not quite identical to its biologic reference product, but it has the same strength, dosage, potential treatment benefits and potential side effects as a biologic medication manufactured by a different company. For more on biosimilars, see page Chapter 10, under Biologic DMARDS.

With the availability of these newer medications, medical professionals have many more options to aggressively treat rheumatoid arthritis and put it into remission.

In addition to medications, a variety of other treatments and interventions may be used to help protect your joints. These include exercise, physical therapy, joint injections, cognitive behavioral therapy and assistive devices. Focusing on certain behaviors, such as healthy eating, maintaining healthy weight and stopping smoking also is key. In some cases, surgery may be necessary.

With proper treatment, many people with rheumatoid arthritis can achieve a state of remission or low disease activity, meaning no symptoms or only minor symptoms. In this way they can avoid the most severe, disabling consequences of the disease.

A CHRONIC DISEASE

When you're first diagnosed with rheumatoid arthritis, it's impossible to predict how severe your condition may become. It may remain mild, or it may progressively worsen. For most people, the disease is chronic, although its symptoms may be more or less severe at different times. Painful flares may alternate with periods of relative remission.

If the symptoms of rheumatoid arthritis are persistent for four or five years, the condition is more likely to pose long-term issues such as heart disease. Your healthcare team will likely need to monitor your RA with regular tests and periodic examinations of your joints.

In some people with RA, the symptoms of inflammation, especially joint swelling, may subside after a number of years. However, joint damage from the previous inflammation may remain, along with some pain.

According to past research, rheumatoid arthritis may reduce life expectancy by up to 10 years. In most cases this is due to the complications of the disease, such as a weakened immune system or the effects of chronic inflammation. But recent developments in treatment are leading to lower disease activity and longer-term well-being in people with RA, so further research is needed.

The prognosis of rheumatoid arthritis has improved significantly, even in the last decade. Medical professionals can diagnose the disease earlier and begin therapies sooner to more rapidly target inflammation and prevent damage to the joints and internal organs. Diagnosis and vigorous treatment at the earliest stages of the disease may help you avoid persistent pain and permanent joint damage and live better, longer.

The degree to which rheumatoid arthritis affects your daily life depends in part on how well you cope with the disease. But with continuing advances in treatment and early detection, many people with RA live long, active lives.

5 Other inflammatory arthritis

In addition to osteoarthritis and rheumatoid arthritis, more than 100 other forms of arthritis can affect the joints. Many of these conditions are uncommon. Some forms are mild and resolve quickly with treatment. Others are widespread throughout the body, affecting multiple organs and blood vessels.

The symptoms can vary considerably, even among people with the same type of arthritis. At the same time, the symptoms of different forms often overlap, making it difficult to diagnose a specific condition.

As with rheumatoid arthritis, genetics plays a role in other forms of arthritis. Some genes have been identified that are associated with particular types of arthritis. But even if you inherit a tendency to develop arthritis, other factors are involved in triggering the disease.

Many forms of arthritis are inflammatory disorders, such as rheumatoid arthritis, with symptoms caused by inflammation in the body. Some are autoimmune disorders, while others are related to infections or how the body processes food. This chapter will discuss some of the more common inflammatory joint disorders apart from rheumatoid arthritis, which was covered in Chapter 4.

SPONDYLOARTHRITIS

Spondyloarthritis (spon-duh-loe-ahr-THRI-tis) refers to a group of autoimmune disorders that cause inflammation in the spine, especially in the sacroiliac joints of the pelvis. It may also affect the joints of the arms, legs and toes. Unlike other types of arthritis, it tends to cause pain at the entheses, which are the points where tendons and ligaments attach to bones.

Diseases in this group include ankylosing spondylitis, reactive arthritis, psoriatic

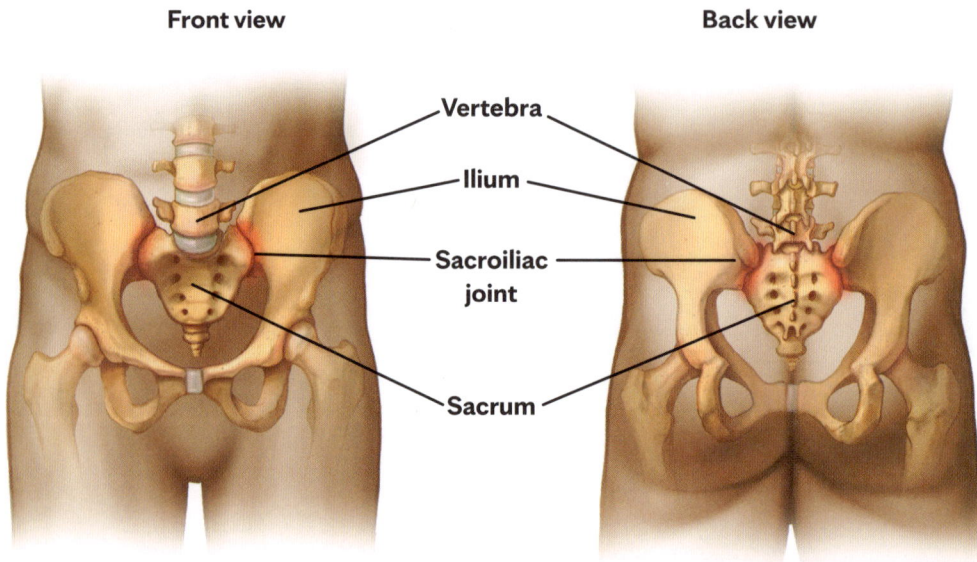

Front view **Back view**

Vertebra

Ilium

Sacroiliac joint

Sacrum

The sacroiliac (SI) joint is the place where two bones — the sacrum and the ilium — come together in your pelvis, forming one SI joint on each side.

arthritis and enteropathic arthritis, which is arthritis associated with inflammatory bowel disease. In addition, some people experience common symptoms of spondyloarthritis but don't have all the distinctive symptoms of any of these four conditions. In this case, the disease is classified as undifferentiated spondyloarthritis.

Like other forms of arthritis, spondyloarthritis appears to stem from a combination of genetic and environmental factors. The human leukocyte antigen B27, also called HLA-B27, is strongly associated with this form of arthritis, although most people with this gene never develop the disease.

People with spondyloarthritis often have low back pain and stiffness from inflam-

mation that causes pain at night, doesn't improve with rest and does improve with exercise. Often, the back pain starts before age 40 and gradually worsens. The knees or ankles may become inflamed, but any joint can be involved. Swelling of the fingers or toes may cause very mild pain or tenderness. Other symptoms may include eye inflammation with a painful red eye that's light-sensitive, a skin rash and bloody stools resulting from bowel inflammation.

A diagnosis is based on your symptoms and a physical exam. An X-ray or an MRI scan may help. For example, an X-ray of your pelvis may show changes typical of this condition. If an X-ray appears typical, an MRI may show evidence of earlier onset of the disease. Blood tests can help rule out other forms of arthritis. You may be tested for the HLA-B27 gene, but having the gene doesn't confirm a diagnosis.

Physical therapy, stretching and range-of-motion exercises can help maintain flexibility in joints and good posture. Several types of medications may be used to control inflammation. These include nonsteroidal anti-inflammatory drugs (NSAIDs), corticosteroids, disease-modifying antirheumatic drugs (DMARDs) and biologic agents, discussed in Chapter 10.

The main types of spondyloarthritis are discussed below.

Ankylosing spondylitis

Ankylosing spondylitis (ang-kuh-LOE-sing spon-duh-LIE-tis) is a chronic disease that primarily causes inflammation in the sacroiliac joints and vertebrae of your spine. It may also affect entheses, where tendons and ligaments attach to bones; the joints of your hips, shoulders, knees and feet; and the joints between your ribs and spine. Your eyes, heart and lungs can be affected as well.

Ankylosing spondylitis is more common in men than in women and typically begins in early adulthood. Many people with this condition carry the HLA-B27 gene. However, HLA-B27 is present in about 6% of the general population in the United States, and most people with the gene never get ankylosing spondylitis. There's often a family history with this condition, and other genes likely play a role.

Symptoms

Many people with ankylosing spondylitis have mild forms that involve only the sacroiliac joints. In others, inflammation involves the entire spine or peripheral joints — or both — leading to physical deformities and other complications.

Early symptoms often include pain and stiffness in your lower back and hips or a dull aching deep in your buttocks. The pain may come and go at first and is often worse in the morning and after periods of inactivity.

Losing flexibility in the lower spine is an early sign of ankylosing spondylitis. Over time, the pain and stiffness may progress up your spine into your ribs and neck.

Ankylosing spondylitis is a chronic condition. As inflammation persists, new bone forms as part of the healing process. The vertebrae may grow or fuse together, forming bony outgrowths and leading to a stiff, inflexible spine. Fusion can also stiffen your rib cage, restricting lung capacity and function.

Many people with ankylosing spondylitis experience eye inflammation, also known as uveitis, and bowel inflammation. In advanced stages, symptoms may include chronic stooping, fatigue, loss of appetite and weight loss.

Diagnosis and treatment

Early diagnosis of ankylosing spondylitis can be difficult if your symptoms are

ARTHRITIS AND INFLAMMATORY BOWEL DISEASE (ENTEROPATHIC ARTHRITIS)

In the United States, an estimated 2.4 to 3.1 million people have Crohn's disease or ulcerative colitis, two common forms of inflammatory bowel disease (IBD). These diseases cause chronic inflammation of the digestive tract. Along with this inflammation, arthritis also develops in certain joints in as many as 25% of people with IBD. This is known as enteropathic arthritis.

Some researchers believe this form of arthritis may result from an immune response to intestinal bacteria in the inflamed bowel. Because people often experience pain and swelling in multiple joints, as well as stiffness in the spine, the condition is considered a form of spondyloarthritis.

mild, since you may attribute the symptoms to more common back problems.

If ankylosing spondylitis is suspected, you may have X-rays to check for changes in your joints and bones, though the characteristic effects of the disease may not be evident early on. If X-rays don't show changes, an MRI can show a more detailed look at the sacroiliac joints and lower spine. Blood tests to check for an elevated erythrocyte sedimentation rate

(sed rate) and for the HLA-B27 gene may help confirm the diagnosis.

Many people with ankylosing spondylitis are able to lead normal, active lives. Effective treatment can decrease pain and may help prevent complications and physical deformities. Stretching and breathing exercises, proper posture and physical therapy are key elements of a treatment program.

NSAIDs can help relieve pain and inflammation from this disease, and medications that block a protein called tumor necrosis factor (TNF) are very effective in improving symptoms and quality of life. (For more on medications, see Chapter 10.)

Reactive arthritis

Reactive arthritis is an inflammatory condition that occurs as a reaction to an infection elsewhere in your body. Many different types of infectious organisms can trigger joint inflammation. This type of arthritis was formerly known as Reiter's syndrome.

What's considered the classic form of reactive arthritis is caused by a bacterial infection in the intestines (GI tract) or the genitourinary tract (GU tract), which includes the urinary and genital organs. The intestinal form is typically caused by foodborne infections from salmonella, campylobacter, shigella or yersinia. Chlamydia, a sexually transmitted infection, can cause the genital form. Reactive arthritis occurs most often in adults between the ages of 20 and 40. While men and women are equally likely to get it from foodborne bacteria, men are more likely to develop this form of arthritis in response to a sexually transmitted infection.

Having a bacterial infection does not mean you'll get arthritis. Reactive arthritis is thought to occur in people who are genetically predisposed to it — many people with the condition carry the HLA-B27 gene. But again, having this gene doesn't guarantee that you'll get reactive arthritis when you experience an infection.

Symptoms

Reactive arthritis typically involves pain and swelling in the knees, ankles, feet and hips. Other joints, such as the wrists and fingers, are affected less often. Inflammation of the tendons, called tendinitis, or inflammation where tendons attach to bones, known as enthesitis, is common. This often results in pain at the heel or back of the ankle (Achilles tendinitis). There may be pain in the lower back and buttocks.

Although joint symptoms are a defining feature of reactive arthritis, the condition can also cause inflammation in your eyes, skin and urethra, which is the tube that carries urine from your bladder. This can lead to eye conditions, skin rashes, increased frequency of urination and a burning sensation during urination. Symptoms generally start 1 to 4 weeks after exposure to a triggering infection. Pain and discomfort may come and go

over a period of several weeks or months. In some people, symptoms subside within a few days. Most people recover within a year. Others may redevelop symptoms after their initial condition disappears.

Diagnosis and treatment

Reactive arthritis can go undetected for some time because symptoms may be mild. Your healthcare team might run tests to see if you have any of the infections associated with reactive arthritis. Blood tests, such as the sed rate, rheumatoid factor and antinuclear antibodies tests, can help determine what type of arthritis you have. You may be tested for the HLA-B27 gene.

Treatment may include antibiotics if your care team suspects a bacterial infection that's ongoing. NSAIDs and corticosteroid medications can help relieve joint pain and inflammation of reactive arthritis. DMARDs such as sulfasalazine and methotrexate or drugs that inhibit tumor necrosis factor also may be prescribed. (For more on medications, see Chapter 10.)

Psoriatic arthritis

Approximately 7.5 million Americans have the skin disease psoriasis, which causes red patches of scaly skin. Among these, as many as 30% to 40% develop a chronic inflammatory arthritis known as psoriatic (sor-ee-AT-ick) arthritis. People with psoriatic arthritis have swollen, painful joints, especially in their fingers and toes, usually in addition to the typical red, scaly skin of psoriasis. They may also develop inflammatory eye conditions.

Psoriatic arthritis affects men and women equally. Most people with the condition have psoriasis long before they develop arthritic symptoms, although sometimes the joint symptoms can occur first. Psoriasis typically develops in adults in their 20s or 30s, while psoriatic arthritis may show up 20 years later. Children also can get psoriatic arthritis.

Both psoriasis and psoriatic arthritis are autoimmune conditions. Most people with psoriatic arthritis have a close relative with the disease, and researchers have identified certain gene mutations that may be associated with it. Among people with a genetic predisposition for psoriatic arthritis, something in the environment, such as a viral or bacterial infection or physical trauma, may trigger the disease.

Symptoms

Psoriasis is a skin condition marked by a buildup of rough, dry, dead cells that form thick scales. These patches, or plaques, of thick, red skin often appear on your elbows, knees or scalp or the lower part of your spine. Your fingernails may become pitted and discolored and may separate from the nail beds.

Psoriasis most commonly develops on the elbows, knees, trunk and scalp. Dry, red patches of skin are covered with silvery scales. Affected joints may become swollen and stiff.

Arthritic symptoms include pain, redness, swelling and reduced motion in your joints, especially the small joints of your fingers and toes. It's common to have morning stiffness lasting more than 30 minutes. You might also feel stiff follow-ing periods of inactivity. Different patterns of psoriatic arthritis cause varying symptoms. The disease might involve joints on one or both sides of your body. Your sacroiliac joints and your spine may be affected, causing inflammatory back pain. Psoriatic arthritis may also cause "sausage-like" swollen fingers or toes.

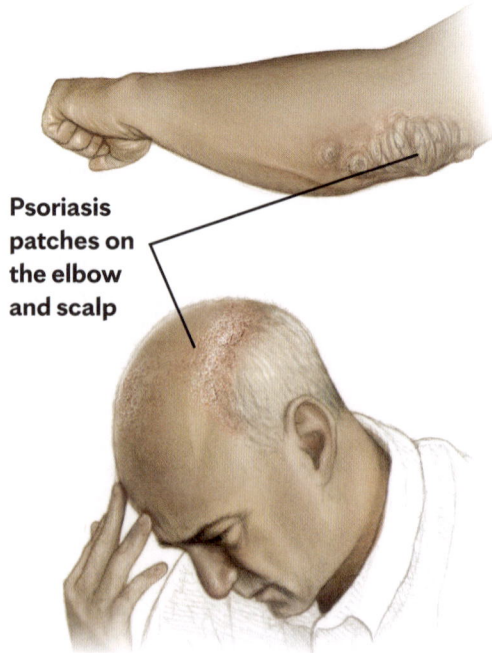

Psoriasis patches on the elbow and scalp

Diagnosis and treatment

To be diagnosed with psoriatic arthritis, you have to have symptoms of both psoriasis and arthritis. Diagnosis can be tricky because in adults, skin problems and joint problems rarely begin at the same time.

You may have blood tests to check your sed rate and test for rheumatoid factor to rule out rheumatoid arthritis. X-rays may show changes in the joints that develop in psoriatic arthritis but not in other arthritic conditions.

If you have a mild form of the disease, a healthcare professional may recommend NSAIDs. If these medications don't control the inflammation, you may be treated with other drugs, such as DMARDs or biologic agents. (For more on medications, see Chapter 10.)

Various treatments, including oral medications, ointments and creams, and ultraviolet light or sunlight, also known as phototherapy, are used to treat skin symptoms.

CONNECTIVE TISSUE DISORDERS

Connective tissue disorders cover a wide range of autoimmune diseases that are often associated with specific auto-antibodies. These conditions often affect multiple organs, including joints. Some of the more common connective tissue disorders are discussed below.

Sjögren's syndrome

Mild decreases in saliva and tear production are normal with aging. If you have Sjögren's (SHOW-grins) syndrome, your saliva glands and tear glands become inflamed and damaged. The result is a dry mouth and a sandy, gritty feeling in your eyes.

Sjögren's syndrome is an autoimmune condition that may occur by itself or along with rheumatoid arthritis, systemic lupus erythematosus, scleroderma or polymyositis.

In Sjögren's syndrome, the immune system attacks the cells of mucous membranes and glands that produce moisture, primarily in your eyes and mouth. The disease may also cause vaginal dryness in women and problems in the muscles, joints, lungs, kidneys and stomach.

Sjögren's syndrome may affect as many as 4 million Americans. The disease is much more likely to occur in women than in men — and is usually diagnosed in people older than age 40.

Experts don't know exactly what causes it. They believe that several factors, including genes and environmental triggers, may contribute to the development of Sjögren's syndrome.

Symptoms

The classic symptoms of Sjögren's syndrome are dry mouth and dry eyes. Your eyes may feel as if dirt specks are lodged in them, and you may have difficulty swallowing or chewing. Other symptoms include:

- Dental cavities
- Prolonged fatigue
- Persistent dry cough or hoarseness caused by dryness in the nose, throat and lungs
- Joint pain, swelling and stiffness
- Mucus-like strands in the eyes, especially in the morning
- Enlarged salivary glands behind your jaw and in front of your ears
- Skin rashes, including purple spots
- Shortness of breath
- Change in your sense of taste
- Nausea, stomach pain or indigestion
- Vaginal dryness
- Raynaud's phenomenon — numbness, pain or skin color changes brought on by cold or stress (see page 64)

Diagnosis and treatment

Your healthcare team may compile a history of your symptoms and do a physical exam, including an eye exam to measure the dryness of your eyes. You might also have blood tests and a lip biopsy, in which a tissue sample containing small salivary glands is removed for analysis. You may also have an ultrasound or other imaging test of your salivary glands to look for changes associated with the disease.

Most people with Sjögren's syndrome can manage symptoms with a self-care plan that includes using artificial tears, avoiding dry environments, sucking sugarless candy and drinking plenty of fluids.

It's important to have your healthcare professional review any medications you take to make sure they aren't contributing to your symptoms. If you have moderate or severe dry eyes, prescription eyedrops such as cyclosporine (Restasis) or lifitegrast (Xiidra) may be recommended. Other medications may be prescribed to help increase the production of saliva and tears, including pilocarpine (Salagen) and cevimeline (Evoxac). In addition, your ophthalmologist may recommend sealing the tear ducts with a plug to prevent tear drainage from your eyes.

To relieve arthritis pain and inflammation, NSAIDs or corticosteroids may be prescribed. If those aren't effective, the DMARD medication hydroxychloroquine (Plaquenil) may help treat Sjögren's symptoms systemwide.

Systemic lupus erythematosus

Systemic lupus erythematosus (er-uh-th-ee-muh-TOE-sus), often called lupus or SLE, is a chronic inflammatory disease that can affect many parts of your body, including your skin, joints, kidneys, blood cells, heart and lungs. There are several other types of lupus that are less common, but the term *lupus* most often refers to SLE.

The most common symptoms of lupus include arthritis and skin rashes. Episodes of lupus tend to come and go throughout your life, and they may make you feel tired and achy. Most people with lupus are women — in fact, the disease affects 7 to 15 times as many adult women as men. It's most commonly diagnosed between the ages of 15 and 45. But it can occur at any age and in either sex. The disease is most common in Black, Hispanic, Asian and Native American women.

Symptoms

No two cases of lupus are exactly alike. Symptoms may come on suddenly or develop slowly. They may be mild or severe, and there may be times when there are no signs or symptoms.

Fatigue, often severe and prolonged, is the most common symptom of lupus, affecting almost everyone who has the disease. You may feel tired even when no other symptoms are present. Arthritis symptoms, including joint pain, stiffness and swelling, especially in your fingers, hands, wrists and knees, are common and may be the earliest indications of the disease.

Other symptoms include:
- Fever
- Butterfly-shaped rash across the bridge of your nose and cheeks or rash on your face, neck or arms
- Sensitivity to sunlight, resulting in rashes, fatigue, fever or joint pain
- Raynaud's phenomenon (see page 64)
- Mouth sores
- Chest pain or coughing
- Hair loss

- Swollen glands
- Swelling in your legs or around your eyes

Diagnosis and treatment

If your medical professional suspects lupus based on your symptoms, the diagnosis may be confirmed with blood tests. One test checks for antinuclear antibodies (ANA), which are proteins produced by the immune system and found in the blood of nearly all people with lupus.

A positive ANA result means you have an active immune system — but not necessarily that you have lupus. People with other autoimmune diseases as well as some healthy individuals also may test positive. You may need further testing for antibodies that are more specific to lupus to confirm the diagnosis.

In addition to ordering blood tests, your healthcare team may evaluate how well your kidney, liver, lungs and heart are functioning.

In the past, lupus was often considered fatal. However, modern treatments have dramatically improved life expectancy with the disease. Your treatment plan will depend on your symptoms and how severe they are. Most treatments aim to reduce inflammation, control joint pain and fatigue, and avoid complications.

Medications used to control inflammation include NSAIDs, the antimalarial drug hydroxychloroquine (Plaquenil), corticosteroids, immunosuppressants such as mycophenolate (CellCept), azathioprine (Imuran), tacrolimus (Prograf) or voclosporin (Lupkynis), and biologics such as belimumab (Benlysta) or anifrolumab (Saphnelo). (For more on medications, see Chapter 10.) Severe symptoms may call for therapies that are more aggressive.

Scleroderma (systemic sclerosis)

Scleroderma (sklair-oh-DUR-muh) means "hard skin." The term refers to a group of rare progressive disorders that cause hardening and tightening of your skin and connective tissues.

Systemic scleroderma is an autoimmune condition that can affect multiple organs. It occurs when your body produces too much collagen, a fibrous protein that makes up connective tissues, including your skin. Researchers aren't sure what causes this abnormal production of collagen. The disease is more common in women than in men and typically affects middle-aged adults. It usually doesn't run in families.

Symptoms

The symptoms of scleroderma vary depending on which form of the disease you have. Skin abnormalities, such as hardening and thickening, are a common feature.

Scleroderma usually causes puffy or tight skin over the fingers. Your skin may lose its elasticity and become shiny as it stretches across the underlying bones and joints. In some people, the skin thickens on the hands, arms, face, chest, feet and legs. When the skin thickening and tightening does not go past your elbows, you are diagnosed with limited cutaneous scleroderma. If the skin thickening and tightening goes past your elbows or involves your chest, you are diagnosed with diffuse cutaneous scleroderma. The terms *limited* and *diffuse* here refer only to the degree of skin thickening and do not refer to the involvement of any other organs.

Often one of the earliest signs of scleroderma is Raynaud's phenomenon, which causes color changes in the fingers and toes — typically from a white to blue to red coloration. This occurs when the small blood vessels in the fingers and toes constrict in response to cold tempera-

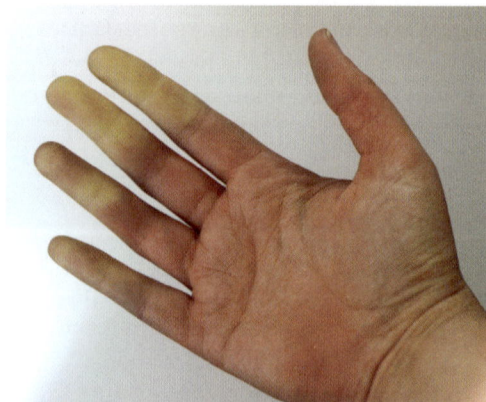

In Raynaud's phenomenon, blood flow to the fingers is reduced when muscle in the artery walls contracts. Skin coloration typically changes from white to blue to red.

tures or to emotional stress. While most people have some blood vessel constriction with cold temperatures or stress, people with Raynaud's phenomenon have an exaggerated response to cold or stress. Some people may develop pitting or sores on their fingertips.

Other symptoms may include stiffness or pain in your joints and curling of your fingers. The disease can also affect your blood vessels and internal organs such as the heart and lungs, causing shortness of breath. If your esophagus or intestines are affected, you might develop digestive problems such as heartburn, bloating or constipation. Your kidneys can also be affected. You will be asked to monitor your blood pressure at home and report any blood pressure changes that could indicate that your kidneys are affected. A systolic (top number) blood pressure increase of more than 20 mm Hg from your baseline, or a diastolic (bottom number) blood pressure increase greater than 10 mm Hg, may be a sign of kidney involvement.

Diagnosis and treatment

Typically, your healthcare professional will review your symptoms and medical history and check your skin for thickened and hardened areas. They will look for changes in your joints and tendons and listen to your heart and lungs.

You may also have blood tests and other imaging or organ function tests, such as a CT scan, a pulmonary function test and an echocardiogram. These can help determine whether your heart or lungs are affected.

There's no cure for scleroderma. However, many treatments can help control symptoms and slow the overproduction of collagen.

For skin changes, anti-itch medications, moisturizers and drugs that suppress the immune system, such as mycophenolate or cyclophosphamide, may be used. Raynaud's symptoms may be treated with medications such as calcium channel blockers (amlodipine or nifedipine) and a phosphodiesterase-5 inhibitor, such as sildenafil, that helps keep blood vessels open. It is also important to keep your hands, toes and core warm to prevent or shorten Raynaud's attacks. Medications also can treat high blood pressure in the arteries in your lungs, known as pulmonary arterial hypertension. Some drugs, including mycophenolate, cyclophosphamide, tocilizumab or nintedanib, may help prevent interstitial lung disease — scarring of the lung tissue. NSAIDs and DMARDs may be prescribed to control joint pain, stiffness and inflammation.

Because scleroderma can cause many different symptoms and can also take a toll on your self-esteem, you may also find it helpful to join a support group or talk with a counselor.

Polymyositis and dermatomyositis

The two rare conditions polymyositis and dermatomyositis are forms of inflammatory myositis, a disease that causes inflammation within muscle tissues. Myositis is also known as inflammatory myopathy (my-AHP-uh-thee).

Polymyositis (pol-e-my-o-SY-tis) causes inflammation and weakness in your muscles. If muscle inflammation occurs along with a skin rash, the disorder is called dermatomyositis (dur-muh-toe-my-o-SY-tis).

Adults between the ages of 30 and 75 are most likely to have these disorders. Dermatomyositis can also affect children, usually between the ages of 5 and 15. Both disorders are more common in women than in men.

It's not known what causes either disease, but they are both autoimmune disorders. Certain inherited genes make you more likely to develop these disorders if you are exposed to specific things in the environment.

However, these environmental risk factors are not always known. When you have an autoimmune disorder, your body's immune system — which is designed to fight off infections — mistakes certain parts of your body tissues as foreign. Then it creates inflammation to fight those tissues.

Symptoms

Muscle weakness is the most common symptom of polymyositis and dermatomyositis. Usually, the weakness begins gradually and gets worse over several months. The weakness is typically felt in muscles on both sides of your body, particularly the muscles closest to the trunk, such as those in the hips, thighs, shoulders, upper arms and neck. You may also have pain and swelling in your joints, leading to stiffness and reduced mobility of joints.

The lack of strength can make it hard to do things such as comb your hair, put on clothes, climb stairs and get in and out of a bed or chair. Entering a vehicle can be challenging. Weakness in the throat muscles can make swallowing difficult and reduce the strength of your voice. Also, lung inflammation may lead to lung problems and cause a dry cough. Lung problems can make it difficult to take in deep breaths while walking or climbing stairs, too.

Dermatomyositis causes several types of rashes. Violet, pink, red or darkened patches of skin may form on the knuckles, fingers, cuticles, elbows, knees, ankles or face, including on the scalp and eyelids. The discolored patches may be accompanied by swelling. Rashes may also appear on the hips, back, neck and arms. These rashes are typically itchy and get worse with exposure to sunlight.

Diagnosis and treatment

Polymyositis and dermatomyositis can be difficult to diagnose. You may have a variety of tests, and your healthcare team may need to see you several times before determining the diagnosis. A physical exam will be done to check for skin changes, joint swelling and lung abnormalities and to test your muscle strength. Blood tests are used to check for elevated levels of certain muscle enzymes, which can indicate muscle inflammation.

If there is concern for lung problems with either polymyositis or dermatomyositis, a pulmonary function test will be done to check for lung function. Your team may order chest imaging studies such as a chest X-ray or a computerized tomography (CT) scan of the lungs.

Other tests you may need to diagnose inflammatory myositis include electromyography, which measures the electrical activity in your muscles, as well as MRIs of certain muscle groups such as thigh muscles, which can show areas of muscle inflammation. A biopsy of muscle tissue also may be done to determine the amount of muscle inflammation and severity of damage.

There is no cure for either condition, but treatment can improve muscle strength and function so that there is little to no disease activity in the skin or muscle. Treatment usually begins with a high dose of a corticosteroid medication either by mouth or by IV to suppress your immune system. The dosage is gradually lowered as symptoms improve, generally within 1 to 3 months.

Your healthcare team may also recommend a DMARD such as azathioprine, methotrexate or mycophenolate mofetil. Because these take a while to become effective in the body, they are often used in combination with corticosteroid therapy, which takes effect quickly. Then the steroids are gradually discontinued as the DMARDs start working. The less time you are exposed to corticosteroids, the less likely you will experience severe side effects from them. If skin, lung or muscle symptoms don't improve, the drug rituximab or intravenous (IV) immunoglobulins — a purified blood product containing antibodies — may be effective.

Topical medications such as topical steroids of various strengths or topical tacrolimus may be used to treat the rashes in dermatomyositis. Medications initially used to treat malaria, such as hydroxychloroquine (Plaquenil), can help resolve the skin rash of dermatomyositis if the rash is mild. However, they don't treat muscle inflammation.

Exercise and physical therapy also are helpful to improve muscle strength and mobility. In addition, people with dermatomyositis should protect themselves from sunlight exposure by using sunscreen, wearing a hat and avoiding the sun during the middle of the day.

VASCULITIS

Vasculitis occurs when there is inflammation of your blood vessels — your veins, arteries and capillaries. There are many types of vasculitis, and most are quite rare. Sometimes vasculitis can cause joint pain. Joint pain is a common symptom of the conditions discussed below.

Giant cell arteritis (GCA)

If you develop new headaches, your temples are tender or painful, and you're more than 50 years old, you may have giant cell arteritis (ahr-tuh-RYE-tis).

This is an inflammation in the lining of your arteries, the blood vessels that carry blood rich in oxygen from your heart to the rest of your body. Giant cell arteritis may also be associated with symptoms of arthritis — pain and stiffness in your neck, arms or hips.

Giant cell arteritis occurs most often in the arteries of your head and especially in your temples. For this reason, the disorder is also known as temporal arteritis or cranial arteritis. It can also cause inflammation in your neck, upper body and arms, or other parts of the body.

Older adults are at the greatest risk of giant cell arteritis. The disease most often occurs in people in their 70s, and it's more common in women than in men. About half of people with giant cell arteritis also have a related inflammatory condition called polymyalgia rheumatica (see page 69).

As with other autoimmune disorders, the inflammation in giant cell arteritis stems from an abnormal immune response. The exact cause isn't known, but researchers believe that both genetic factors and aging play a role. An unknown factor may trigger the onset.

Giant cell arteritis often involves the arteries of the scalp and head, especially those over the temple.

Symptoms

Giant cell arteritis frequently causes headache, weight loss, fever and fatigue. Most people with the condition develop a new, severe headache. Other symptoms include:

- Double vision or sudden, painless loss of vision in one or both eyes
- Tender, thickened artery in the temple
- Scalp tenderness
- Jaw pain when chewing, known as claudication
- Throat or tongue pain
- Pain and stiffness in shoulders, neck, arms or hips (symptoms of poly-myalgia rheumatica)

Note that pain is usually worse in the morning and improves with activity. If giant cell arteritis is left untreated, it can

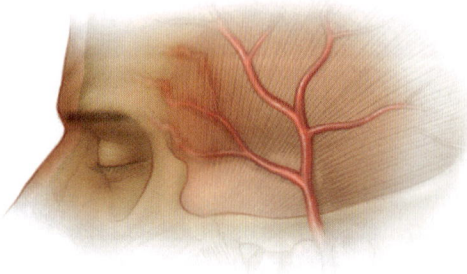

Giant cell arteritis often involves the arteries of the scalp and head, especially those over the temple.

lead to permanent blindness, a stroke or an aneurysm because of the arteries that are damaged by inflammation.

Diagnosis and treatment

To diagnose GCA, a medical professional may start with your medical history and do an exam. They may also order blood tests to check for inflammation, including tests for sed rate and C-reactive protein. These levels are usually high in people with GCA. If arteries in your chest, arms and neck are thought to be affected, your care team might order an imaging test. Advanced imaging tests such as color Doppler ultrasound or positron emission tomography (PET) can produce detailed images of your larger blood vessels and show areas of inflammation.

To confirm the diagnosis, a small tissue sample, or biopsy, may be taken of a temple artery. If you have giant cell arteritis, the sample usually shows signs of inflammation and abnormally large cells (giant cells), which give the disease its name.

Because GCA can cause vision loss, immediate treatment is needed. In fact, you may be started on medication even before the diagnosis is confirmed. Treatment of GCA consists of high doses of a corticosteroid drug. The biologic medication tocilizumab (Actemra) also has been shown to be effective in treating GCA. This reduces the risk of a disease flare and may allow you to take lower doses of steroids. Once your inflamma-

tion is under control, the steroid dosage prescribed will be gradually reduced to the lowest dose needed to keep inflammation down.

People who take steroids over the long term should be counseled on protecting their bones, as steroids can make bones brittle, leading to osteoporosis. Talk with your healthcare professional about calcium, vitamin D and weight-bearing exercise. Occasionally, members of your healthcare team might prescribe other medications to treat osteoporosis or to reduce the risk of complications from swollen blood vessels.

POLYMYALGIA RHEUMATICA (PMR)

Polymyalgia rheumatica (pol-e-my-AL-juh rue-MAT-ih-kuh) is an inflammatory disorder that occurs in people over the age of 50.

The name of this condition comes from the Greek for "pain in many muscles." It causes widespread muscle aches and joint stiffness, especially in your neck, shoulders, thighs and hips. You might have inflammation in other areas of your body as well.

Just what triggers PMR isn't known, but aging and genetic and environmental factors probably play a role. PMR affects older adults almost exclusively — the age at onset is most often in the 70s. Women are more likely than men to develop PMR, and people of northern European and Scandinavian descent are at higher risk.

Symptoms

PMR typically causes pain and stiffness in the muscles of your shoulders, neck, upper arms, lower back, thighs and hips. Stiffness is usually worse in the morning or after sitting or lying down for long periods. A slight fever, fatigue and unexplained weight loss also may occur.

Symptoms may come on abruptly or gradually. In some people, pain may appear almost overnight. Other people might develop a gradual worsening of aches, stiffness and fatigue over weeks or longer.

About 10% to 15% of people with PMR may also have giant cell arteritis (see page 68) either before or after having PMR. The two disorders can also occur at the same time.

Diagnosis and treatment

If your symptoms suggest that you may have polymyalgia rheumatica, your healthcare team might order blood tests. The sed rate and C-reactive protein levels are usually elevated in people with PMR, while markers for rheumatoid arthritis are usually negative.

Aspirin and NSAIDs such as ibuprofen can help treat mild symptoms. However, the usual treatment is a daily dose of a corticosteroid drug, which generally provides immediate and complete relief from symptoms. PMR may require a prolonged course of treatment with corticosteroids. A newer biologic medication, sarilumab

(Kevzara), may be sometimes used to reduce the risk of disease flares and to allow tapering of corticosteroids.

CRYSTALLINE ARTHRITIS

Some forms of arthritis are related to how the body breaks down, or metabolizes, food. When certain substances build up in the body after food is metabolized, they can form crystals that lead to inflammation of the joints. The two most common crystal diseases that cause joint problems are discussed in the following sections.

Gout

Gout is a painful form of arthritis that's been recognized since ancient times. It causes sudden severe attacks of pain, tenderness, redness, warmth and swelling in some joints. It usually affects one joint

Uric acid deposits, called tophi

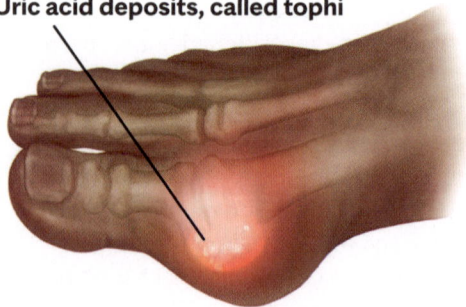

Gout occurs when you have an excessive amount of uric acid in your system. Tiny crystals form in the joints, commonly in your feet, and can cause intense pain, inflammation and redness.

at a time — typically the large joint of the big toe. But it can also occur in your feet, ankles, knees, hands and wrists. Fortunately, gout is treatable, and there are ways to reduce the risk that it will recur.

The prevalence of gout has been increasing over the last few decades, now affecting more than 8 million people in the United States. Although men are generally more likely than women to get gout, women become more susceptible to it after going through menopause.

Gout is caused by having too much uric acid in the bloodstream. Normally, uric acid — a waste product — dissolves in blood and is filtered through the kidneys. From there, it enters your urine and is excreted from your body. But sometimes your body produces too much uric acid, or, more commonly, your kidneys don't filter it adequately. When uric acid builds up in your blood, it can form microscopic urate crystals in a joint or surrounding tissue. The crystals are sharp and needle-like. This sets off an intense inflammatory reaction.

Symptoms

Gout attacks usually happen suddenly, often at night. You may go to bed feeling fine but then wake up in the middle of the night feeling like your big toe is on fire, with severe pain and swelling. The affected joint may be red or purple, hot, and extremely tender. The pain typically lasts 5 to 10 days, then disappears completely. You may have a period with no symptoms at all, followed by a painful

episode. An episode of gout can be triggered by drinking too much alcohol, eating too much of certain foods, surgery, severe illness or joint injury.

If gout isn't treated, it may lead to persistent swelling, stiffness, pain and damage in one or more joints after a number of years. The uric acid crystals may build up into large deposits called tophi (TOE-fie), which look like lumps beneath the skin around the joints. A high level of uric acid in the blood can also contribute to many conditions, including kidney disease, obesity, diabetes, high blood pressure (hypertension), cardiovascular disease and kidney stones.

Diagnosis and treatment

Gout is diagnosed by identifying uric acid crystals in a sample of fluid taken from an inflamed joint. This process is called aspiration. Different treatments can be used during the acute swelling, including medications such as NSAIDs, colchicine and prednisone as well as steroid injections into the involved joint.

Once an acute attack is under control, your healthcare professional may prescribe a drug to reduce the risk of future episodes. Preventive medicines, which include allopurinol (Zyloprim), febuxostat (Uloric) and probenecid, can help keep the level of uric acid within a normal range. The goal level of uric acid in the blood is <6.0 milligrams per deciliter (mg/ dL). If your gout cannot be controlled or if the uric acid level does not normalize with these medications, pegloticase

(Krystexxa) may be recommended. You may also need to watch your diet by avoiding too much protein from animal sources, limiting alcohol and drinking plenty of water.

Pseudogout

A second type of crystal also can cause joint problems. Pseudogout (SOO-doe-gout), also known as acute calcium pyrophosphate crystal arthritis, occurs when crystals of calcium pyrophosphate dihydrate (CPPD) build up in the lining of a joint, called the synovium, setting off an episode of pain and swelling. Although the symptoms are similar to those of gout, pseudogout typically affects a joint such as your knee, wrist or ankle, whereas gout most often affects the big toe.

Pseudogout occurs most often in adults in their 60s or older. The disease can occur with no obvious cause or during recovery from acute illness or surgery. Genetic factors may play a role. Joint injury, osteoarthritis, hyperparathyroidism, low magnesium levels or excess storage of iron also can contribute.

Symptoms

Attacks of pseudogout can occur abruptly, causing severe pain, swelling and warmth in the affected joint.

PSEUDOGOUT AND GOUT: WHAT'S THE DIFFERENCE?

Disease	Cause	Symptoms	Who does it affect?	Treatment
Pseudogout	Deposits of calcium pyrophosphate dihydrate crystals in joints	Pain and swelling, usually in large joints such as the knee	Typically older adults	NSAIDs, steroids, colchicine
Gout	Deposits of uric acid crystals in joints	Pain and swelling, usually in the big toe	Typically older men	NSAIDs, steroids, colchicine, allopurinol, febuxostat, probenecid, pegloticase

Diagnosis and treatment

Like gout, pseudogout can be diagnosed by examining a sample of fluid from an affected joint to see whether CPPD crystals are present. An X-ray can reveal evidence of joint damage, along with crystal deposits in the joint cartilage, known as chondrocalcinosis.

NSAIDs (ibuprofen, naproxen, indo-methacin) can reduce pain and inflammation but will not rid your joint of the CPPD crystals. When large joints are involved, such as the knee, aspirating the joint fluid and injecting the joint with a corticosteroid may help relieve pain and pressure. To prevent further attacks, low doses of colchicine or NSAIDs may help.

SEPTIC (INFECTIOUS) ARTHRITIS AND INFECTION-RELATED ARTHRITIS

As discussed earlier in this chapter, inflammation in your joints can develop in response to a bacterial infection elsewhere in your body. The name for this is reactive arthritis. Other types of infections can trigger arthritis symptoms, too. Sometimes an infection gets into the joint itself, leading to pain, swelling and warmth of one or more joints. This is known as infectious arthritis or septic arthritis.

Most often septic arthritis is caused by bacteria, but it can also be due to viruses or fungal infections. Usually the infection travels through the bloodstream into the involved joint. In some cases, a deep wound may allow an infection into the joint. If the infection isn't treated, the joint can become damaged.

Septic arthritis often causes sudden symptoms in the affected joint, including pain, stiffness, swelling, warmth and fever. The knee, wrist, ankle and hip are most often involved. If a septic joint is suspected, fluid will be aspirated from the joint with a needle and syringe. The sample is then sent to the lab to check for infection. If you have a fever, a blood test may be done to see if the infection is in the blood.

Several types of infections that can cause arthritis symptoms are discussed below.

Bacterial infections

Infectious arthritis can occur if a bacterial infection in your blood vessels spreads through the blood to a joint. It can also develop if a wound or other injury allows bacteria into the joint through the skin.

Staph bacteria is the most common type to cause septic arthritis. If not treated promptly, septic arthritis due to staph can destroy a joint. Another type of septic arthritis, a gonococcal joint infection, is caused by the sexually transmitted bacteria that causes gonorrhea. People with this type of infection tend to have painful inflammation in the wrists, fingers, ankles and toes. Often, they have a fever and feel unwell. They may also have a skin rash.

Your risk for septic arthritis is higher if you take medications that suppress the immune system, such as chemotherapy, steroids or drugs for rheumatoid arthritis. Having an artificial heart valve or joint replacement also raises your risk of developing a joint infection. Only about 0.5% to 1% of people with a replaced joint develop an infection. Unfortunately, artificial joint infections are hard to treat. A structure called a biofilm develops within the joint, and it can act as a kind of shield to the bacteria. This makes it difficult for the bacteria to be found and destroyed by the immune system or by medications.

To treat bacterial septic arthritis, antibiotics are typically given through a vein in your arm. Later you may be able to switch to antibiotic pills. Sometimes the joint needs to be drained to remove the infected fluid. A severe infection may require surgery to clean out the joint.

Viral infections

Many viruses may cause joint pain or inflammation. Typically, viruses affect the same joints on both sides of the body. The pain begins suddenly and is often accompanied by a rash and fever. Some viruses can be diagnosed through lab tests.

Common viruses that can cause joint pain include:

Parvovirus This virus causes a "slapped cheek" appearance in children (Fifth disease). In adults, it causes pain in multiple joints that is sometimes confused with rheumatoid arthritis.

Hepatitis B and hepatitis C These viruses are transmitted through blood from one infected individual to another.

Human immunodeficiency virus (HIV) This sexually transmitted infection usually causes flu-like illness within a month or two after the virus enters the body. Symptoms including joint pain may last for a few weeks.

Epstein-Barr virus This virus, also known as mononucleosis, causes prolonged fatigue and achiness mostly in young people.

Mumps This virus causes swelling of the cheeks and achy joints.

Chikungunya This virus causes a high fever, rash, headaches, joint pain and severe pain with walking.

Viral arthritis usually resolves on its own within six to eight weeks. Treatment generally involves pain medications to relieve symptoms. For a few viruses, such as hepatitis C, an antiviral treatment can help to clear the virus from your body.

Lyme disease

Lyme disease is caused by a type of bacteria that lives in the digestive tract of deer ticks. If you're bitten by a tick that stays attached for 36 hours or more, the bacteria can transfer into your skin.

One of the hallmarks of Lyme disease is a reddish, oval- or disk-shaped rash known as erythema migrans. This is followed by flu-like symptoms, a fever, chills, sore throat and fatigue.

Without treatment, the bacteria may spread to the joints and other parts of the body. Weeks later, you may develop stiffness, sharp pain and swelling in your joints. The pain may affect one joint for a few days and then go away and reappear in another joint. Even if bacteria don't enter the joints, Lyme disease may cause an inflammatory response in your body that leads to joint inflammation.

A medical professional can diagnose Lyme disease with a physical exam and blood and synovial fluid tests. Treatment with antibiotics should start as early as possible. Left untreated, Lyme disease can lead to chronic joint inflammation (Lyme arthritis), particularly in your knee. Other organs, such as your heart or brain, may be affected as well.

Rheumatic fever

Rheumatic fever is an inflammatory disease that can affect the heart, joints, skin or brain. It can develop if strep throat or scarlet fever isn't properly treated. Strep throat and scarlet fever are both caused by an infection with streptococcus bacteria. While the infection itself doesn't enter the joints, the immune system's reaction in rheumatic fever causes inflammation that can lead to joint pain. Symptoms can occur several weeks after the initial infection.

Anyone can get rheumatic fever, although it primarily affects children between ages 5 and 15. The disease is rare in developed countries, including the United States, but it remains common in many developing countries.

Sometimes rheumatic fever causes heart valve damage and heart failure. This is known as rheumatic heart disease, and it may not be discovered until years later. Treatments can reduce tissue damage and lessen symptoms.

Symptoms

If rheumatic fever develops after a strep infection, the symptoms usually begin two to four weeks after infection. Symptoms vary and can change during the course of the disease. They may include:
- Fever
- Joint pain and tenderness, most often in the knees, elbows, wrists and ankles
- Red, hot or swollen joints
- Chest pain and shortness of breath
- A new heart murmur
- Fatigue
- Uncontrollable, jerky movements of your limbs and face or more subtle movement difficulties, such as problems with handwriting
- Areas of pink rash with clear centers
- Pea-sized lumps under your skin, usually over bony areas

Rheumatic fever usually affects several joints in quick succession, each for a short time. Pain may seem to move from one joint to another.

Diagnosis and treatment

Diagnosis typically includes a physical exam, listening for abnormal heart rhythms, simple movement tests and blood samples to test for evidence of recent strep infection. Your healthcare team may also order other blood tests, as well as an electrocardiogram (ECG) of the heart, which checks for abnormal heartbeats.

Penicillin or another antibiotic is typically prescribed to kill the strep bacteria. To control a fever, joint pain and inflammation, aspirin, an NSAID or a steroid medication also may be prescribed. Anticonvulsant medications can help control jerky movements.

MOVING FORWARD

Even though these inflammatory disorders are chronic diseases, you may be able to avoid their most severe consequences and maintain an active, productive life. Both professional care and self-care are essential elements.

Many people find that they can reduce the impact of these diseases by following a carefully planned, individualized treatment program outlined by their healthcare team. Diet, exercise, and knowing when to stop and rest are all important parts of this approach to successfully managing inflammatory joint pain.

6 Back pain and spine disorders

Most people experience back pain at some point in their lives. Often this pain lasts just a few days to a few weeks. Pain in the lower part of the back, also known as the lumbar region, is the most common because this area bears the most body weight and stress.

Back pain can have many causes, from poor posture to cancer. The most common cause is an injury to a muscle or ligament (strain), usually the result of putting too much force on your back or overusing the back muscles in repetitive tasks. An injured muscle may "knot up" into a spasm.

Other causes of back pain include osteo-arthritis, a herniated or ruptured disk, spinal stenosis, and ankylosing spondylitis.

Most back pain disappears with self-care, although it may take a few weeks. Pain

and soreness usually start to improve within the first 72 hours after they begin. If this doesn't happen, consult your medical professional. It's also a good idea to seek medical care for back pain if you are over age 50, if you have a history of back pain or cancer, or if you notice any of the red flag symptoms listed on page 81.

Your healthcare professional will examine your back and look at how you sit, stand, walk and lift your legs. Diagnostic tests such as blood or fluid tests generally aren't needed to confirm the cause of back pain.

If a tumor, fracture, infection or other serious problem is suspected, you may need to have imaging tests. An X-ray, magnetic resonance imaging (MRI) scan, computerized tomography (CT) scan or bone scan can help identify the cause of pain. Another type of test called electro-myography (EMG) can help detect the

Vertebral column

Cervical

Thoracic

Lumbar

Sacrum

Coccyx

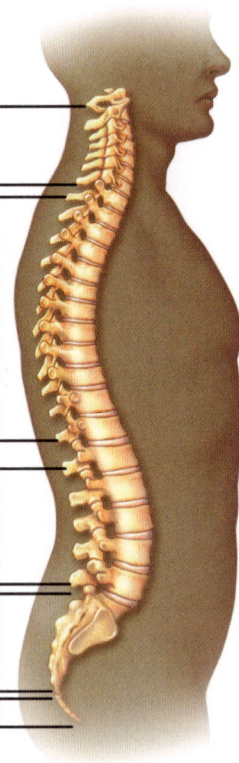

source of numbness or tingling, often related to underlying nerve disorders.

Many back problems respond well to home treatments such as taking anti-inflammatory medication like ibuprofen or naproxen. Applying ice or heat or gently massaging the area also can help. Studies show that most cases of back pain improve in a matter of weeks, regardless of the type of treatment you use. If your back pain hasn't resolved within four weeks, your healthcare team may suggest muscle relaxants, electrical stimulation or physical therapy.

Although back pain is more common as you get older, it's not an inevitable part of aging. You can reduce your risk of developing painful back problems by doing exercises that strengthen the muscles that support your back and practicing good posture and adopting work habits that protect your back. Staying active in general can help to maintain your back strength and function.

DIFFUSE IDIOPATHIC SKELETAL HYPEROSTOSIS (DISH)

Diffuse idiopathic skeletal hyperostosis (hi-pur-ahs-TOE-sis), or DISH, is a hardening of ligaments and tendons where they attach to bone. The tissue forms bony growths at these points, usually around the spine. These bone spurs, as the bony growths are called, may also form in the shoulders, elbows, hands, hips, knees, ankles or heels.

DISH often goes undiagnosed until it causes pain or other problems. It's more common in males and in people over 50, and it has been associated with obesity and diabetes mellitis. Your risk may also be higher if you've taken retinoid medications such as isotretinoin, which is used to treat acne and other skin conditions.

Signs and symptoms

Most people with DISH show no symptoms. DISH may be found when having X-rays or another imaging test for a different condition. When symptoms do occur, they tend to include stiffness and

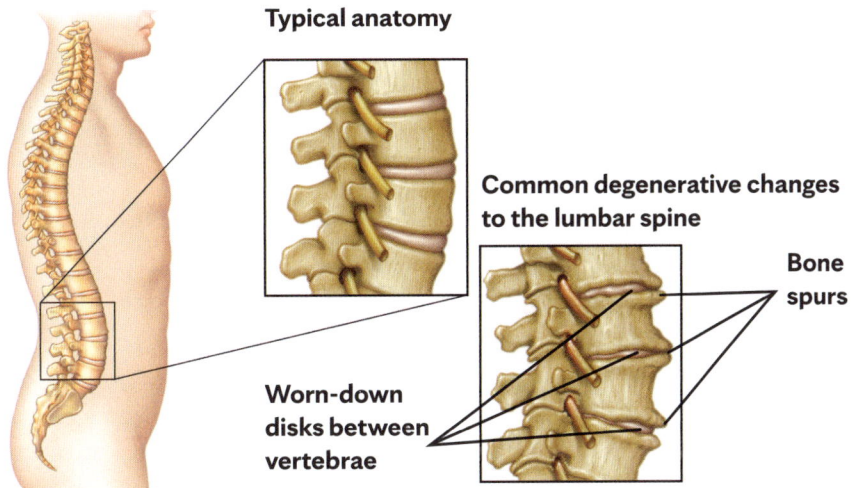

Typical anatomy

Common degenerative changes to the lumbar spine

Bone spurs

Worn-down disks between vertebrae

pain, most often in the upper back. Pain can develop when bone spurs begin pressing on the body parts around them. If DISH develops in your neck, you might have difficulty swallowing or your voice may become hoarse.

Diagnosis and treatment

Your healthcare professional can diagnose DISH based on X-rays or another imaging test of the spine. They may begin with a physical exam, pressing lightly on your spine and joints to feel for abnormalities and to check your range of motion.

There is no cure for DISH, but you can take steps to reduce the pain and stiffness. Treatments may include physical therapy, heat, pain medications and steroid shots. If you have bone spurs on your heels, shoe inserts may help. Staying as active as possible also helps

reduce stiffness and keeps your muscles strong.

HERNIATED DISK

Between the bones of the spine, known as the vertebrae, are disks that act like cushions, with a tough outer covering and a jellylike center. Sometimes a tear can develop in the outer covering, allowing the jelly material inside to push out. This is called a herniated disk and is usually the result of age-related wear and tear. It's also sometimes called a slipped disk or a ruptured disk.

Signs and symptoms

Herniated disks cause symptoms when the jellylike material pushes out and presses on nearby nerves. The most common symptoms are pain, numbness and tingling that spread down one arm or leg,

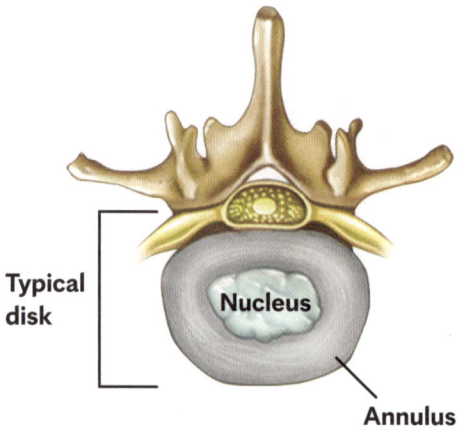

Typical
disk

Nucleus

Annulus

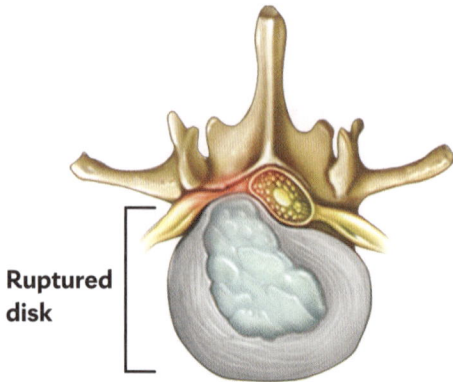

Ruptured
disk

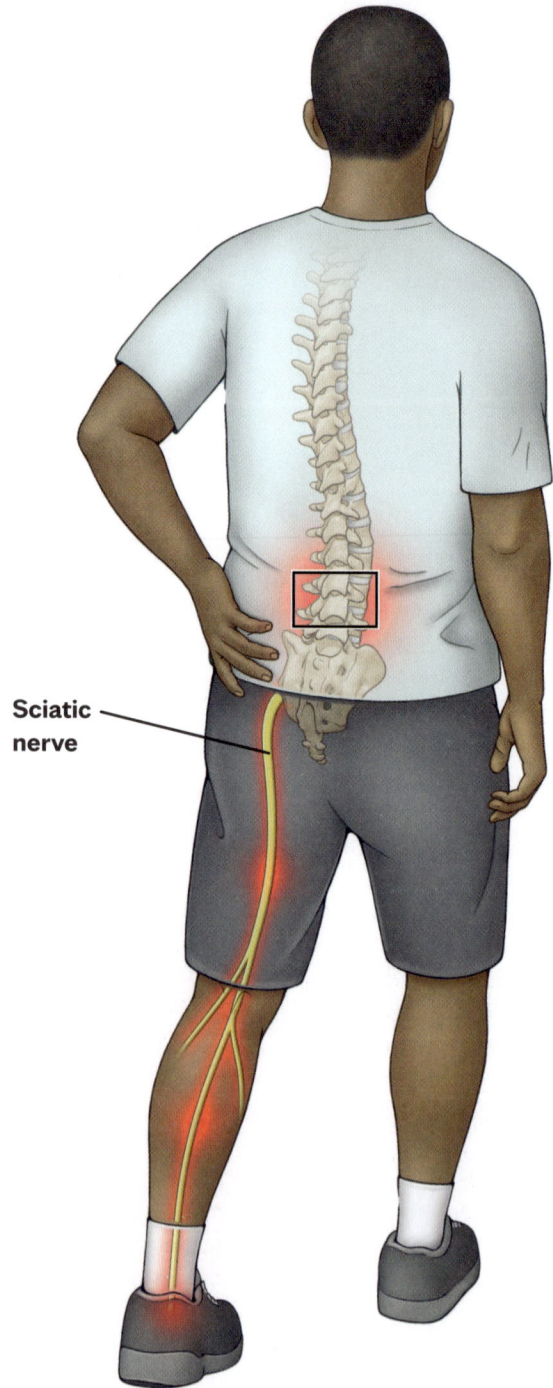

Sciatic
nerve

RED FLAGS: SIGNS AND SYMPTOMS YOU DON'T WANT TO IGNORE

Most of the time, back pain is an annoying problem that improves over time. But in some cases, back pain may be a symptom of a serious problem that needs medical treatment. Get care immediately if you experience any of the following:

- Fever with new back pain
- New bowel or bladder problems with back pain
- Pain from a fall or a blow to your back

You should also contact your healthcare team if your pain:

- Is constant or intense, especially at night
- Spreads down one or both legs
- Occurs with weakness, numbness or tingling in one or both legs
- Includes abdominal pain or throbbing
- Coincides with unexplained weight loss

depending on which disk in the spine is affected. You may also experience muscle weakness. However, sometimes a herniated disk doesn't cause any symptoms.

In rare cases, a herniated disk can cause serious complications. Seek emergency care if you have back pain and have a fever, have trouble going to the bathroom or controlling your bowel or bladder, or experience foot drop, which is when you can't flex your feet.

Diagnosis and treatment

Usually, a healthcare professional can diagnose a herniated disk based on your medical history and a physical exam. They will check for tenderness and may also check your reflexes, muscle strength and ability to feel light touches.

Symptoms usually improve on their own within four to six weeks. Meanwhile, conservative treatments such as pain medication, exercise and avoiding painful movements may help. If the symptoms don't improve, imaging tests such as an MRI or CT scan may be needed to help identify the problem.

Treatment for a herniated disk can include pain medications, muscle relaxants, injections, physical therapy, spinal traction, acupuncture and massage. A small number of people may need surgery to get relief.

Staying as active as possible is an important part of treatment, even if you have some pain or discomfort. Although bed rest was once recommended, researchers now know that long periods of rest can make spine pain worse.

CERVICAL SPINE DISORDERS

The vertebrae of the neck make up the upper portion of the spine; this area is called the cervical spine. As in the back, the vertebrae are stacked one on top of another, with disks between them that function as cushions. Ligaments cover the bones and the disks, helping to stabilize and protect the spine. The spinal cord runs down through the vertebrae and connects to other nerves. The muscles surrounding the spine are responsible for holding the head upright.

Neck pain can result from problems with any of these parts, including muscle or ligament irritation, arthritis, or a pinched nerve. Many people — up to half or more of all adults — experience neck pain at some point. Regardless of the cause, most people recover with conservative therapies.

It's often difficult to know for sure what exactly is causing neck pain. Your symptoms and the degree of pain may not correlate with the severity of the problem. In other words, you may have strong pain from a small change in the spine, or you may feel only mild symptoms from a more significant problem.

Many of the causes of neck pain, such as changes to the vertebrae, cannot be repaired or undone. This makes it all the more important to work on the factors you can control. Your posture, muscle strength, sleep habits, proper teeth alignment and the amount of tension in your head can all help relieve neck pain or contribute to it.

Some of the more common causes of neck pain include the following:

Cervical strain An injury to the neck muscles can cause muscle spasms and pain.

Cervical spondylosis This condition involves age-related wear and tear of the bones and disks in the cervical spine.

Cervical discogenic pain A problem with the disks between the vertebrae, such as irritation or degeneration of the disks, is one of the most common causes of neck pain. The pain is worse when the neck is held in one position for long periods of time (for example, while driving).

Cervical facet joint syndrome This type of arthritis affects the facet joints, located on both sides of the vertebrae. You use these joints when moving your neck and head.

Whiplash injury This condition is usually caused by the trauma of an abrupt forward or backward movement of the neck, such as often happens in a car accident.

Cervical myofascial pain Tight areas of neck muscle may feel tender and painful.

DISH This is a hardening of ligaments and tendons where they attach to bone (see page 78).

Cervical spondylotic myelopathy This pinching of the spinal cord in the neck is due to changes from degenerative arthritis, and it keeps the spinal cord from functioning properly. This condition may cause weakness, make walking difficult, decrease bowel or bladder control, and bring about sexual dysfunction.

Cervical radiculopathy A nerve root in the neck may become irritated or pinched where it leads out from the spinal cord. When this occurs, it can cause pain or tingling in the shoulder and arm.

Diagnosis and treatment

A medical professional will examine your neck by moving your head to the left and right, forward and backward, and side to side. Imaging tests also may be needed to confirm a diagnosis, depending on your symptoms.

Most of the time, the pain resolves with a conservative treatment such as taking acetaminophen (Tylenol, others) or anti-inflammatory medications. Sometimes a muscle relaxant or antidepressant may be prescribed to help treat pain.

Self-care treatments such as ice and heat may also help reduce pain. Massage can help relieve muscle spasms, and stretching exercises may help loosen and strengthen the muscles. Because emotional stress can increase neck tension, reducing stress may help prevent neck pain. In addition, good neck posture can lessen tension across the muscles. Sleeping with a small pillow under the nape of your neck keeps your neck in a neutral position. When carrying heavy items, carry them close to your body rather than with outstretched arms to lower the risk of straining your neck or back.

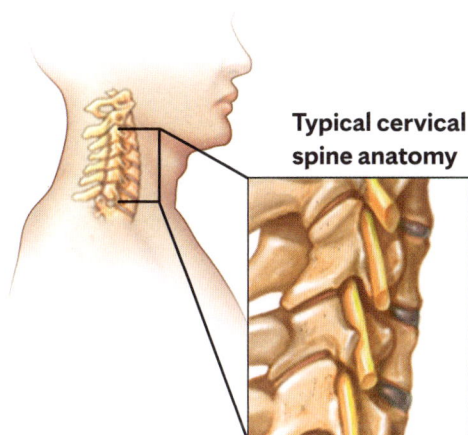

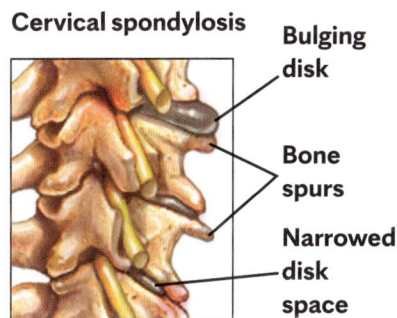

Typical cervical spine anatomy

Cervical spondylosis

Bulging disk

Bone spurs

Narrowed disk space

Other treatments may include acupuncture, a neck brace, steroid injections, electrical stimulation and biofeedback, which is a method of learning to regulate your response to pain.

Chiropractic therapy, physical therapy, and assisted stretching and lengthening of the neck (cervical traction) are sometimes helpful as well. Surgery isn't usually needed. However, if a nerve is being pinched by a herniated disk and doesn't respond to conservative therapy, surgery may be an option.

MECHANICAL LOW BACK PAIN

Almost everyone experiences back pain at some point. In most cases, the back pain isn't serious, and it usually resolves on its own. However, if you have any red flag symptoms (see page 81) with persistent pain, see a healthcare professional.

Your lower back, like your neck, is made up of vertebrae, shock-absorbing disks, the spinal cord and other nerves, muscles, tendons and ligaments. One or more of the tissues in the lower back may become painful when irritated. For example, this can occur with bulging or torn disks, a vertebra out of place, narrowing in the spinal canal or other changes.

Pain from these issues is called mechanical — due to pain sensors within the mechanical working parts of the spine. Often it's difficult to determine the specific location and cause of the irritation and pain. Back pain also may be due to arthritis of the spine joints or, less often, a tumor or infection.

Diagnosis and treatment

A physical exam may be all you need to get a diagnosis. Imaging tests usually aren't necessary unless your back pain doesn't improve after four to six weeks.

Staying active, even through mild pain, is a key part of treatment. Sometimes treatment will also involve pain medications, physical therapy, low back or lumbar spine traction, acupuncture,

massage, measures to reduce stress or steroid injections.

Low back pain can be a recurring problem, so it's important to stay active and learn exercises that help strengthen and stretch your back. When lifting objects, lift from your legs instead of with your back. And avoid sitting or standing in the same position for too long. Following these tips can help protect you from future injuries.

SCHEUERMANN'S KYPHOSIS

A humped back, known as kyphosis, can result from changes in the spine. Scheuermann's kyphosis, also known as juvenile kyphosis, occurs when the vertebrae develop a wedged shape,

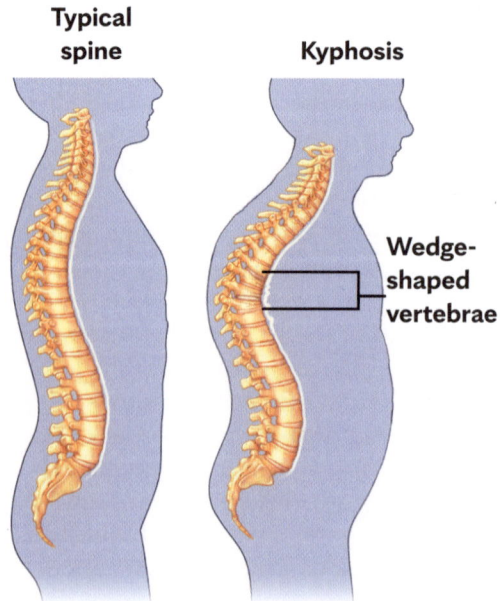

Typical spine

Kyphosis

Wedge-shaped vertebrae

causing the spine to curve forward. It occurs in some children during a growth spurt, when the growth plates in the spine haven't yet hardened into solid bone.

The curve tends to form in the upper or middle back and may sometimes be taken for poor posture. The difference is that the curve doesn't disappear when you stand up straight or lie flat on your back.

Evidence shows that genetics predisposes some people to Scheuermann's kyphosis. But other factors likely also affect the bone growth.

Signs and symptoms

Along with a humped back, this condition often causes back pain around the time of puberty. The pain is typically worse after activities and improves with rest. Later in adolescence, as bone growth slows down, the pain usually improves.

Diagnosis and treatment

Scheuermann's kyphosis is diagnosed with X-rays. Your healthcare team will look for at least three vertebrae in a row with a wedge shape to confirm the diagnosis.

Conservative treatment is usually recommended. This may include exercising the muscles around the spine, managing the pain and avoiding activities that make the pain worse. In rare cases of a significant curve, you may need to wear a back brace or have surgery to correct the spinal curve.

SPINAL STENOSIS

Spinal stenosis (stuh-NO-sis) is the narrowing of one or more areas in your spine. This narrowing puts pressure on the spinal cord and roots of the spinal nerves.

The spinal cord is a bundle of nerves and nerve cells that extends the full length of your spine. The cord is housed in a canal within the vertebrae. Smaller nerves branch off from the spinal cord, forming an intricate communication network between your brain and the rest of your body.

Spinal stenosis doesn't always cause problems. In cases where the narrowed spinal canal puts pressure on the spinal cord, a wide range of symptoms can result. It may cause pain, cramping or numbness in your legs, back, neck, shoulders or arms. Inflammation also can contribute to your symptoms.

Spinal stenosis typically affects adults over age 50. Most often, the spinal narrowing results from osteoarthritis. But an injury, cancer or another disease can also lead to it.

As the disks between the vertebrae age and bone spurs or other changes of arthritis form, the spaces between the bones may decrease or disappear. These changes can cause vertebrae and soft tissue to push inward into the spinal canal.

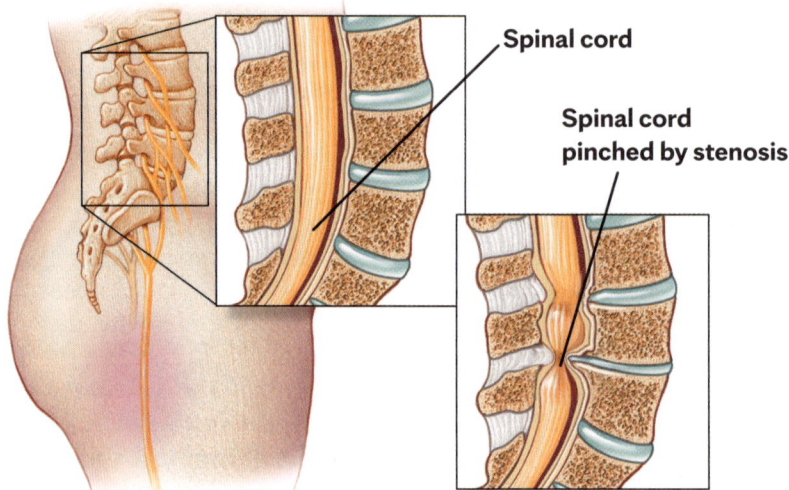

Spinal cord

Spinal cord pinched by stenosis

Spinal stenosis may result when the spinal canal becomes narrowed by osteoarthritis or some other cause. It usually affects the neck or lower back. If the spinal cord or nerve roots in the lower back are pinched, stenosis may cause pain, numbness and tingling in your hips, buttocks and legs.

Signs and symptoms

Symptoms of spinal stenosis vary, depending on where in the spine the narrowing occurs and which nerves are affected. If the narrowed area does cause symptoms, they often start gradually and get worse over time. They may include:

- Pain that runs down the back of your leg
- Numbness, tingling, cramping or weakness in your hand, arm, foot or leg
- Loss of balance
- Diminished bowel and bladder control

The pain of spinal stenosis usually improves if you lean forward, crouch or sit down. You'll likely notice pain more when you walk downhill. This is different from leg pain that occurs as a result of poor circulation, which is usually worse when you walk uphill and improves when you stop walking.

Diagnosis and treatment

Spinal stenosis can be difficult to diagnose because leg pain is often the main symptom. In addition to a physical exam, you'll also likely undergo imaging tests, such as a spinal X-ray, MRI or CT.

Many people with spinal stenosis find effective relief with pain relievers, rest, physical therapy, exercise and other conservative treatments.

If you have severe pain that interferes with your ability to walk or do other activities, increasing leg weakness, or reduced bladder or bowel control, surgery may be recommended to relieve the pressure and maintain the strength and integrity of your spine.

SPONDYLOLYSIS AND SPONDYLOLISTHESIS

Spondylolysis (spahn-duh-LOL-ih-sis) is a crack or separation in the thin section of bone that connects the back and front parts of a vertebra. It affects about 7% of people, most often during adolescence. It's more likely to occur with overuse activities or an injury (trauma). It's more commonly seen in sports that put a lot of stress on the lower back, especially by bending backward, during growth spurts in young athletes. For example, dancers, gymnasts, figure skaters, wrestlers, divers and football linebackers are particularly at risk. However, the condition can affect anyone.

Spondylolysis can occur on one or both sides of the vertebra, and in one or more bones. When fractures occur in both sides of a vertebra, the bone may slip forward out of alignment. Spondylolisthesis (spon-duh-loe-lis-THEE-sis) occurs when there is "slippage," known in

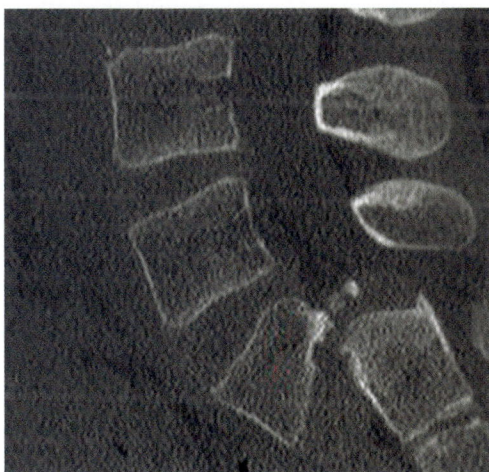
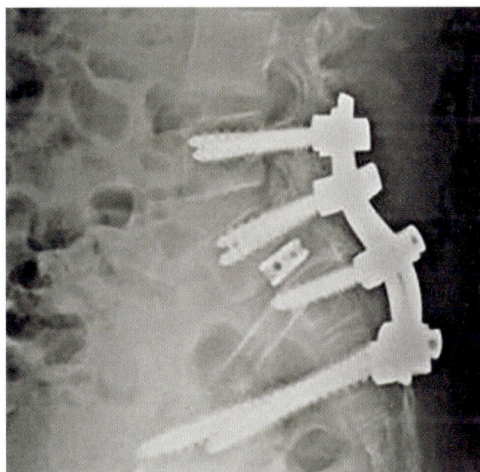

A CT scan (left) shows an extreme case of spondylolisthesis in the lower back. The L5 vertebra, the lowest bone in the lumbar spine, is almost completely off the S1 vertebra below it. An X-ray (right) shows the corrected spine, with rods and screws in place, after surgery to fuse the L5 with the bones above and below it. In most people with spondylolisthesis, the slippage is less severe and surgery isn't needed.

medical terms as *listhesis,* of one vertebra on another. This can put pressure on the nerves and lead to symptoms that are more severe.

Signs and symptoms

Children who develop spondylolysis early in life usually have no symptoms. The condition is found when X-rays or other images of the spine are taken for other reasons. In adolescent athletes, symptoms often develop gradually. The most common symptom is lower back pain during activities, particularly when bending backward.

Children with spondylolisthesis develop pain that spreads across the lower back and into the buttocks or the back of the legs. A slipped vertebra can lead to numbness, tingling and weakness if it presses on nerve roots. Athletes may experience sharp pain with back extension during activities — for example, kicking a soccer ball or striking a volleyball.

Diagnosis and treatment

Spondylolysis is diagnosed with a physical exam and X-rays or other imaging tests. In people with no symptoms, a fracture may be found when imaging tests are done for another reason.

There is limited evidence regarding the best treatment options for these conditions. In addition, treatment varies depending on symptoms and whether the bone has slipped out of alignment. For most adolescents with a fracture or a bone that has slipped only partially, several months of rest from activity may be the most effective way to allow symptoms to improve. Back braces have been used in the past but usually aren't needed for healing.

If someone has a severely slipped vertebra or doesn't respond to nonsurgical therapies, surgery may be needed to fuse the bones of the spine in the correct position.

7 Childhood arthritis

Nearly all children have a hurt limb or joint at some point. Usually, the pain improves with limited intervention. Joint pain in children may be caused by inflammation within the joint or other conditions related to the bones and muscles. Some conditions are associated with changes to the bones and joints that occur as children grow. These may even resolve on their own with time.

However, nearly 300,000 children in the United States have some form of chronic, inflammatory arthritis, the majority occurring as some form of juvenile idiopathic arthritis. As in adults, arthritis in children can take many different forms, with various causes, symptoms and risks. Whatever the cause, most joint pain in children can be improved with the right diagnosis and modern treatments.

JUVENILE IDIOPATHIC ARTHRITIS

Juvenile idiopathic arthritis (JIA) is a chronic autoimmune disease that causes joint inflammation in children, defined as symptoms beginning at age 16 and younger. The word *idiopathic* means that the cause is unknown — and the exact cause of JIA is unclear. But, like adult rheumatoid arthritis, juvenile idiopathic arthritis is an autoimmune disease and involves both genetic and environmental factors.

There are several distinct subtypes of JIA based on features of the disease. The following sections give information on each type.

Oligoarticular JIA

This is the most common form of JIA, affecting four or fewer joints — typically the larger joints, such as the knees and ankles. Often only one knee is affected, which can make diagnosis challenging, as there are usually no other symptoms. Girls are more likely to have this form of JIA than are boys.

Oligoarticular JIA most commonly occurs in very young children, often before the age of 4. Many children with this form can achieve remission, with no symptoms of arthritis. Remission can exist for some time, even off treatment.

Polyarticular JIA

Poly means many, and this form of arthritis affects five or more joints — typically small joints, such as those in the hands and feet in addition to larger joints. It often affects the same joint on both sides of the body, such as both wrists, but can also affect the spine, such as in the neck. Polyarticular JIA can begin at any age and affects girls more often than boys.

This subtype of JIA most resembles adult rheumatoid arthritis. Certain test results, including a positive rheumatoid factor (RF) or a positive cyclic citrullinated peptide (CCP) antibody count, can help characterize polyarticular JIA as essentially a childhood-onset form of rheumatoid arthritis. However, these tests are rarely positive in children, as this is one of the least common subtypes. It is known to have a more difficult course and be more difficult to treat.

Enthesitis-related arthritis (ERA)

This subtype of JIA is closely related to adult forms of spondyloarthritis. The main feature is inflammation — called enthesitis — that occurs at the sites where tendons or ligaments attach to bones near a joint. It is also accompanied by arthritis, usually involving the ankles, feet, spine and pelvis.

Children with ERA can have back pain and stiffness around their sacroiliac joints, where the spine connects to the pelvis. An MRI may show inflammation much earlier in the disease course than a plain X-ray and is useful in identifying arthritis in this body area. Children who have arthritis mainly in these joints may be diagnosed with juvenile anky-losing spondylitis. This is often considered a type of ERA with features similar to those of ankylosing spondyli-tis in adults.

ERA usually occurs in children over age 6 and is more common in boys than in girls. In addition, about 60% of children with ERA have a gene called human leukocyte antigen B27 (HLA-B27). But having this gene doesn't mean you have or will get the disease. About 6% of the general U.S. population has the gene.

Psoriatic arthritis

Psoriatic arthritis can affect children as well as adults and is more common in girls than in boys. Psoriasis is a red, scaly and flaky skin rash that can also cause pitted nails. Not every patient with psoriasis will have arthritis, but when they do, the arthritis usually affects multiple joints. This can look different than other forms of arthritis, such as when the fingers or toes become swollen, known as dactylitis ("sausage digits"). Older children and teens with psoriatic arthritis may have back or hip pain. Rarely, this condition can cause inflammation of the eye, a condition known as uveitis.

Psoriasis and psoriatic arthritis are strongly linked to family history. Because of this, a child with JIA may be diagnosed with psoriatic arthritis if they have a family member with psoriasis. The child doesn't need to have a personal history of psoriasis in order for the condition to be characterized as psoriatic arthritis.

Systemic JIA

Systemic JIA (formerly called Still's disease) is a unique and rare form of JIA. It is the only form of JIA that can be directly life-threatening. The disease is characterized by a recurring high fever that typically appears in the afternoon and evening and is often accompanied by a faint pink rash that can come and go on any part of the body. The arthritis in systemic JIA usually affects multiple joints. It may appear along with the initial fevers or rash, or it may not show up until months after the onset of fevers.

True to its name, systemic JIA can affect many areas of the body, not just the joints. It is the only form of JIA that affects internal organs. Children with this condition may develop an enlarged liver and spleen, swollen lymph nodes, or heart or lung disease. Some disease flares can create excessive amounts of inflammation causing a storm of inflammatory chemicals called cytokines. This condition, macrophage activation syndrome (MAS), is life-threatening, and patients may experience it once, multiple times or never during the course of their disease.

Symptoms

Symptoms of JIA vary from one child to another even when the subtype is the same. They can fluctuate from day to day and even throughout the same day. They may include:

- *Joint swelling with stiffness and achy pain.* Children may not complain of joint pain or swelling. Rather, you may notice them limping, being less active than usual, or favoring one arm or leg over the other. You may notice difficulty in the way your child crawls, walks, jumps, colors, ties shoes, eats, or holds a cup or spoon. Discomfort may be more pronounced in the morning or after a nap and then improve with some activity. Arthritis in JIA is chronic, however, and though day-to-day variability is seen, on a physical exam the changes are always evident once it has set in, until treatment occurs.
- *Bone and joint changes.* If arthritis in children is severe or goes untreated for a long period of time, a joint may lose its range of motion.

This typically improves once the inflammation is treated, but it may require physical therapy. Joint inflammation in children can also cause growth changes, leading to uneven leg or arm lengths.

- *Eye inflammation.* Eye inflammation or uveitis occurs with several subtypes of JIA, most commonly with oligoarticular JIA. The uveitis associated with oligoarticular JIA often doesn't cause any signs or symptoms. In some forms like ERA and psoriatic arthritis, it may cause eye pain, redness and increased sensitivity to light. Routine eye examinations are recommended because eye inflammation can be difficult to detect, and it may lead to decreased vision. The frequency of eye exams is determined by the subtype of JIA and other risk factors.
- *Rash.* Certain forms of JIA can include skin changes. A constant scaly red rash could be psoriasis, related to psoriatic arthritis. But a faint pink rash that comes and goes (with a fever) could be a sign of systemic JIA.
- *Fever.* A recurring high fever is a characteristic sign of systemic JIA that is not present or associated with other forms of JIA. However, other autoimmune diseases also include arthritis as a symptom or feature, and fever may also occur in these autoimmune diseases, including lupus, dermatomyositis, vasculitis and inflammatory bowel disease.

Like other forms of arthritis, JIA includes times when symptoms are present, called flares, and times of remission.

Diagnosis and treatment

The diagnosis of JIA is based on a medical history and physical examination. There is no single laboratory test that can diagnose JIA — or exclude JIA as a diagnosis. Blood tests can help exclude other causes of symptoms, pinpoint the type of arthritis or clarify another diagnosis. These tests may include:

- *Complete blood count (CBC).* This important test can suggest an infection, cancer or certain autoimmune diseases if white blood cell levels are highly elevated or decreased. If the test shows significant anemia, this could suggest inflammatory bowel disease or celiac disease as a cause of arthritis.
- *Erythrocyte sedimentation rate and C-reactive protein (CRP).* As with adult rheumatoid arthritis, an elevated sed rate or CRP can indicate the presence of inflammation. These tests may be used to determine how severe the inflammation is and to rule out other conditions. In children, these lab tests are not always abnormal, even with active arthritis.
- *Antinuclear antibodies (ANA).* These are proteins produced by the immune system among people with certain autoimmune diseases, including arthritis. Antinuclear antibodies are present in about 40% of children with JIA. This test does not diagnose JIA or show if arthritis or JIA is likely to develop later. However, children with diagnosed JIA who have a positive ANA test are at increased risk for uveitis.

- *Other antibody tests.* Rheumatoid factor (RF) and CCP antibody tests are positive in some children with polyarticular JIA, but only in a minority. Abnormal testing isn't required for a diagnosis of JIA.

In addition to lab tests, X-rays may be taken to rule out conditions such as fractures, tumors, infections and birth defects. X-rays may also be used after diagnosis to monitor bone development and possible joint damage. Additional blood tests may be done to look for infections and other conditions associated with bone and joint pain.

The healthcare professional may also remove some fluid from your child's swollen joint to test for an infection that could cause arthritis. Removing fluid may temporarily relieve pain and improve joint mobility, and during the process corticosteroids can be injected into the joint as treatment.

Treatment for JIA depends on the type of arthritis your child has and on the symptoms observed. For all children, treatment aims to control the arthritis with the goal of remission — when no arthritis is detectable. With or without remission, the focus is on maintaining a normal level of physical and social activity. Your healthcare team may recommend a combination of strategies that help relieve pain and swelling, maintain joint movement and strength, and prevent complications. The treatment program may include medications, procedures, exercise, eye care, dental care and good nutrition.

In addition to relieving pain and swelling, medications for JIA can slow the progress of the disease and help with normal bone growth. Initial treatment often includes nonsteroidal anti-inflammatory drugs (NSAIDs), such as ibuprofen or naproxen. Joint injections with corticosteroids also may be used to control inflammation at a specific joint.

Disease-modifying antirheumatic drugs (DMARDs) and biologic drugs are frequently prescribed when the risk of joint damage or disease progression is higher, as in children with polyarticular and systemic JIA. Because these medications suppress the immune system, it's important to talk through the risks and benefits with your child's healthcare team. Certain types of JIA are beginning to benefit from developed therapeutics specific to those subtypes, including new treatments for systemic JIA, ERA, and psoriatic arthritis.

Parents can help children with JIA by encouraging physical activity, normal routines and positive outlooks. Family members should also be prepared to help children cope with the emotional aspects of having a chronic disease.

OTHER INFLAMMATORY JOINT CONDITIONS

Some types of inflammatory childhood arthritis cause symptoms similar to those of JIA but don't fit under the same umbrella. These diseases may be associated with other chronic conditions, or they may develop as a temporary overactive immune response.

Enteropathic arthritis

Arthritis that's associated with inflammatory bowel disease (IBD) is called enteropathic arthritis. Children and teens who have IBD, an autoimmune disease, experience inflammation of the intestines and colon. Crohn's disease and ulcerative colitis are the two most common types of IBD.

About 10% to 20% of people with IBD develop enteropathic arthritis. The large joints are most commonly affected, but the pelvis and sacroiliac joints also can be involved. It's not unusual for a child with IBD to develop arthritis first with intestinal symptoms occurring later. Thus, if a child has arthritis, as well as diarrhea, bloody stools, fevers, weight loss or belly cramps, IBD may be the cause. Treating the underlying bowel inflammation often improves the joint symptoms.

Reactive arthritis

This type of arthritis is not a chronic autoimmune disease. Rather, it usually occurs after an infection of the gut or urinary tract. Inflammation that's part of the immune response can set off a reaction in the joints, causing redness, swelling and stiffness. However, the infection itself is not in the joints, and it can occur even after the initial symptoms of infection are gone.

Reactive arthritis causes pain and swelling of one or just a few joints. The knees and ankles are most commonly affected. This condition can also cause inflamma-

tion of the outer layer of the eye, a condition known as conjunctivitis. Reactive arthritis can affect the skin in various ways, but this occurs less often than in adults. Children may have pain with urination if urethritis develops, which is when the urinary tract becomes inflamed.

Reactive arthritis is often a self-limited condition, meaning it goes away on its own after running its course. Usually NSAIDs are the only treatment needed to control the pain and swelling. The original infection may need to be treated if it hasn't resolved. However, antibiotics usually aren't helpful in improving joint symptoms if there's no lingering active infection.

Transient synovitis

Transient synovitis is a specific type of reactive arthritis that's isolated to the hip. It occurs most often in children between the ages of 3 and 8 and is more than twice as likely to affect boys than girls. Transient synovitis causes relatively sudden pain and a limited range of motion in the hip. Usually only one hip is involved, and a child may limp or refuse to bear weight on the affected side. The cause of the disease isn't clear. But since it typically occurs soon after a mild infection, it's considered a type of abnormal immune response.

When this condition is suspected, imaging tests such as an ultrasound often show extra fluid in the hip joint. Most children with transient synovitis don't seem ill and don't have a fever. NSAIDs are used to reduce inflammation and relieve hip pain. Symptoms resolve within a few days to a few weeks, and most children return to normal activities.

Your doctor may want to rule out an active bacterial hip infection as the cause of pain, especially if the child looks ill, has a fever or has abnormal lab tests. This may be done by extracting fluid from the hip joint for testing.

CONNECTIVE TISSUE DISEASES

Connective tissue diseases are a group of autoimmune illnesses that tend to affect the skin, muscles and certain internal organs. They are seen as distinct from other autoimmune illnesses that primarily cause inflammation in the joints, spine and ligaments. However, arthritis is frequently seen as a possible symptom in these conditions as well. The following connective tissue diseases may be a source of joint pain in children.

Juvenile dermatomyositis

An autoimmune response in the body can cause inflammation of the muscles. This is called inflammatory myopathy, and it typically leads to muscle weakness. When it affects children, it's usually caused by dermatomyositis, which occurs with characteristic skin rashes. When children have muscle weakness, you may notice them having difficulty getting up off the floor, getting into and out of a vehicle, or climbing stairs. Activities such as washing

their hair or feeding themselves also may become difficult. In more severe cases, dermatomyositis can affect the child's voice and ability to swallow or breathe comfortably.

There are several classic skin signs of dermatomyositis in children. One is the appearance of Gottron's papules, raised red spots over the knuckles, elbows or knees. Another indicating development is redness over the chest, known as a shawl sign. A third symptom is redness around the base of the fingernails or a heliotrope rash, which manifests in a bluish purple discoloration around the eyes. The rashes are typically worse after sun exposure.

Blood tests can help diagnose dermatomyositis by showing evidence of inflammation and elevated levels of muscle enzymes. Sometimes a healthcare professional may order a nerve test called electromyography (EMG), or a biopsy of the muscle may be taken to confirm the diagnosis. An MRI may be a less invasive way to check for muscle inflammation. There's no cure for this disease, but DMARDs and biologics can control symptoms in the muscles and skin. Some children may experience prolonged remission even without therapy.

Systemic lupus erythematosus

Systemic lupus erythematosus, or lupus, is a systemic autoimmune disease. It can occur at any age, but in children it's most likely to occur near puberty and is much more common in girls than boys. Lupus can cause many symptoms in children, including a rash, mouth sores, hair loss, arthritis and skin sensitivity to the sun. Lupus can also affect internal organs such as the kidneys, heart and liver.

Diagnosis and treatment of lupus are similar for both children and adults, involving different tests and medications based on symptoms. See page 62 for more information on lupus.

VASCULITIS

Vasculitis is inflammation of the blood vessels from autoimmune activity. It can cause blood vessels to become weak, narrowed, blocked, enlarged or scarred. A damaged blood vessel may not function normally, affecting blood flow to the tissues.

Several forms of vasculitis occur in children, and all may include arthritis as a symptom. The two most common conditions in childhood are discussed below.

IgA vasculitis (formerly Henoch-Schönlein purpura)

This type of vasculitis primarily affects children. It causes inflammation and bleeding in the small blood vessels in the skin, joints, intestines and kidneys. This leads to abdominal and joint pain and a rash of purplish marks. If the kidney is affected, the urine may become bloody or darkly colored, almost like tea or coffee. Most commonly, the large joints may develop arthritis and can become quite swollen.

A diagnosis of IgA vasculitis (IgAV) is based on the symptoms and an exam. Your healthcare team will do blood and urine tests and may also do imaging tests. Occasionally, a skin or kidney biopsy is done to rule out other possibilities.

The disease frequently goes away on its own within several weeks. Resting, drinking enough water, maintaining a healthy diet and controlling blood pressure may help symptoms improve.

Kawasaki disease (KD)

This vasculitis occurs almost universally in children and is most common in young children between the ages of 1 and 3. It can affect blood vessels of all sizes, but most notably it can cause inflammation of the arteries in the heart. These arteries supply oxygen-rich blood to the heart muscle.

Features of Kawasaki disease include a high fever lasting for more than five days; redness and pain of the eyes, also called conjunctivitis; red, dry lips and a swollen tongue; swollen lymph nodes in the neck; and red or painful palms and soles. Joint pain is a symptom in up to 1 in 4 children with the disease, although this usually doesn't lead to joint damage. Peeling skin is another sign of the disease as it advances.

The most concerning symptoms occur when the heart vessels are involved. One of the first signs may be an increased heart rate. The disease can also cause bulges in the artery walls, known as aneurysms, raising the risk of heart attack or internal bleeding.

A medical professional can diagnose KD based on the symptoms and by ruling out other diseases with similar symptoms. Your healthcare team will likely order an echocardiogram, which is an ultrasound imaging test of the heart, to determine if the heart vessels are inflamed. Once a diagnosis of KD is made, treatment with intravenous immune globulin (IVIg), a potent anti-inflammatory, will be started. This significantly reduces the risk of aneurysm. Steroids are usually avoided, as they may worsen bulging arteries.

ORTHOPEDIC CONDITIONS

When children have joint pain, it's often not from autoimmune causes. Rather, it's due to abnormalities of the bones or joints as their skeletons are growing and changing. These conditions may cause discomfort, a limp or limited range of motion. Some of the common orthopedic causes of joint pain in children are discussed below.

Congenital hip dysplasia

Hip dysplasia is the medical term for a hip socket that doesn't fully cover the ball portion of the upper thigh bone — the femur. Most children with this condition are born with it. As the hip joint develops, the socket part of the joint doesn't form normally, and the hip joint is too loose. The ball of the hip can then slip out of the joint easily.

In younger infants, hip dysplasia doesn't usually cause any symptoms since the joints are not weight-bearing. It may be found on routine examination. Symptoms may occur as children start to walk. They may have pain, or they may limp or walk in an uneven manner. Milder cases may not show symptoms until the teenage years.

When this condition is suspected, an X-ray may be taken to look directly at the hip joint. Treatment depends on the child's age. Loose hips are expected in babies less than 2 weeks old. But if the looseness continues, the baby may need to wear a soft brace to hold the hip joint in place so that the bones can grow normally. The brace is usually worn for 2 to 3 months. For babies older than 6 months, surgery may be necessary to correct the hip joint position, followed by a cast for 3 to 4 months. If the hip joint isn't positioned correctly, pain or damage in the joint may develop as children get older.

Legg-Calvé-Perthes disease

Legg-Calvé-Perthes (LEG-kahl-VAY-PER-tuz) disease occurs when the blood supply to the ball part of the hip joint, known as the femoral head, is temporarily interrupted and the bone begins to deteriorate. This condition usually affects children between 3 and 12 years of age and is more common in boys. As the bone weakens, it breaks apart and can lose its round shape. The bone eventually heals itself, but if it has changed shape, it can cause pain and stiffness. Children may start having hip pain or a limp that can begin either suddenly or slowly.

The loss of blood supply to the hip joint, called avascular necrosis, is sometimes due to an underlying medical condition such as obesity, infection or steroid use. There may be a family history. But many times, the underlying cause isn't clear.

Early in the disease, X-rays of the hip may appear normal. Other imaging studies such as a bone scan or MRI may help identify changes in the bone.

Treatment involves keeping the ball in the joint socket so that it can heal in its round shape. This may require activity restrictions or crutches for younger children or a cast or surgery for older children. The long-term outcome depends on the damage to the joint as well as the child's age. Children less than 6 to 8 years of age have a better prognosis.

Osgood-Schlatter disease

Osgood-Schlatter disease causes pain on the front of the knee, in the area just below the kneecap called the tibial tuberosity. It usually affects children ages 9 to 14, often after a growth spurt. It's also seen in children who do a lot of running or jumping. Pain may occur in one or both knees. It usually gets worse over time and can be severe. The pain is typically worse with running, kneeling, jumping, climbing stairs and walking uphill, while it improves with rest.

The condition can usually be diagnosed during a physical exam. Ice or over-the-counter (OTC) medications such as ibuprofen (Advil, Motrin IB) or acetamin-ophen (Tylenol, others) may help ease the pain. A physical therapist can recommend stretches and strengthening exercises for the leg muscles to help with pain, too. Most children can continue their normal activities, including sports, as long as the pain is not severe and improves with rest. Occasionally, a kneepad or brace may be needed to cushion the front of the knee.

Symptoms tend to resolve on their own as the child's growth slows, which may take 6 to 18 months. Knee problems from this disease don't usually continue into adulthood.

Slipped capital femoral epiphysis (SCFE)

Slipped capital femoral epiphysis (SCFE) is the most common hip disorder in adolescence. It usually occurs in children 12 or 13 years of age who are overweight. Most children with SCFE will complain of groin pain, but sometimes it causes knee or thigh pain.

This condition limits the range of motion of the hip. It's caused by changes in the head of the femur — the ball-shaped top of the thigh bone — that sits in the hip socket. Normally the femoral head sits atop a growth plate that connects it to the rest of the bone. In SCFE, it slips out of position on the growth plate, like ice cream slipping off a cone. This causes pain in the hip joint and a limp. SCFE may occur after minor trauma.

If your doctor suspects SCFE, X-rays usually can confirm the diagnosis. Most children with SCFE will need surgery to stabilize the slipping bone.

GROWING PAINS

Growing pains often occur in children, usually between ages 3 and 12. They are the most common cause of intermittent joint pain in children. The pain is most often felt deep in the legs and in the muscles and joints on both sides of the body. Typically, a child will wake up at night or during naps with pain but won't have any symptoms of other musculoskeletal conditions. The pain usually occurs at least once a month for three months or more. It may be worse after days when the child is more active.

The cause of growing pains isn't clear. Possible factors include bone density, overuse of the muscles and emotional disturbances. Often, there is a family history of similar pains.

Your healthcare professional can diagnose growing pains with a physical exam and by ruling out other causes. With growing pains, the physical exam and any lab tests and X-rays taken will be normal. Sometimes, the diagnosis can be made based on the history of symptoms, as growing pains characteristically cause pain late in the day or during sleep.

Massage, heat or OTC pain medications can help relieve the pain. If symptoms keep recurring, stretching or in some cases physical therapy may help. Growing pains usually resolve within a year or two. Meanwhile, children should be encouraged to continue normal activities.

8 Different causes of pain

Pain is a common experience. If you have arthritis, you already likely know how debilitating pain can be. But pain can be a symptom of many other conditions, too.

Pain is a significant cause of disability and a major contributor to healthcare costs. Pain that lasts for more than three months is called chronic pain, and it affects up to 2 out of every 5 Americans. Pain that's short-term, called acute pain, affects millions more. Acute pain is associated with a specific cause and is the most common reason people seek medical care — ankle sprains are a good example. Chronic pain, on the other hand, is now seen as a health condition in its own right.

Because pain is a major problem in the United States and worldwide, researchers are dedicated to understanding it and finding the best ways to treat it. In recent years, for example, experts have learned

much more about fibromyalgia and conditions that have different causes of pain. This new understanding, in turn, has changed the way some types of pain are managed.

This chapter offers insight into what's known today about pain, both in arthritis and in other conditions.

WHAT CAUSES PAIN?

Pain can have many different causes. Acute pain is the body's short-term response to injury such as from a broken bone, a cut or scrape, or surgery. In time, acute pain goes away as the injury heals. Chronic pain lingers long after the time it should take for an injury to heal, and it sometimes occurs without a clear cause. Most injuries should heal within around three months, so pain that persists beyond this time frame is considered to be chronic.

Pain that is defined as chronic is broken down into one of three groups: nociceptive, neuropathic or nociplastic pain. While nociceptive and neuropathic pain are associated with evidence of injury to the body or disease affecting nerves involved in sensing pain, nociplastic pain describes a form of pain that occurs when the nerves involved in sensing pain are behaving differently but aren't damaged or affected by a disease. Nociceptive and neuropathic pain are most associated with pain that starts outside the brain and spinal cord in the peripheral nervous system — for example, in a damaged joint. Nociplastic pain is often linked to changes in signaling in the brain or spinal cord — this can be thought of as central pain.

Nociceptive pain

This is the kind of pain we feel from things like cuts, burns or sprains. It happens when our body's pain sensors — nociceptors — detect damaged tissues and send signals to the brain, which results in a pain experience. It is normally a protective mechanism and is the body's way of saying, "There is something wrong here, protect this area so that it can heal." This type of pain can also persist when there is ongoing inflammation, for example, due to an inflamed joint in rheumatoid arthritis or long-lasting damage such as in osteoarthritis. It is usually a sharp or aching pain and tends to occur in a localized area.

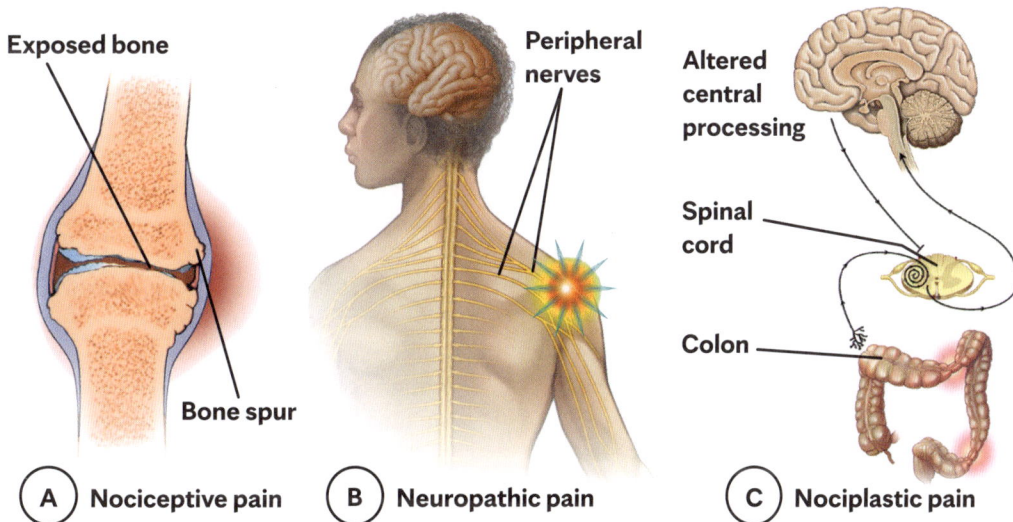

A. Tissue damage or inflammation, from disease (such as osteoarthritis) or injury, causes pain signals that are sent to the brain. **B.** Neuropathic pain results from signals from damaged nerves. A pinched nerve is one example. Diabetes and other diseases also can cause nerve damage. This type of pain may feel like stabbing, tingling or burning. **C.** Pain occurs due to changes in how the brain or nerves process sensory signals. Signals may translate to widespread aching pain or get "turned up" so that mild sensation feels extreme.

Neuropathic pain

This type of pain occurs when nerves are damaged or affected by a disease. As an example, nerve damage is often seen in diabetes. It can also occur in conditions like sciatica. It usually feels different than nociceptive pain and can be burning, tingling, or shooting or feel like electric shocks.

Nociplastic pain

This category of pain was added to capture situations where pain is present but there is no evidence of direct injury to the body or any nerve damage. It occurs due to changes in how the brain and nerves process pain, which can be seen on research brain scans and sensory tests but is not captured by current clinical tests. Fibromyalgia is the best example of nociplastic pain, but it can also be present in many other conditions, too, including some types of chronic back pain, pelvic pain and headache, to name a few. Although nociplastic pain can be caused by nerves anywhere in the body, it is most commonly due to nerves in the brain and spinal cord processing signals differently than is typical. When this amplifies the signals, it is known as central sensitization. The pain can feel like aching pain, is often widespread, and can also feel like a mix of lots of different types of pain and sensations that can move around the body and change.

Here's how it works. Your body is covered in tiny sensor cells that monitor what you feel, taste, touch and smell. These sensor cells take the information they gather and send it to your brain.

When your brain gets these messages, it decides what to do about them. For example, if your brain gets the message that you're cold, it triggers shivering, and you may respond by grabbing a blanket or turning up the heat.

With central sensitization, the messages sent from these sensor cells to your brain

CAN YOU HAVE MORE THAN ONE TYPE OF PAIN?

Although pain is broken down into these three types, you can have more than one type of pain at once, and this can also change over time. In fact, as many as 2 out of 5 people with osteoarthritis, rheumatoid arthritis, and other joint diseases that cause pain and swelling in a joint have nociceptive and nociplastic pain.

This can make it hard to tell where the pain started. For example, if you've had arthritis but feel as though you hurt all over, are tired all the time and don't always have achy joints, you may have fibromyalgia.

An honest and thorough conversation about your symptoms can help your healthcare team uncover the true source of your pain and treat it appropriately.

get turned up, much like the volume on a radio. A slight chill may make you feel like you're freezing, for example. Lights may seem brighter, sounds may seem louder — and pain hurts more than it should. Even a light touch can hurt.

Mayo Clinic experts have found that nociplastic pain and central sensitization are linked to many symptoms and syndromes:

Pain Muscle or joint pain that isn't caused by inflammation is common.

Fatigue Fatigue is usually present all the time with central sensitization, and it doesn't get better after sleep. It may get worse with physical or mental activity. Fatigue is said to be chronic when it lasts for six months or more and isn't caused by another medical issue.

Numbness or tingling These sensations can appear with or without pain.

Headaches Both migraines and tension headaches can be symptoms of nociplastic pain. Tension headaches may cause pain and pressure in the head. Migraines can cause other symptoms, too, including nausea, vomiting, weakness, numbness, and sensitivity to light and sound.

Sleep problems Sleeping too much, being unable to sleep or not feeling refreshed after sleeping are all symptoms of central sensitization. Sleep apnea may need to be ruled out.

Dizziness or lightheadedness These feelings may happen all the time, or they may occur only upon sitting or standing too quickly.

Weakness A general sense of weakness can be a sign of central sensitization.

Brain fog, memory issues and short attention span Some people say they feel like their memory isn't as good as it used to be, or they have trouble paying attention.

Sensitivities The body may overreact to food, medication or changes in the environment. Sensitivities can increase in number and become more intense over time.

Temporomandibular joint (TMJ) disorder This disorder involves pain in the jaw joint and the muscles that control your jaw. People usually cannot point to a prior injury to explain the pain.

Irritable bowel syndrome This condition affects the large intestine and often causes cramping, belly pain, bloating, gas, diarrhea and constipation.

Interstitial cystitis Pain and pressure in the bladder, pelvic pain and the frequent urge to void are all symptoms of this disorder. It's linked to central sensitization when there's no tissue damage or infection to explain the symptoms.

Chronic pelvic pain This is sometimes referred to as pain below the belly button. In women, it can happen with menstrual problems, so a healthcare professional will usually rule out other causes of the pain first.

Restless legs syndrome Symptoms of this disorder can be mild or severe and tend to get worse at night. Restless legs syndrome can lead to poor sleep, as well as fatigue during the day.

Postural orthostatic tachycardia syndrome (POTS) POTS is a condition that causes lightheadedness, fainting and a rapid increase in heart rate. This happens when a very low amount of blood goes to the heart after someone stands up after lying down. Symptoms are relieved by lying down.

Depression and anxiety Depression and anxiety can lead to as well as be symptoms of nociplastic pain.

Fibromyalgia This widespread pain disorder is commonly linked to nociplastic pain. Fibromyalgia affects the way the brain processes pain signals, causing even the slightest pain to hurt more. Aside from pain, fibromyalgia can cause fatigue and issues with sleep, memory and mood. Learn more about fibromyalgia below.

FIBROMYALGIA: EXAMPLE OF NOCIPLASTIC PAIN

According to some estimates, 10% to 15% of people have a chronic widespread pain disorder, the most common of which is fibromyalgia. As you learned earlier in this chapter, fibromyalgia is a common syndrome linked to nociplastic pain.

Pain isn't the only symptom of fibromyalgia. It also causes fatigue and issues with sleep and mood. Although there's no one way to describe what fibromyalgia feels like, some say they hurt all over, while others say they feel as if they always have the flu.

Fibromyalgia affects between 2% and 4% of people worldwide. It is more common in women than in men. Researchers have learned that several factors may contribute to fibromyalgia:
- Genetic factors
- Maternal stress
- Low birth weight
- Adverse childhood experiences
- Social and developmental context
- Physical inactivity
- Obesity
- Whiplash and other forms of physical trauma
- Sleep disorders
- Mood disorders
- Emotional trauma
- Painful conditions
- Multimorbidity
- Frailty

Signs and symptoms

The main symptom of fibromyalgia is chronic, widespread pain that persists for at least three months. Fatigue and sleep problems are also core symptoms. Sleep problems may include trouble falling asleep, waking up during the night, or waking up unrefreshed or exhausted.

The pain with fibromyalgia may be a deep ache, a tingling sensation or soreness. It may vary depending on the time of day, your activity level, the weather, lack of sleep, and stress or anxiety. Most people

DO YOU HAVE CHRONIC WIDESPREAD PAIN?

If you've had pain in several different areas or all over for at least three months in a row, you may be experiencing chronic widespread pain due to nociplastic pain. Before making a diagnosis, your healthcare team will likely try to rule out other causes. Your team may check to see if you have pain in your joints or in the soft tissues of your body. You may be asked to show where you feel pain and how long you've been feeling it. You may have a blood test and other tests that check your muscle strength and tone, reflexes, and coordination. You'll also want to report if you're having other symptoms that could be causing your pain, such as fatigue or sleeplessness.

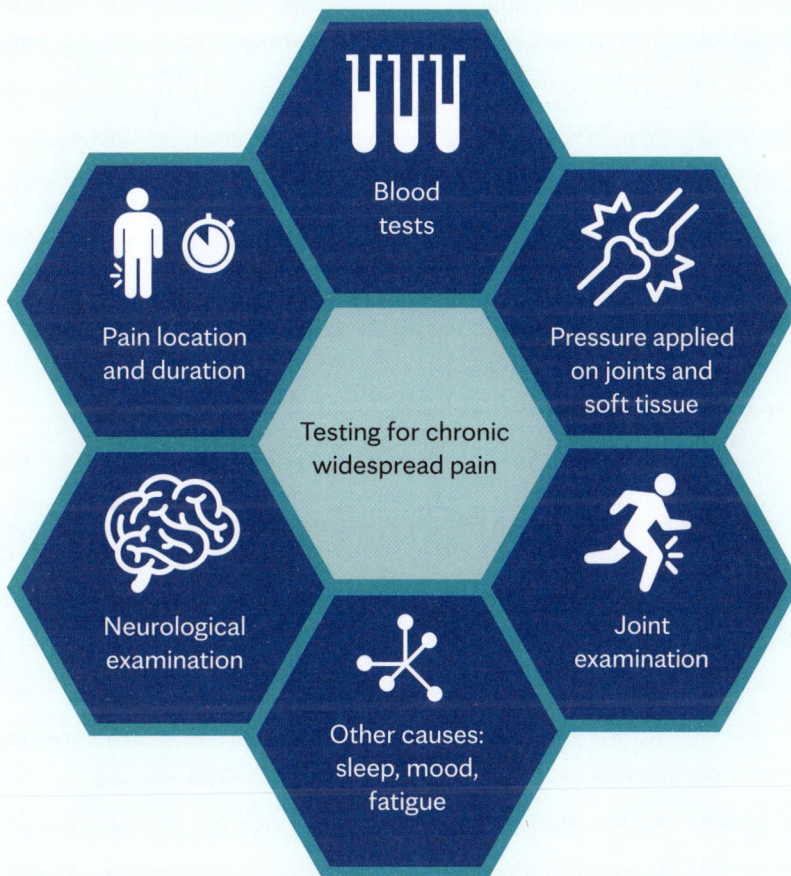

Blood
tests

Pain location
and duration

Pressure applied
on joints and
soft tissue

Testing for chronic
widespread pain

Neurological
examination

Joint
examination

Other causes:
sleep, mood,
fatigue

FIBROMYALGIA VS. ARTHRITIS

Fibromyalgia has been linked to arthritis for many years. Although they share pain as a symptom, they're two different but potentially overlapping disorders. Fibromyalgia pain isn't caused by swelling or damage to the joints. Instead, it is largely due to the increased sensitivity of pain sensors, and it may hurt just about everywhere. And unlike arthritis, fibromyalgia doesn't cause inflammation in the joints or tissues, like in tendinitis or bursitis, but it can produce very similar symptoms.

Some very early studies have suggested that fibromyalgia may be caused by altered responses in the immune system, but this work has not been confirmed in large-scale studies or studies with human subjects, and there is no good evidence to say that fibromyalgia is an autoimmune condition. Some of the symptoms can feel like there is inflammation all over your body or as if you are developing flu, but there is no evidence that using immunotherapy helps in fibromyalgia. However, research has shown a connection between different types of arthritis and the presence of fibromyalgia. Around 20% to 40% of people with a rheumatic condition also have fibromyalgia, which is much more common than in the general population. Research studies have been able to show that patients who have different types of arthritis alongside fibromyalgia and those who just have fibromyalgia alone experience similar changes in brain activity.

Even with these possible connections, it's important to keep in mind that fibromyalgia and arthritis are separate conditions with different causes. They're also managed differently. If you have symptoms that lead you to suspect that you have either condition, it's best to talk with your healthcare team about it.

feel some degree of muscle pain all the time. And the pain may move all over your body.

Aside from pain, other signs and symptoms of fibromyalgia include:

- Stiffness
- Pain in the jaw or face
- Digestive problems, including belly pain, bloating, constipation or diarrhea
- Numbness or tingling in the hands and feet
- Depression, anxiety or mood changes
- Sensitivity to weather and temperature changes
- Sensitivity to odors, noises, bright lights and touch
- Irritable bowel syndrome
- Headaches
- Not being able to think clearly

- Problems with attention and short-term memory
- Difficulty recalling specific words
- Pelvic pain and pressure
- Feeling the need to empty the bladder often or urgently
- Sensitivity to foods and medications

These symptoms may look familiar — as they're all symptoms of nociplastic pain.

Diagnosis and treatment

There's no standard lab test to show if someone has fibromyalgia. Instead, your healthcare team will generally ask about your medical history, the medications you're taking, and the symptoms you're experiencing, what they're like and how long you've had them. You'll also likely have tests to rule out other causes for your symptoms.

Medical professionals used to look for tender points to tell if someone had fibromyalgia. Tender points are areas of the body that hurt or are sensitive to the touch when pressed. Although tender points are no longer part of today's fibromyalgia guidelines, some healthcare workers still look for them in people who may have fibromyalgia. Researchers have found, though, that people with fibromyalgia don't always have tender points. Likewise, having tender points doesn't always mean that someone has fibromyalgia.

Instead of relying on tender points, today's fibromyalgia guidelines focus on having widespread pain for at least three months alongside important non-pain symptoms like fatigue and sleep disturbance.

The lack of a diagnostic test for fibromyalgia can be frustrating for patients and clinicians alike. Sometimes people can feel like their symptoms are being dismissed, that it is only diagnosed when everything else has been ruled out and that it is "all in their head." It is important to remember that this collection of apparently unrelated symptoms is very typical, and it is often the non-pain symptoms that most help to reach the right diagnosis. We have lots of evidence to show that the pain is very real and that there are clear changes in the way the brain and nerves are functioning.

Although fibromyalgia is chronic, it isn't directly life-threatening and doesn't necessarily get worse over time. It doesn't damage the body like arthritis can, which means that you can regain normal function. With support, you can manage its symptoms.

While certain medications are approved by the U.S. Food and Drug Administration to treat symptoms of fibromyalgia, no one medication can relieve every symptom all the time. And often, medication may not help at all or may even make you feel worse. Learn more about medications in Chapter 10.

Instead of relying on medications, current guidance based on the evidence advises focusing on education, lifestyle changes and overall well-being, including:

- Learning about fibromyalgia — in particular, that it is a real condition with a real cause and that it's treatable
- Getting regular physical activity that you increase slowly over time
- Pacing yourself by balancing periods of activity with periods of rest
- Moderating your activities so you're not doing too much — or doing nothing at all
- Taking steps to manage mood, including stress, anxiety and depression
- Setting a regular block of sleep time to ensure that you're going to bed at the same time and waking up at the same time every day
- Following a healthy diet
- Reaching and maintaining a healthy weight
- Connecting with others

Special treatment programs that focus on all these self-management steps — and more — can help. These types of programs are offered at Mayo Clinic campuses in Rochester, Minnesota, and Jacksonville, Florida.

9 Evaluation for arthritis and other joint pain

Arthritis has many different signs and symptoms, causes, and outcomes. When you have a joint problem, identifying the cause and the best way to manage it may be a complex process.

Initially, your healthcare professional will take a complete medical history and do a physical exam to sort out whether the joint problem is inflammatory or noninflammatory in nature. In the exam, they'll examine your tender joints and muscles and listen to your description of your symptoms.

With a hands-on approach like this, a healthcare professional can usually get a good idea of what's going on inside your body to address the symptoms, make a diagnosis and decide treatment options.

Sometimes tests are needed to confirm a diagnosis. Lab tests and imaging studies may also be done to monitor disease progress, check medication effectiveness

or determine if the drugs you're taking are causing harmful side effects. Most lab tests will require a simple blood draw. Other tests may need a sample of urine, joint fluid, or small pieces of skin or muscle tissue.

This chapter outlines the process of evaluating joint pain and the lab tests, imaging tests, procedures and specialty consultations you're likely to encounter. While lab tests and X-rays aren't needed for every form of arthritis, they are very important to confirm or rule out the presence of some diseases.

LABORATORY TESTS

Lab tests are essential to the diagnostic and treatment process. The right tests, along with your healthcare team's observations and your honest feedback, can help you get the safest and most effective treatment for your disease.

Still, lab tests have their limitations. Some may show negative results even when a person has the disease being tested for — this is called a false negative. For example, many people with rheumatoid arthritis (RA) test negative for rheumatoid factor. Other tests may be positive in people who don't have a particular disease — this is a false positive. Your healthcare team can talk with you about what the results of each test may mean.

Anti-cyclic citrullinated peptide (anti-CCP) antibody

This test, like the test for rheumatoid factor (RF), checks for a particular antibody that is present in approximately 60% to 80% of people with rheumatoid arthritis. While most people with anti-CCP antibodies also test positive for rheumatoid factor, the RF antibody can occur in people with many other conditions besides rheumatoid arthritis. Thus, a positive anti-CCP antibody test is more specific to RA. The anti-CCP antibody may be present years before rheumatoid arthritis develops.

Antinuclear antibody (ANA)

This test detects antinuclear antibodies in your blood. A positive ANA test generally shows that your immune system is creating antibodies that have the potential to attack your own tissue. ANA is commonly found in the blood of people who have lupus, but it can also suggest the presence of polymyositis, scleroderma, Sjögren's syndrome, juvenile idiopathic

arthritis or rheumatoid arthritis. It is also found in many people who are healthy, particularly people over age 65. Certain medications or infectious diseases may also lead to a positive ANA test.

When the test is negative, the result is still useful in that it helps your healthcare team rule out certain connective tissue diseases. If the ANA test is positive, antibody tests that are more specific may be ordered to check for underlying connective tissue disorders. The ANA test does not need to be repeated, as the result doesn't change with disease activity.

C-reactive protein (CRP)

This test, like the sed rate (see below), is a blood test that measures inflammation in your body. It measures a substance produced by the liver that increases with inflammation in the body. If you have an inflammatory type of arthritis, you may have this test periodically so that your healthcare professional can monitor your inflammation levels.

Creatinine test

This test is used to determine how well the kidneys are functioning. It measures the level of creatinine, which is a normal waste product of the muscles, in the blood. A high level of creatinine means that the kidneys are not removing waste products from the body well enough. This test is ordered to check for underlying kidney disease, which can occur with some types of arthritis. The test may also be used to monitor kidney function when people are on certain medications that can be toxic to the kidneys.

Erythrocyte sedimentation rate (ESR)

This test, often called the sed rate, measures how fast red blood cells (erythrocytes) fall and settle, like sediment, in the bottom of a glass test tube over the course of an hour. Inflammation can cause the cells to clump together, and these dense clumps fall faster than other cells. The higher the sed rate, the greater the amount of inflammation. Many different conditions can cause an elevated ESR, including infection, inflammation and cancer, as well as increasing age and pregnancy.

Hematocrit (HCT) and hemoglobin (Hgb)

These tests measure the number and quality of your red blood cells. A low quantity of red blood cells, a condition known as anemia, may suggest that your medications are causing gastrointestinal bleeding. Alternatively, an underlying disease may be the cause of the anemia.

Human leukocyte antigen (HLA) typing

This test detects the presence of certain genes, specifically genetic markers, in the blood. The genetic marker HLA-B27 is often present in people with ankylosing spondylitis or other spondyloarthropathies. About 6% of the general population has the HLA-B27 genetic marker, so having the gene doesn't mean you have or will have one of the associated types of arthritis.

Liver enzyme tests

These tests measure levels of liver enzymes in the blood, such as serum glutamic-oxaloacetic transaminase (SGOT), serum glutamic-pyruvic transaminase (SGPT) and alkaline phosphatase. They can help doctors determine if certain medications have caused damage to the liver. Liver enzymes can be elevated due to underlying liver disease or from medications that are toxic to the liver.

Lyme serology

This test detects an immune response caused by the bacteria that cause Lyme disease. By confirming this immune response, the test can be used to diagnose Lyme disease, which can cause fatigue, stiffness and joint pain.

Muscle enzyme tests

When muscles are damaged by inflammation in some rheumatic diseases, the muscles release enzymes, such as creatine phosphokinase (CPK) and aldolase. Blood tests can detect these enzymes and measure the amount of muscle damage. Monitoring muscle enzyme levels can also determine how well medication has reduced the inflammation that caused the muscle damage.

Platelet count

Platelets are a substance in blood that helps the blood to clot. A low number of platelets is a concern because bleeding may be harder to stop. Medications, infections and certain diseases may lower the platelet count.

Rheumatoid factor (RF)

This test measures the level of an antibody (rheumatoid factor) that can attack healthy tissue in your body. Rheumatoid factor acts against the blood component gamma globulin, mistaking it for a foreign invader. This test is often positive in people with rheumatoid arthritis. However, it can be seen in healthy people as well as those with other conditions, such as chronic infections, cancer or other inflammatory disorders. Because of this, this test may be considered along with other test results in making a diagnosis.

In the early stages of rheumatoid arthritis, only 1 in 4 people with the condition may test positive for RF. Some people with rheumatoid arthritis have a negative RF throughout the course of the disease. Where this is the case, the condition is called seronegative rheumatoid arthritis.

Uric acid

Most people with gout will have an elevated uric acid level. Gout is a condition that occurs when excess uric acid crystallizes and forms deposits in the joints and other tissues, causing inflam-mation and severe pain. However, the uric acid level may be normal in 25% or more of people with gout. In addition, having an elevated uric acid level doesn't mean you have gout, as many people have elevated uric acid levels without any joint complaints. When gout is diagnosed, the treatment goal is to reduce the uric acid level to less than 6.0 milligrams per deciliter (mg/dL). Medications are often needed to reduce the uric acid level.

White blood cell count

White blood cells help fight infection. A blood test showing a low number of white blood cells suggests that your body will have a harder time fighting an infection. You may have a low white blood cell count because of certain medications or an underlying disease.

PROCEDURES

In addition to various blood tests, your healthcare team may request certain procedures to evaluate your joint symptoms. Some of the more common procedures are outlined here.

Electromyography (EMG)

Electromyography measures the electrical activity of muscle fibers to detect the cause of nerve or muscle problems. This diagnostic procedure uses a needle and electrode stickers to measure activity within a muscle as well as signals traveling between two or more points. It may be ordered for further evaluation of people with nerve or muscle complaints such as numbness, tingling, weakness, or pain radiating down one arm or leg.

Joint fluid tests

If you have a swollen joint and the cause is unknown, withdrawing the fluid from the joint to have it analyzed in a lab may be helpful. This procedure is especially important if your healthcare professional thinks the joint may be infected.

The healthcare professional inserts a needle into a joint space and removes fluid into a syringe. The joint fluid, called synovial fluid, can be examined under a polarizing microscope to look for uric acid crystals, seen in gout, and calcium pyrophosphate crystals, seen in pseudo-gout. The fluid also can be sent to a lab to identify an infection. And the number of white blood cells in the synovial fluid sample will help your healthcare team determine whether the fluid is inflammatory or noninflammatory.

Muscle biopsy

In some people, joint and muscle symptoms may include weakness and the elevated presence of CPK or aldolase, which are muscle enzymes. A muscle biopsy may be necessary to confirm the type of muscle disease. A surgeon can use a needle or make a small cut to take a sample of the muscle. The tissue can then be examined in a lab for signs of damage

to the muscle fibers. Findings can confirm a diagnosis of muscle disease, such as polymyositis, or inflammation of the blood vessels, called vasculitis, or another condition.

Skin biopsy

If you're experiencing joint pain along with a rash, your healthcare team may order a skin biopsy. A small sample of skin is taken and examined under a microscope. This can help the healthcare team diagnose forms of arthritis that involve the skin, such as lupus, vasculitis and psoriatic arthritis.

IMAGING (RADIOGRAPHIC) STUDIES

Often, imaging tests may be helpful in evaluating musculoskeletal complaints. Different imaging technologies create pictures in various ways, showing bones, joints and soft tissue with different levels of detail. Each technique can be useful in certain cases. For example, a simple X-ray may be all that's needed to confirm a diagnosis of osteoarthritis, while magnetic resonance imaging (MRI) may be the best option in diagnosing a problem with a tendon or ligament.

Arthrography

This X-ray procedure uses radiopaque dye, which is designed to stand out against radiation. The dye is injected into a joint space before the X-ray is taken so that it will outline structures such as ligaments inside the joint. Arthrography can be used to view a torn ligament or fragmented cartilage in the joint, which would otherwise not show up on a regular X-ray. However, MRI is now generally used in place of arthrography.

Bone mineral density (BMD)

The most accurate way to evaluate bone density is with a test for bone mineral density known as dual energy X-ray absorptiometry. This test is needed when screening for or diagnosing osteoporosis or osteopenia, a less severe condition of low bone mass. A BMD test is also used to predict a person's risk of fracture or to monitor the improvement during treatment for osteoporosis.

This test is quick and painless and involves very little radiation. X-rays of the lower spine and hip are used to measure how many grams of calcium and other bone minerals are packed into a segment of bone. Measurements of bone density at these sites are typically very accurate.

Bone scan

Bone scanning is a type of nuclear imaging test that is highly sensitive to certain changes in bone. For the scan, a small amount of a radioactive substance is injected into a vein in your arm and is absorbed by any healing bone. The substance is then detected by a bone-scanning device, which creates an image of the bone that can be viewed on a computer screen.

A bone scan can be used to diagnose a fracture, particularly if a suspected fracture isn't showing on other tests, such as plain X-rays and CT or MRI. It may also be helpful to rule out a bone infection or a tumor that has spread from a cancer in another part of the body. However, while a bone scan can help reveal a problem in the bone, it may not show whether the problem is a fracture, tumor or infection.

Computerized tomography (CT) and dual energy CT

Standard computerized tomography (CT) scanners use X-rays to take pictures of the body in cross-sectional "slices." This technology is best for imaging bone. Dual energy CT is a newer technology that combines the conventional X-ray and a second, less powerful X-ray to make the images. This helps show a wider range of materials in the image, such as calcium deposits that will show up differently from bone. It gives advantages over standard CT for a wide range of tests and procedures. Dual energy CT can be helpful in diagnosing gout by assessing the amount of uric acid crystals present, especially when a joint aspiration can't be done.

A CT scan, like a conventional X-ray, exposes people to ionizing radiation. This form of radiation can potentially increase the risk of cancer or affect tissue in other ways. However, the risks with a CT scan are generally very low and are usually far outweighed by the benefits of the test. Your healthcare team can explain the risks of CT or other medical imaging.

Magnetic resonance imaging (MRI)

Magnetic resonance imaging (MRI) creates highly detailed pictures and may be used to determine the extent and exact location of damage in the body. While CT scans use X-rays to create a "slice" image, an MRI uses a magnetic field and radio waves to take many high-resolution slices. It then combines them to create a 3D picture.

Like CT, MRI can be used to detect fractures that aren't visible on plain X-rays. MRI is especially valuable for imaging muscles, ligaments and tendons. MRI may be used if the cause of pain is thought to be a soft tissue problem — for example, rupture of a major ligament or tendon or damage to structures inside the knee joint. MRI can be used to detect inflammation of the joints or tendons. MRI can be more helpful than CT in detecting some abnormalities, such as small fractures or inflammation of the hip and pelvis.

MRI is more expensive than CT and takes more time — from 15 minutes to an hour or more. Some people may feel claustrophobic inside the MRI unit, which is typically a large tube open on both ends. An open-sided MRI can be used, but the image may not be as clear.

Ultrasonography

In recent years, ultrasound has been used more frequently to identify inflammation in and around joints and tears or inflammation of tendons.

Ultrasonography is also used as a guide when a needle is inserted into a joint, for example, to inject medication or remove joint fluid. As an alternative to CT and MRI, ultrasound is less expensive. And unlike CT, it involves no exposure to radiation.

However, ultrasonography is not always available, and it requires highly skilled medical professionals to perform and interpret the scan.

X-rays

Plain (conventional) X-rays are typically the first imaging studies done when sorting out a musculoskeletal disorder. They are usually ordered to help evaluate painful, deformed or abnormal areas of bone. Your healthcare professional may diagnose fractures, tumors, injuries, infections and deformities from X-ray images.

X-rays can show changes that confirm a certain kind of arthritis. For example, in rheumatoid arthritis or other inflammatory arthritis, an X-ray will show that bone has eroded in one or more joints. In osteoarthritis or other noninflammatory conditions, X-rays may show the joint space narrowing and bone spurs developing.

X-rays are most valuable for detecting breaks or changes in bone. Plain X-rays do not show soft tissues such as muscles, bursae, ligaments, tendons or nerves. Imaging tests that are more specific, such as MRI or ultrasound, may be needed to see those tissues.

SPECIALTY EVALUATIONS

If you see your medical provider for joint pain, the evaluation process is often complex. Depending on your symptoms, you may need to see medical professionals in several different subspecialty groups. Your healthcare team may refer you to the following medical specialties to help diagnose and manage your condition.

Cardiology

A cardiologist specializes in heart conditions and often sees people with symptoms including shortness of breath, chest pain or dizzy spells. Sometimes a person without symptoms of heart trouble is referred to a cardiologist after a heart murmur is heard during a physical exam.

You may see a cardiologist if you have inflammatory arthritis. The inflammation of this type of arthritis can affect the blood vessels, putting you at higher risk of heart disease.

Dermatology

A dermatologist evaluates abnormalities of the skin, hair, nails and mucous membranes. You may need to see a dermatologist if you have certain joint conditions that occur with a rash. Sometimes, a dermatologist may need to take a biopsy of the rash for testing.

Endocrinology

An endocrinologist is a clinician who is specially trained in conditions affecting the glands, including the pituitary, thyroid, adrenals, ovaries, testes and pancreas. If you have inflammatory arthritis, you may need treatment with the corticosteroid prednisone, which can lead to diabetes and low bone mass, known as osteoporosis. You may need to see an endocrinologist to monitor those conditions. Rarely, the thyroid gland, adrenal glands and other glands can be involved with inflammatory conditions.

Gastroenterology

A gastroenterologist is a physician with dedicated training in conditions of the gastrointestinal system — the esophagus, stomach, small intestine, colon, rectum, gallbladder and liver.

People with inflammatory bowel disease (Crohn's disease and ulcerative colitis) may have an associated inflammatory arthritis, needing care for both conditions. Taking nonsteroidal anti-inflammatory drugs (NSAIDs) for arthritis pain also may cause esophagus or stomach issues. A gastroenterologist can help manage these side effects.

Hematology

A hematologist is a specialist in blood disorders. A low red blood cell count (known as anemia), platelet disorders and white blood cell disorders are occasionally seen in people with arthritis as a result of the disease or as side effects of medications.

Infectious disease

An infectious disease specialist focuses on diagnosing and managing infections. People with arthritis may see this type of specialist if they take immunosuppressive medications, which weaken the immune system and raise the risk of infection. Steroids, disease-modifying antirheumatic drugs (DMARDs) and biologics all weaken the immune system.

Nephrology

A nephrologist evaluates and treats kidney disease. Various kidney diseases can be seen in people with certain types of arthritis. Many arthritis medications can affect the kidneys as well.

Neurology

A neurologist specializes in nervous system disorders. These include problems in the brain and spinal cord, collectively called the central nervous system, as well as the peripheral nervous system. Several types of arthritis may affect the nerves. Imaging studies of the brain or spinal

canal may be necessary. Nerve tests, known as electromyography, may be ordered for people who have symptoms of a nerve being pinched. Compression of a nerve can occur due to joint swelling or bone spurs from arthritis.

Neurosurgery

A neurosurgeon specializes in the diagnosis and surgical treatment of nervous system disorders. If you have symptoms of a compressed nerve in your neck or low back that don't respond to conservative therapy, you may need a neurosurgery consultation to discuss surgery as a treatment option.

Ophthalmology

An ophthalmologist specializes in eye and vision abnormalities. People with inflammatory arthritis are at higher risk of inflammation of their eyes. Certain medications such as hydroxychloroquine (Plaquenil) also may affect the eyes, so if these medications are part of your treatment, you'll need regular eye examinations.

Orthopedics

Orthopedic surgeons diagnose and manage musculoskeletal conditions. In most cases, these problems are treated first with nonsurgical options such as medications, physical therapy and exercise. If these treatments fail to resolve the problem, surgery may be necessary. An orthopedic surgeon can review surgical treatment options with you.

Physiatry (physical medicine and rehabilitation)

Physiatrists diagnose and treat a wide variety of medical conditions affecting the brain, spinal cord, nerves, bones, joints, ligaments, muscles and tendons. Also known as physical medicine and rehabilitation (PM&R), this specialty focuses on helping people to regain function.

People with arthritis may benefit from the expertise of PM&R specialists in guiding their rehabilitation to regain the strength or movement needed for everyday activities. Physical and occupational therapy is an important treatment regimen for maintaining function in arthritic conditions.

Psychiatry

A psychiatrist focuses on the diagnosis, treatment and prevention of mental, emotional and behavioral disorders. Many people with arthritis also have anxiety and depression symptoms due to their pain and decline in health, as well as related sources of stress such as financial costs. A psychiatrist can help manage these symptoms to improve overall health.

Pulmonary medicine

A pulmonologist evaluates diseases of the lungs. Many forms of inflammatory arthritis can affect the lungs. Problems may include scarring or lumps, known as nodules, on the lung tissue, as well as inflammation and buildup of fluid or mucus. In addition, some medications used to treat inflammatory arthritis, such as methotrexate, can affect the lungs. A pulmonologist may help diagnose issues with the lungs and guide treatment.

Rheumatology

A rheumatologist specializes in the diagnosis and treatment of musculoskeletal diseases and systemic autoimmune conditions. Together these are known as rheumatic diseases. Rheumatic disease can affect the joints, muscles and bones, leading to pain, swelling and stiffness. Over time, rheumatic diseases can cause abnormally shaped bones or joints. If you have arthritis, a rheumatologist is often the main healthcare professional you'll see for your related symptoms after being referred by your primary care provider. The rheumatologist will coordinate care with other specialists if needed.

10 Medications for arthritis

Just as there's a wide range of symptoms among people with different kinds of arthritis, a broad array of medications is available to help control these symptoms. It's important that you work with your healthcare professional to find the best drug treatments for you.

Medications can help relieve pain, make joint movement easier and prevent further damage from inflammation. Some medications can be purchased without a prescription, sometimes called over-the-counter, at convenience stores. Others are powerful drugs that can only be obtained with a medical prescription. Some medications can be used to treat several kinds of arthritis, while others are used for a single type of arthritis.

Medications may help you feel better and allow you to lead a more active life. Like all drugs, though, arthritis medications can cause side effects, including dry mouth and upset stomach as well as an

increased risk of infection, heart attack or stroke. The benefits of a particular drug must be weighed against its side effects. You and your healthcare professional can discuss these risks in relation to your needs and circumstances.

For most people with arthritis, medications play a central role in their treatment plans, which may also include other therapies and lifestyle changes. In the past, rheumatoid arthritis and other forms of the disease were considered disabling and difficult to manage. But newer medications and combinations of treatments have greatly improved the overall well-being and outlook for many people with joint pain.

Because there are so many different types of medications to treat arthritis, and there may be different brand names of each, this chapter will refer to medications by their generic names for ease of reading. For the list of brand names, information on how a drug is given, and a summary of the benefits and risks for each, see the medication guide on page 127.

DIFFERENT TREATMENT STRATEGIES

The treatment plan you and your healthcare team decide on will depend largely on the type of arthritis you have and the severity of your symptoms. Other important factors include your level of pain, how much your symptoms affect your daily life, and your personal preferences about medications and other therapies.

Treating osteoarthritis and other noninflammatory arthritis

The main treatment goal for osteoarthritis or other noninflammatory arthritis is to manage the pain and inflammation and improve joint function.

Part of your treatment plan will include a healthy balance of exercise and rest. Exercise helps strengthen your joints and the muscles that support them, while rest can prevent pain and inflammation from getting worse. If you're overweight, your healthcare professional may also recommend weight loss to reduce stress on your joints.

Your treatment plan may include oral medications, particularly for pain relief. For mild to moderate pain, the pain reliever acetaminophen is often a first choice. Topical pain relievers in the form of creams, gels and ointments also can be applied to painful joints.

For moderate to severe pain, or if you have signs of inflammation, you might take one of many medications that fall under the category of nonsteroidal anti-inflammatory drugs (NSAIDs).

If your joints are still painful despite using pain relievers, you may benefit from injections of medication directly into the joints. These medications may include corticosteroids or hyaluronic acid derivatives, which contain a substance similar to natural joint fluid. (For more on injections, see Chapter 14.)

For pain that isn't controlled by other therapies, your healthcare professional may recommend a short-term course of opioid medications. These are potent pain relievers. Their big drawback, as you may know from headlines in recent years, is that they can lead to dependency if used regularly over long periods of time. They can also make you drowsy or constipated and make your skin itchy.

If your symptoms are persistently severe, your healthcare team may refer you to an orthopedic surgeon to consult on surgeries that might help. (For more on surgical options, see Chapter 11.) Unfortunately, there is no medication to stop the progression of osteoarthritis.

Treating rheumatoid arthritis and other inflammatory arthritis

Treatment for rheumatoid arthritis has changed dramatically over the last several decades. The same is true for other inflammatory arthropathies, such as psoriatic arthritis and spondyloarthritis. Medical professionals used to start out with mild pain relievers and then progress to more powerful drugs if symptoms worsened — similar to the way osteoarthritis is treated. However, treatment for these types of arthritis is now more aggressive upfront.

Studies demonstrate that damage can occur in a joint within the first year or two of disease onset. Fortunately, there are now multiple treatment options to lessen or halt the inflammation that causes joint damage, and healthcare professionals will use the most effective medications available right away. Quick action stalls the inflammatory process in the early stages of the disease before serious damage to the joint can occur. This approach helps to prevent potentially lifelong symptoms or make them less severe.

Nonsteroidal anti-inflammatory drugs (NSAIDs) and steroids

Healthcare professionals typically use NSAIDs to help reduce day-to-day pain in people with these conditions. They may also consider steroids, especially if someone has a significant disability from the disease. Sometimes a steroid injection into the joint may offer a significant benefit. Or your healthcare professional may prescribe a low dose of an oral steroid as a "bridging therapy." The aim is to quickly reduce inflammation until the right medication, or combination of medications, is found to control the inflammation over the long term.

Disease-modifying antirheumatic drugs (DMARDs)

These synthetically produced drugs are the mainstay treatment for inflammatory arthritis. They work by slowing down or suppressing your immune system, which has been hijacked by the disease to increase inflammation in your joints. Early intervention with DMARDs can also improve your quality of life and life expectancy with the disease.

Many different DMARDs are available.

Conventional DMARDs such as hydroxychloroquine, methotrexate, leflunomide or sulfasalazine are typically prescribed first. Each of these medications works differently and has its own unique set of side effects. The downside to all DMARDs is that they take time to work — usually 3 to 6 months. A low dose of a steroid may be needed until the DMARD becomes effective.

Shots of a gold solution used to be prescribed but are no longer used, as DMARDs work better, faster and with fewer side effects. Other medications, such as the antibiotic minocycline, also may help to treat rheumatoid arthritis. Minocycline acts as an adjunct, or booster, to the DMARD, but it isn't effective enough to use by itself.

Studies have shown that, in certain situations, a combination of disease-modifying drugs (combination therapy) provides more benefits than taking just one — with no added side effects.

While you're taking these drugs, your healthcare team will monitor you for any signs of infection or disruption of organ function. Basic blood and urine tests may also be ordered. This is because DMARDs can inhibit your immune system and interfere with certain organs, such as your liver, lungs or kidneys.

Biologics

If a DMARD or combination of DMARDs doesn't effectively treat your inflammatory arthritis symptoms, your healthcare professional may recommend adding or switching to a newer category of medications called biologic DMARDs. They are also referred to as biologic agents or simply biologics. Like conventional DMARDs, they can relieve pain and stiffness and protect joints from damage by slowing or halting the inflammatory process. They differ from conventional DMARDs in that they typically contain large molecules derived from living sources, such as cell cultures, while conventional DMARDs usually contain small molecules that are made by way of a chemical process.

Biologic DMARDs are designed to work against specific targets. Some interfere with the action of immune substances

TNF, AN EXAMPLE OF CYTOKINES IN THE IMMUNE RESPONSE

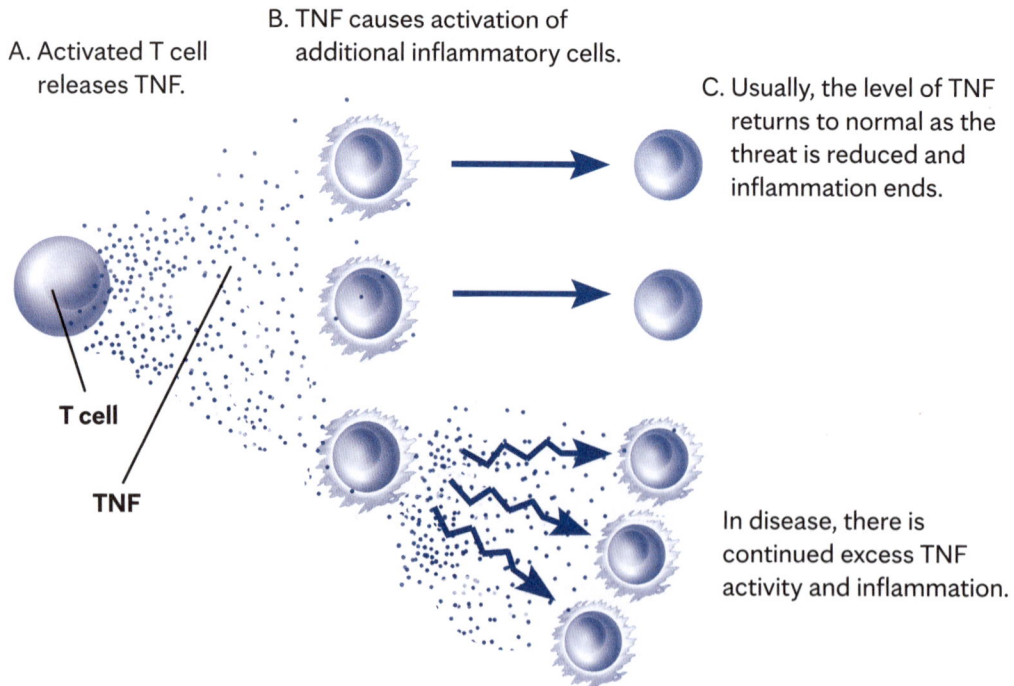

A. Activated T cell releases TNF.

B. TNF causes activation of additional inflammatory cells.

C. Usually, the level of TNF returns to normal as the threat is reduced and inflammation ends.

T cell

TNF

In disease, there is continued excess TNF activity and inflammation.

called cytokines. Cytokines mobilize immune cells that fight off an infection or another perceived threat. With an autoimmune disease such as rheumatoid arthritis, where healthy cells are wrongly seen as threatening, cytokines contribute to the inflammatory reaction. (See diagram on page 122.) Biologics can stop or slow this response.

The largest group of biologics works against a cytokine called tumor necrosis factor-alpha (TNF-alpha). Others target a type of cytokine called interleukin (IL). Specific targets include IL-1, IL-6, IL-17, IL-12/IL-23 and IL-23.

Some biologics disrupt the activation of certain T cells. These cells coordinate your body's immune response to invaders. Other biologic medications work to deplete B cells, which produce antibodies that perpetuate the immune reaction. Antibodies are helpful when you're fighting an infection, but they're part of the problem in an autoimmune reaction.

The newest class of medications used for inflammatory arthritis is targeted DMARDs. These drugs interfere with specific signaling pathways, such as the Janus kinase pathway, inside immune cells.

TREATMENT WITH INFLIXIMAB, A TNF INHIBITOR

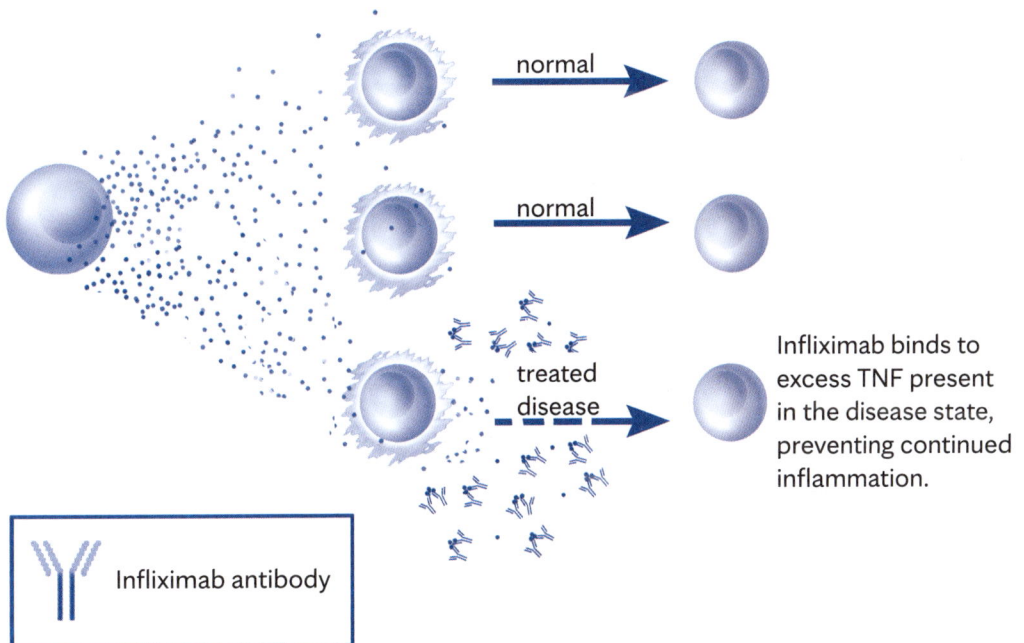

normal

normal

treated disease

Infliximab binds to excess TNF present in the disease state, preventing continued inflammation.

Infliximab antibody

Biologics are often used along with conventional DMARDs such as methotrexate to treat inflammatory arthritis. And some biologic medications are approved for the treatment of other inflammatory diseases, such as psoriatic arthritis, ankylosing spondylitis and inflammatory bowel disease.

While conventional DMARDs are taken by mouth, most biologics are not. Some biologics may be injected subcutaneously — under the skin — which can be done at home. Others are given by intravenous (IV) infusion, which is usually done at a clinic or hospital. The kinase inhibitors are small molecules and therefore can be taken by mouth.

Biologics can weaken your body's ability to fight infection, so your healthcare professional will want to make sure you don't already have an underlying infection, such as tuberculosis or pneumonia. Having another illness can put you at an increased risk of infection. Existing infections should be treated before you receive a DMARD or biologic agent, since these medications can make the infection worse. It's also very important that you're up to date with your vaccinations.

Because of the increased risk of serious infection, experts generally recommend against combining two or more biologic DMARDs.

For some biologic medications, biosimilars can be substituted. A biosimilar is a biologic drug that is almost an identical copy of an original drug that is manufactured by a different company. Why

almost? Since these drugs are produced from living sources, there are naturally small variations in the molecules of the active components. Like generic drugs, biosimilars can be produced when the original product's patent expires. In the United States, they still must be officially approved by the Food and Drug Administration (FDA).

If you've had inflammatory arthritis for a long time, your healthcare professional may focus less on disrupting the inflammatory process, which is likely to be less active at this point, and more on relieving pain and other symptoms.

Treating gout

Gout is treated differently depending on where it is in its progression — during an attack of acute gout or in between attacks to prevent future attacks. When someone develops acute gout, one or more joints will have swelling, redness and warmth. A joint may need to be drained — a process called aspiration — to confirm gouty crystals in the joint fluid. Confirming these crystals is an important part of distinguishing gout from infections and other conditions.

An acute attack of gout can be treated with medications that reduce inflammation. Your healthcare team might prescribe NSAIDs unless you have a history of stomach issues, bleeding, kidney disease or other conditions or using a blood thinner. Steroids also can help and can be taken either by mouth or through a joint injection. Colchicine is another option. This drug can stop the inflammation from gout and help prevent attacks. However, it may cause nausea and diarrhea. Anakinra, an IL-1 inhibitor, may be used if you can't receive other treatments because of certain medical conditions or if other treatments haven't helped. It is typically reserved for people who are hospitalized with multiple conditions. Icing the area over the inflamed joint can be helpful, too.

If you've been diagnosed with gout and you have more than two attacks a year, you'll need long-term treatment to lower the uric acid load in the body.

TYPICAL TREATMENT OF GOUT

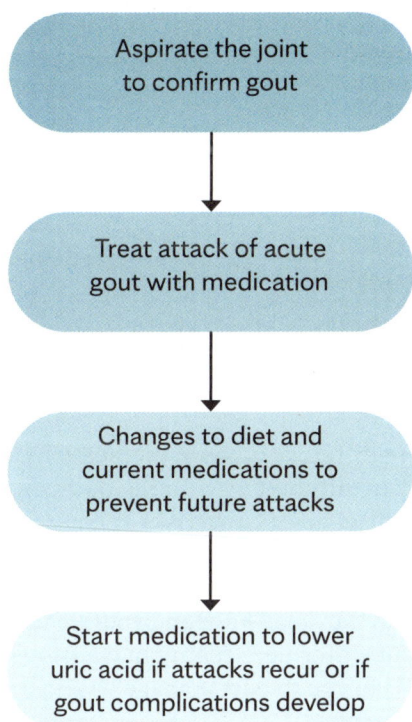

Aspirate the joint to confirm gout

↓

Treat attack of acute gout with medication

↓

Changes to diet and current medications to prevent future attacks

↓

Start medication to lower uric acid if attacks recur or if gout complications develop

The goal is to bring your uric acid level below 6.0 milligrams per deciliter (mg/dL) or, in some severe cases, less than 5.0 mg/dL. Several medications may be used. For people who develop hard masses of uric acid crystals, called tophi, the IV drug pegloticase may be helpful.

When you start a urate-lowering medicine, there's a higher risk of a gout flare until the uric acid level stabilizes. Therefore, your healthcare team will likely have you take another medication — such as an NSAID, a low-dose steroid or colchicine — for 3 to 6 months to prevent an attack.

The following different types of medications may be used to treat acute gout symptoms:

Gout medications

Generic	Brand
NSAIDs: ibuprofen, naproxen, celecoxib, others	(multiple)
Steroids: prednisone, others	(multiple)
colchicine	Mitigare, Gloperba, others
anakinra	Kineret

Some medications may reduce your risk of gout by limiting the amount of uric acid your body makes. This group, called xanthine oxidase inhibitors (XOIs), includes the drugs allopurinol and febuxostat.

XOI medications

Generic	Brand
allopurinol	Zyloprim
febuxostat	Uloric

Uricosuric and uricase medications also work in different ways to lower the amount of uric acid in the body. They help your body to remove more uric acid. These drugs include probenecid and pegloticase.

Uricosuric and uricase medications

Generic	Brand
probenecid	(generic)
pegloticase	Krystexxa

Like all medications, each of these carries risks of certain complications. Before starting any of these drugs, it's best to talk with your healthcare team to make sure you understand the risks and any precautions you should take.

Treating fibromyalgia

Fibromyalgia is a complex pain disorder, which is discussed more in Chapter 8. Typically, treatment of fibromyalgia includes improving sleep, reducing stress, and developing a slow and progressive exercise program. These steps can ease the pain and other symptoms.

Medications can be a helpful part of treatment. Various medications are used to help with sleep, stress and pain in people with fibromyalgia. Currently, only three drugs are FDA-approved for use in fibromyalgia. These include two antidepressants (duloxetine and milnacipran) and an anti-seizure drug (pregabalin).

However, depending on your symptoms and circumstances, your healthcare team might recommend off-label medications. These are drugs that haven't been approved by the FDA for the specific use of treating fibromyalgia but may help relieve your symptoms. For instance, tricyclic antidepressants are frequently used to improve pain, fatigue and deep sleep.

The drugs currently approved by the FDA for treating fibromyalgia include:

Fibromyalgia medications

Generic	Brand
duloxetine	Cymbalta
milnacipran	Savella
pregabalin	Lyrica

These different types of medications work in different ways in the body, and each drug has its own risks and precautions. As always, talk with your healthcare team about your treatment options, the effects they may have and your needs. Making informed treatment decisions can help you to best manage your fibromyalgia.

ARTHRITIS MEDICATION GUIDE

The following pages give more information about many of the most common medications used in treating arthritis. Still more may be available to you, as new research and drug innovation continue to change the landscape. If you have questions about medications or treatment, make sure to discuss them with your healthcare team.

Where a brand is listed as (generic), only generic versions of the medication are available.

ARTHRITIS MEDICATION TYPES AT A GLANCE

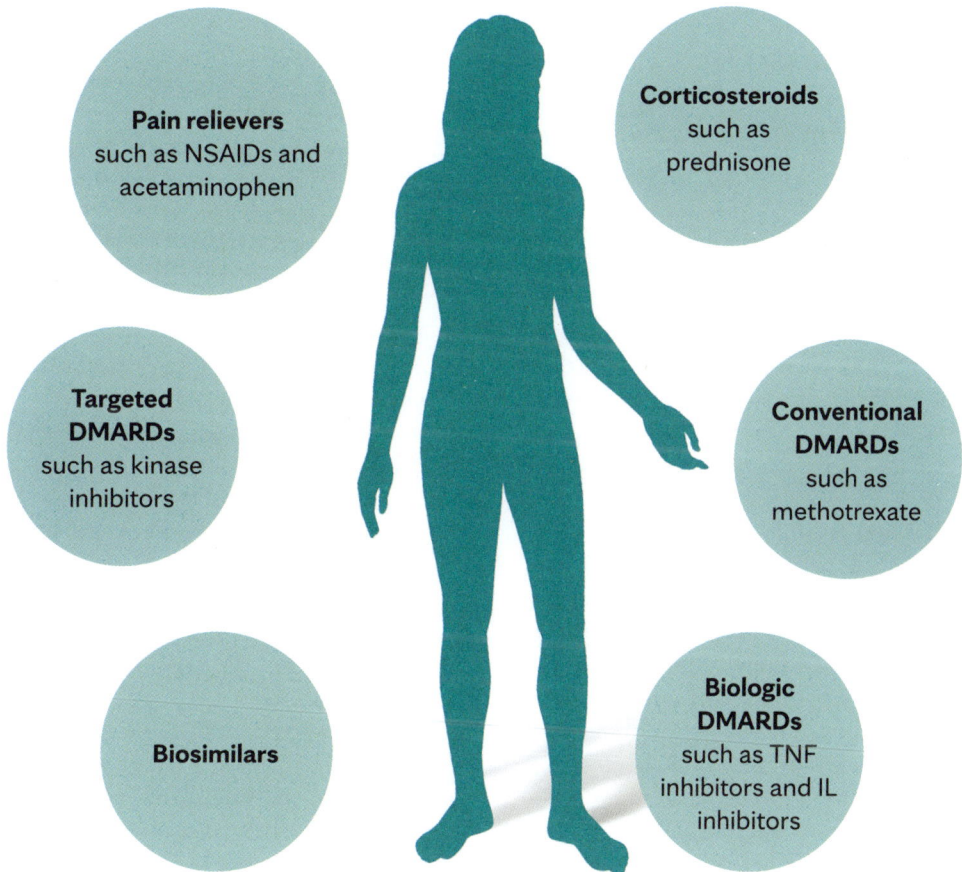

Pain relievers
such as NSAIDs and
acetaminophen

Corticosteroids
such as
prednisone

**Targeted
DMARDs**
such as kinase
inhibitors

**Conventional
DMARDs**
such as
methotrexate

Biosimilars

**Biologic
DMARDs**
such as TNF
inhibitors and IL
inhibitors

PAIN RELIEVERS

When arthritis makes your joints hurt, you naturally want quick relief. A number of different types of pain relievers can help. Some are available over-the-counter (OTC), while others will need to be prescribed by your healthcare professional.

A note of caution: These drugs can have serious side effects. In some cases, the risks include the potential for you to become dependent on or addicted to them.

Your body can also develop a tolerance to some pain relievers. So the longer you take them, the higher the dose you'll need to get the same relief.

In addition, by masking pain, these drugs may trick you into thinking that you can be more active than you should be, increasing the risk of additional damage or injury. Talk with your healthcare team about the risks of any medications you take.

NSAIDs and aspirin

The medications in this group are effective pain relievers that also help ease the stiffness and swelling caused by inflammation. Despite minor differences among different types of these drugs, they all work against inflammation in a similar way. They inhibit an enzyme called cyclooxygenase (COX), which is responsible for the production of prostaglandins. Prostaglandins are hormone-like chemicals that help send pain messages to your brain and are key to the inflammation process.

A larger dose of these drugs is required to reduce inflammation than is needed to relieve pain. If you have osteoarthritis, you may be able to take a smaller dose, because inflammation typically isn't severe and the pain may come and go.

With rheumatoid arthritis or another inflammatory joint disease, however, you may need a larger dose to feel relief.

Many different types of these drugs are available. This group of medications includes OTC medicines such as ibuprofen (Advil, Motrin IB) and aspirin, as well as other drugs available by prescription. Every person with arthritis is different, so

NSAID and aspirin medications

Generic	Brand
diclofenac	Lofena, others
diclofenac and misoprostol	Arthrotec
ibuprofen	Advil, Motrin IB, others
indomethacin	Indocin
meloxicam	Mobic, others
naproxen	Aleve, Anaprox DS, Naprosyn, others
piroxicam	(generic)
sulindac	(generic)
celecoxib (COX-2 inhibitor)	Celebrex
aspirin	(multiple)

the best choice of medication varies. What works for a friend or relative may not work for you.

Drugs in this group can cause an upset stomach, gastrointestinal bleeding, cardiovascular problems, and liver and kidney damage. Older people are at highest risk of complications. Because of the risk of side effects, your healthcare team will prescribe the lowest effective dose of these medications for the shortest time needed.

A subset of NSAIDs works by inhibiting only the cyclooxygenase-2 (COX-2) enzyme. COX-2 inhibitors relieve joint pain just as well as other NSAIDs yet cause fewer ulcers and less gastrointestinal bleeding. However, they may be more expensive and may increase your cardiovascular risks.

Based on your overall health — including your gastrointestinal and heart health — your care team can help determine which type of medication in this group might provide the most benefits for you with the fewest risks.

How they're usually given:
- By mouth

Benefits:
- Provide mild to moderate pain relief
- Ease inflammation and joint stiffness

Risks:
- Upset stomach, abdominal pain, nausea
- Internal bleeding
- Heartburn, stomach ulcers
- Skin reactions
- Headache, dizziness, fatigue
- Ringing in the ears, hearing loss
- Constipation, diarrhea
- Kidney problems

Precautions:
- Use them with caution or consider other therapies if you have ulcers, gastrointestinal bleeding, asthma or cardiovascular disease. Talk to your healthcare team first.
- Don't take two or more different NSAIDs at the same time.
- Talk to your healthcare team about NSAID use in children, including OTC brands.
- Risks, especially kidney and stomach problems, are greater if you're older than age 65.
- NSAID use with blood-thinning medications increases bleeding risk.
- Before any surgery or dental work, inform the surgeon or dentist if you are taking any of these medications.
- Consult your healthcare professional before giving aspirin to children or teenagers. Aspirin use in children has been linked to Reye's syndrome.

Acetaminophen

Acetaminophen is a pain reliever used to treat common headaches, muscle aches, toothaches and sore throats. It is widely available over-the-counter and is often

Generic	Brand
acetaminophen	Tylenol, others

combined with other drugs in medications to treat multiple symptoms, such as for cold or flu relief.

Acetaminophen works by interfering with how the body processes pain. Because the drug has a limited effect on inflammation, it's appropriate for arthritis that causes pain but little inflammation — as is often the case in osteoarthritis — and for people who are unable to take NSAIDs.

Many people with arthritis find that acetaminophen can ease their pain as well as an NSAID can. If you have mild pain from osteoarthritis or other types of noninflammatory pain, your healthcare team may recommend acetaminophen as the first choice for pain relief. It is inexpensive and usually doesn't cause side effects as long as you don't take more than the recommended dose.

High doses of acetaminophen taken over a long period of time can lead to liver problems, especially if you consume alcohol daily or take other medicines containing acetaminophen.

How it's usually given:
- By mouth

Benefits:
- First choice for mild pain relief
- Works fast

Risks:
- High doses can lead to liver damage, especially if the medicine is consumed with other medications or with alcohol.

Precautions:
- Check the labels of other medications you take to see if they contain acetaminophen.

Tramadol

If acetaminophen or an NSAID doesn't completely relieve your pain, your healthcare team may recommend a medication called tramadol. This drug is a less potent opioid that can be used alone or along with acetaminophen or an NSAID.

Studies show that taking tramadol can provide pain relief similar to other stronger opioids such as codeine.

Tramadol may not make you as sleepy as codeine can, though it may increase the possibility of headaches.

How it's usually given:
- By mouth

Benefits:
- Provides moderate to high pain relief
- May cause less drowsiness than other opioids

Tramadol medications

Generic	Brand
tramadol	ConZip, Odolo
tramadol with acetaminophen	(generic)

REDUCE YOUR RISK OF STOMACH PROBLEMS FROM NSAIDS

Nonsteroidal anti-inflammatory drugs can make life easier by helping control the pain and inflammation of arthritis. Unfortunately, they can also give you an upset stomach or even an ulcer.

Gastrointestinal bleeding is a potentially serious side effect of NSAIDs. In addition to suppressing prostaglandins associated with inflammation and pain, NSAIDs decrease production of a chemical that protects your stomach lining. This allows stomach acid to erode the lining and cause bleeding and ulcers.

Because bleeding and ulcers in the stomach can occur with no warning, it's important to get regular checkups. If you're taking NSAIDs regularly, your blood count and liver enzyme level should be checked periodically. Your healthcare team may also suggest that you take a medication, such as a proton pump inhibitor (PPI), to decrease some of the gastrointestinal side effects. PPIs are drugs that reduce the amount of stomach acid.

If you regularly take traditional NSAIDs, here are steps that may help you minimize the risk of stomach problems:
- Take NSAIDs with food and water or milk.
- Avoid alcohol, since this increases the risk of gastric bleeding.
- Take the lowest possible dose to reduce symptoms.
- Take your medication later in the day if possible. If you take an NSAID once a day, doing so in the afternoon or evening may be easier on your stomach.
- Don't take more NSAIDs, or take them more often, than are prescribed.
- Don't take other NSAIDs or medications containing NSAIDs, whether prescription or non-prescription, at the same time.
- Talk to your healthcare team or pharmacist about other medications you take that may interact with NSAIDs and increase your risk of stomach problems.

Risks:
- Drug abuse or dependency, especially when used for extended periods
- Nausea, stomach pain
- Constipation, diarrhea
- Lightheadedness, dizziness
- Drowsiness

Precautions:
- Avoid taking tramadol with alcohol, including with medicines containing alcohol.
- This medication can increase your risk of seizures.
- Serotonin syndrome may occur when using this medication with certain

other medications (antidepressants, certain migraine drugs). Let your healthcare team know immediately if you experience agitation, hallucinations, irregular heartbeat or lack of coordination.
- Withdrawal symptoms can occur if this medication is stopped abruptly.
- Long-term use during pregnancy may result in neonatal withdrawal symptoms.
- This medication may increase suicidal thoughts.

Opioids

Opioids are powerful pain relievers that block pain signals traveling to the brain. However, these drugs can be addictive and cause drowsiness. Because of this, they're prescribed mainly for a short duration and for intense pain. In certain cases, when other pain control methods aren't working or aren't an option, some medical professionals may prescribe an opioid medication to treat severe arthritis pain.

With the increasing use of opioids in recent decades, cases of opioid abuse and drug dependency have become more common. If your healthcare professional suggests an opioid as part of your treatment, make sure you understand the risks and how to take it safely.

How they're usually given:
- By mouth

Benefits:
- Provide relief for moderate to severe pain

- Work well for pain that hasn't responded to other therapies

Risks:
- Drug abuse or dependency, especially when used for extended periods
- Lightheadedness, dizziness
- Drowsiness
- Constipation
- Upset stomach, nausea

Precautions:
- Breaking, chewing or crushing opioid medications that are extended release (ER), slow release (SR) or controlled release (CR) can lead to rapid and potentially fatal absorption of the drug.
- Avoid taking opioids with alcohol, including medicines containing alcohol.

Opioid medications

Generic	Brand
codeine with acetaminophen	Tylenol No. 3, others
fentanyl	Duragesic, others
hydrocodone with or without acetaminophen	Norco, Vicodin, others
hydromorphone	Dilaudid
meperidine	Demerol
morphine	(multiple)
tapentadol	Nucynta
oxycodone with or without acetaminophen	OxyContin, Percocet, others

- You can develop a tolerance to these medications, which will result in larger and larger doses being necessary to achieve the same amount of pain relief.
- Withdrawal symptoms can occur if these medications are stopped abruptly.
- Long-term use of opioids during pregnancy may result in neonatal withdrawal symptoms.

Topical pain relievers

Topical pain medications are absorbed through your skin. The most common varieties are creams or gels that you rub into the skin over your painful joints. Others come in the form of a spray or a patch that sticks to your skin. Some are available by prescription from your healthcare team, but others are available over-the-counter.

Because the ingredients are absorbed through the skin, topical preparations

Topical medications

Generic	Brand
capsaicin	Zostrix, others
diclofenac (NSAID)	Voltaren gel, Pennsaid, others
lidocaine	Lidoderm, Salonpas Lidocaine, others
menthol	Bengay, Icy Hot, others
salicylates	Aspercreme, others

usually have fewer side effects compared with medications that are taken by mouth and absorbed through your bloodstream.

For adults over age 75 with osteoarthritis of the hands or knees, the American College of Rheumatology recommends topical NSAIDs instead of oral NSAIDs.

The active ingredients in topical pain medications may include:

Capsaicin

Capsaicin (kap-SAY-ih-sin) creams inhibit a chemical that's important for sending pain messages. Capsaicin comes from chili peppers.

For some people, the creams work well to relieve joint pain. But others dislike the burning or stinging sensation that can occur when they apply the cream. With continued use, the burning and stinging often lessens.

Salicylates

Salicylates (suh-LIS-uh-lates) contain the pain-relieving substance found in aspirin. Although people with arthritis may use these creams, these products have not been studied specifically for their ability to relieve arthritis symptoms.

Menthol

Menthol produces a sensation of hot or cold that may temporarily override your ability to feel arthritis pain. As with salicylate-based topicals, menthol-based preparations haven't been rigorously studied in the specific context of arthritis.

NSAIDs

Some studies indicate that NSAID creams and gels may work as well as their oral counterparts. In the United States, the FDA has approved several versions of prescription gels and liquid drops containing the NSAID diclofenac to treat osteoarthritis in the hands, wrists, elbows, feet, ankles and knees. A topical patch containing diclofenac also is available.

Lidocaine

In some situations, healthcare professionals may prescribe lidocaine patches for joint pain. The patches are approved in the U.S. to treat a painful complication of shingles, but a healthcare professional may also prescribe them for other forms of pain such as arthritis pain. This is called an off-label use. The lidocaine patches are placed on the skin over the painful joint for 12 hours at a time. The medication numbs the area.

When using topical pain relievers, be careful to wash your hands thoroughly after use, especially before you rub or touch your eyes. Don't use these pain relievers on broken or irritated skin or in combination with a heating pad, bandage, wrap or dressing.

If you're allergic to aspirin or you are taking an anticoagulant blood thinner, check with your healthcare professional before using topical medications that contain salicylates.

How they're usually given:
- Topically — through your skin — via a cream, gel, spray or patch

Benefits:
- Provide local pain relief

Risks:
- Itching
- Stinging or burning sensation
- Rash

Precautions:
- Avoid rubbing or touching your eyes after using the medication until you've thoroughly washed your hands.
- Don't rub the medication into skin that is broken or irritated.
- Check with your healthcare team before using topical medications that contain salicylates if you're allergic to aspirin or are taking a blood thinner.
- Don't cover the medication with a bandage or wrap or use it in combination with a heating pad.

CORTICOSTEROIDS

Corticosteroids are another group of medications used to fight inflammation caused by arthritis. Also called steroids or glucocorticoids, corticosteroids are artificial versions of a hormone called cortisol.

These drugs work by blocking your body's production of prostaglandins, hormone-like substances that cause inflammation. Corticosteroids also suppress the immune system to control inflammation.

Corticosteroids fight inflammation effectively and quickly. They ease symptoms of stiffness, pain and fatigue, and they reduce swelling, helping protect your joints and other affected areas. In the short term, corticosteroids can make you feel dramatically better.

Corticosteroids can be injected directly into a sore or inflamed joint. This allows the medication to go directly to the needed area without affecting the entire body. Relief can last for several months, and injections can be repeated in the future, although usually no more than 2 to 4 times a year.

Certain corticosteroids such as prednisone and other similar drugs can also be taken by mouth. They offer widespread relief of inflammation due to rheumatoid arthritis, usually in a matter of days.

However, taken in high doses over long periods of time, these drugs can have many side effects, including mood changes, weight gain, muscle weakness, loss of bone density, diabetes, cataracts, increased risk of infection and high blood pressure.

As a result, oral corticosteroids are generally reserved for treating acute symptoms or flare-ups. In rheumatoid arthritis, oral corticosteroids may be used to tide you over while you wait for other medications, such as a DMARD, to become fully effective. Once the DMARD kicks in, the corticosteroid can be slowly decreased and eventually discontinued.

How they're usually given:
- By mouth, by injection into the affected joint, intravenously

Benefits:
- Provide fast relief for severe pain
- Ease inflammation
- Relieve flare-ups and sudden worsening of symptoms

Risks:
- Nausea
- Difficulty sleeping (insomnia)
- Increased appetite
- Anxiety and irritability
- Changes in mood
- Swelling of the hands, legs and feet
- Changes in vision
- Increased blood sugar
- Increased blood pressure

Corticosteroid medications

Generic	Brand
betamethasone	Celestone Solus-pan
dexamethasone	(generic)
methylprednisolone	Depo-Medrol, Medrol, Solu-Medrol
prednisolone	Pediapred, Orapred ODT
prednisone	(generic)
triamcinolone	Kenalog-10, others

GENERIC AND BIOSIMILAR VS. BRAND-NAME

Many drugs used to treat arthritis are available as both brand-name and generic medications. And increasingly, biosimilars may be an option alongside biologics. What's the difference?

A drug that's discovered or developed in a laboratory begins with a generic name selected by experts and governmental agencies. After extensive research and testing of the drug's safety and effectiveness, the company that developed the drug typically takes it to market with a brand name and sells it exclusively for a fixed period. When the patent rights on the drug expire, any other drug company can manufacture and sell the drug under its generic name or another brand name. In any case, the FDA still must approve the new versions before they can be sold.

Generic versions are available for many drugs on the market. For consumers, that's good news because generics often cost considerably less than their brand-name counterparts. Generic drugs have the same active ingredients, strength and method as the brand-name versions. They also carry the same risks and benefits.

When patent rights on a biologic DMARD expire, other drug companies may produce a biosimilar medication. The active components of biosimilars are not exactly identical to the original drugs. This is because of natural variation in producing these medicines. Manufacturers must do thorough studies of the biosimilars they make that show that the biosimilar medicines are as safe and pure as the reference products. And they also must be as effective. See page 122 for more on biosimilars.

Your doctor or pharmacist can determine whether you should use a brand-name medication or a generic or biosimilar version, based on your medical needs, the specific drug and its availability.

- Weight gain
- Osteoporosis

Precautions:
- Avoid live virus vaccines while taking corticosteroids.
- Corticosteroids may increase your risk of infection. Wash your hands frequently and avoid people who are ill.
- These medications should not be stopped abruptly if used for an extended period.

CONVENTIONAL DISEASE-MODIFYING ANTIRHEUMATIC DRUGS (DMARDS)

If you have an inflammatory arthritis, such as rheumatoid arthritis, your healthcare professional will likely recommend that you take one or more DMARDs — sooner rather than later.

All these drugs work to slow or stop the inflammatory process that's characteristic of rheumatoid arthritis and other rheumatic diseases, such as psoriatic arthritis, ankylosing spondylitis and forms of juvenile arthritis. By halting the disease process, DMARDs help prevent further damage to your joints.

Methotrexate

Methotrexate is one of the first DMARDs doctors turn to for established rheumatoid arthritis. It was originally used to treat cancer, but in lower doses it can treat rheumatic diseases. The drug relieves painful and swollen joints and prevents further joint damage. It inhibits an enzyme, interfering with cell division and slowing down the immune system. Side effects are typically manageable, and its cost is relatively low.

Methotrexate is often combined with other drugs, such as another DMARD.

Generic	Brand
methotrexate	Trexall, Rasuvo, others

Using methotrexate as the cornerstone of combination therapy often results in better control of rheumatoid arthritis than can be achieved with methotrexate alone, with no increased side effects from combining medicines.

Methotrexate can be taken by mouth or by injection, typically as a single dose once a week. If taking it by mouth bothers your stomach, you might fare better with an injection. Taking regular doses of folic acid also can help minimize the side effects of nausea and gastrointestinal discomfort.

Liver damage is a potential but rare side effect of taking methotrexate. Before prescribing the drug, your healthcare professional will likely have you tested for hepatitis B and C to make sure there's no existing liver inflammation. While taking the drug, it's important to limit alcohol consumption to avoid increasing your risk of liver injury.

Drugs such as methotrexate can also reduce the infection-fighting potency of your white blood cells, making you more vulnerable to infection. These drugs may lower the number of platelets in your blood, with the result that you bruise or bleed more easily. They can also lower your red blood cell count, causing fatigue. Lung damage is another rare side effect.

At the low doses used for rheumatoid arthritis, these side effects are unlikely. But call your healthcare team immediately if you develop a fever or shortness of breath. Also tell your healthcare team if you experience unexplained bruising, fatigue or any other side effects.

If you take methotrexate, you'll need to have your blood tested regularly to help ensure that the drug doesn't produce unwanted changes in your liver and bone marrow. Visits with your healthcare team can help address any side effects quickly.

How it's usually given:
- By mouth or subcutaneous injection

Benefits:
- A common first choice in rheumatoid arthritis drug therapy

Risks:
- Upset stomach, nausea
- Loss of appetite
- Mouth sores
- Serious infections
- Blood cell deficiencies, resulting in bleeding and bruising more easily than normal, fatigue, weakness

Precautions:
- Methotrexate isn't recommended if you're pregnant, as it can harm the baby. If you hope to become pregnant, discuss potential alternatives with your healthcare professional.
- Methotrexate may not be right for you if you have an existing infection, blood disorder, kidney, liver or lung disease, history of lymphoma, peptic ulcer, or ulcerative colitis.
- While taking this medication, your blood cell counts and kidney and liver function will be monitored regularly.
- If you experience any reaction to the drug, contact your healthcare team right away.
- Don't drink alcohol when taking this medication.
- Discuss your vaccinations with your healthcare team before starting this medication.

DRUG INTERACTIONS

Many people use more than one medication. Unfortunately, the action of one drug can be altered by the action of another, either decreasing or increasing the desired effect or producing a potentially dangerous reaction. Even vitamins and herbal supplements can sometimes cause serious interactions with other drugs.

When taking medications for arthritis, be sure to tell your healthcare professional about every drug you use, including nonprescription medications, vitamins, minerals, herbal supplements and alternative remedies.

Bring all current medications with you to a doctor's visit. That way, the proper dosages can be determined for both prescription and nonprescription drugs you take. Your medical professional or pharmacist also can create a schedule for taking your medications. This way you can take the drugs you need, but minimize the chance of harmful interactions.

Leflunomide

If you need an alternative to methotrexate, your healthcare professional may recommend leflunomide, an immunosuppressant that reduces pain, stiffness, inflammation and swelling. It may also slow or halt joint damage associated with rheumatoid arthritis.

Similar to other immunosuppressants, leflunomide inhibits certain substances — in this case, a type of enzyme — made by your immune system. It can be used alone or in combination with methotrexate to increase the benefits of DMARD therapy.

Leflunomide may cause a range of side effects, including nausea, diarrhea, skin rash, upset stomach, weight loss and hair loss. As with methotrexate, it can also increase your risk of liver damage and infection, so most of the same precautions apply. You'll undergo regular blood tests to monitor your red and white blood cell counts and platelet counts.

Your healthcare team will test your liver function before you begin taking the medication and will conduct regular tests from then on. If you already have a liver condition, you may not be able to take leflunomide.

If you develop liver problems while taking the drug, you may need to change the dosage or stop the medication altogether. Minimizing your alcohol intake can help reduce your risk of liver damage.

Avoid leflunomide if you're pregnant, breastfeeding or hoping to become pregnant. It can harm the developing fetus and may cause serious side effects in nursing infants. (Men hoping to become fathers may want to avoid this drug as well. Check with your medical professional.)

This medication stays in your body for a long time. It can take many months to completely eliminate leflunomide from your system. If necessary, your healthcare professional can prescribe a drug called cholestyramine to speed up the elimination of leflunomide from your body.

How it's usually given:
- By mouth

Benefits:
- May be an alternative to methotrexate
- May be combined with methotrexate for rheumatoid arthritis that is hard to treat

Risks:
- Diarrhea
- Nausea
- Rash
- Hair loss
- Hypertension

Precautions:
- It's important to avoid pregnancy while on this medication and during

Generic	Brand
leflunomide	Arava

the time the drug is being eliminated from your body.

- Leflunomide isn't recommended if you already have a liver disorder, as the medication can make it worse.
- Screening for infections such as tuberculosis and hepatitis B and C is recommended before starting the medication.
- While taking this medication, you'll be monitored regularly for changes in your blood cell counts and kidney and liver functions.
- If necessary, elimination of the drug from your body can be sped up by taking the drug cholestyramine. Without this procedure, it may take up to two years to clear the drug from your system.
- Discuss your vaccinations with your healthcare team before starting this medication.

Sulfasalazine

If your rheumatoid arthritis symptoms are mild to moderate, your healthcare professional may recommend sulfasalazine, a drug that's also used to treat inflammatory bowel disease.

Research suggests that sulfasalazine may be more effective than the medication hydroxychloroquine at treating active inflammation. It's also useful in combination therapy.

Generic	Brand
sulfasalazine	Azulfidine

Your healthcare team will likely order periodic blood tests to monitor the effect of this drug on your blood cells. Side effects are uncommon. Some people have stomach discomfort, which usually goes away after reducing the dose or switching to delayed-release tablets.

If you're allergic to sulfa or aspirin, sulfasalazine probably isn't for you, because it's derived from these ingredients. It could cause an allergic reaction, such as skin rash, wheezing, itching or fever.

How it's usually given:
- By mouth

Benefits:
- Effective for early, mild rheumatoid arthritis

Risks:
- Upset stomach
- Headache
- Rash
- Nausea, vomiting, loss of appetite

Precautions:
- Tell your healthcare professional if you experience sore throat, fever, paleness, easy bruising, or a yellowish cast to the eyes or skin, as any of these may indicate a serious blood disorder.
- Caution is recommended with a serious blood disorder or liver or kidney disease.
- Urine or skin may change in color to mild yellowish orange.

Hydroxychloroquine

Originally a treatment for malaria, hydroxy-chloroquine has also been found to be effective for rheumatoid arthritis — although how it works to reduce joint damage isn't clear. It takes about six months for this drug to become effective. If you have early, mild rheumatoid arthritis, your healthcare professional may recommend starting out with hydroxychloroquine, reserving more potent DMARDs, such as methotrexate and leflunomide, for later if your symptoms get worse.

Hydroxychloroquine is a common choice for use in combination with other DMARDs or in combination with cortico-steroids. Using it in this way can reduce the amount of steroids you need to take.

Hydroxychloroquine has few side effects, but at high doses it may increase the risk of damage to parts of the eyes, such as the retinas. The dose prescribed for rheu-matic diseases generally isn't that high. Still, your healthcare team will probably want you to have an eye exam before starting the medication and regularly thereafter, to catch any changes.

Hydroxychloroquine is used to treat lupus and other rheumatic diseases as well.

How it's usually given:
- By mouth

Generic	Brand
hydroxychloro-quine	Plaquenil

Benefits:
- Effective for early, mild rheumatoid arthritis and lupus

Risks:
- Upset stomach, nausea
- Rash
- Dizziness
- Headache
- Vision changes

Precautions:
- Before starting the medication, you will need a baseline eye exam. If you remain on this drug for more than five years, an annual eye exam is recommended thereafter to monitor for vision changes.
- Caution is recommended when liver disease or alcoholism is present.

BIOLOGIC DMARDS

Biologics are recommended for early, severe rheumatoid arthritis or rheuma-toid arthritis that hasn't responded to methotrexate or combination therapy. These targeted drugs can also be com-bined with DMARDs, NSAIDs and corticosteroids.

Because of how they work, biologics limit your ability to fight infections. (For more explanation, see page 326.) If you have an acute infection, your healthcare team will want to treat the infection before starting you on a biologic medication. In addition, you should be tested for tuberculosis to check for latent disease that could become active.

Tumor necrosis factor (TNF) inhibitors

Tumor necrosis factor (TNF) inhibitors appear to be as effective as the DMARD methotrexate in treating rheumatoid arthritis. For rheumatoid arthritis that doesn't respond well to either methotrexate or a TNF inhibitor, a combination of the two drugs may be more effective than using either drug alone.

When injected into the body, TNF blocking agents such as infliximab, adalimumab, certolizumab and golimumab attach to circulating TNF-alpha molecules — a type of cytokine — via an antibody. They neutralize the TNF-alpha molecules before the molecules can set off an immune reaction. Etanercept works by blocking the receptor that TNF attaches to.

Because TNF inhibitors can weaken the immune system, your risk of infection is increased, especially if you're also taking methotrexate or corticosteroids. Your healthcare team will monitor you for signs of infection. Let your care team know if you have symptoms of infection, such as a fever, or if you aren't feeling well.

TNF inhibitors

Generic	Brand
adalimumab	Humira
certolizumab pegol	Cimzia
etanercept	Enbrel
golimumab	Simponi
infliximab	Remicade

Some people have developed symptoms of disorders such as lupus or multiple sclerosis while taking TNF inhibitors. An increased risk of lymphoma, a type of cancer, has also been reported. However, studies suggest that this increase is a complication of rheumatoid arthritis rather than an effect of the biologic medication.

If you have congestive heart failure, your health professional may recommend against TNF inhibitors because they can worsen your heart function.

FDA-approved uses:
- Rheumatoid arthritis
- Psoriasis, psoriatic arthritis
- Ankylosing spondylitis
- Inflammatory bowel disease
- Juvenile idiopathic arthritis (JIA)
- Uveitis

How they're usually given:
- Subcutaneous injection, intravenous (IV) infusion

Benefits:
- They target TNF-alpha, an immune substance that plays a major role in the chronic inflammatory cascade that characterizes rheumatoid arthritis.

Risks:
- Mild reaction at injection site (redness, pain, itching, swelling or bruising), infusion reaction
- Headache
- Abdominal pain
- Upper respiratory tract infection
- Can cause a lupus-like reaction

- May exacerbate multiple sclerosis
- May increase risk of new or worsening heart failure
- May increase risk of serious infection
- May increase risk of skin cancer
- May cause new or worsening psoriasis

Precautions:
- Prior to receiving a TNF inhibitor, you'll be screened for tuberculosis and hepatitis B and C. If necessary, an infection will be treated before you start therapy.
- Your healthcare team will monitor you closely for signs of infection while you're taking a TNF inhibitor. Call your healthcare professional right away if you have a fever, don't feel well or experience unexplained weight loss, excessive sweating, coughing or difficulty breathing.
- Vaccination with live vaccines isn't recommended while taking a TNF inhibitor.
- TNF inhibitors may not be appropriate if you have chronic or recurring infections or if you have a history of heart failure.
- These medications may damage the protective coating that surrounds nerve fibers in the brain and spinal cord.
- Biologics can affect certain blood cells, so let your care team know if you experience bleeding, bruising, fatigue or weakness more easily than normal while taking these medications.
- TNF inhibitors are likely safe during pregnancy and breastfeeding, but talk with your healthcare team about the risks and benefits.

Interleukin-1 inhibitors

IL-1 inhibitors are biologics that bind with cell receptors normally reserved for the cytokine interleukin-1. By taking the immune protein's spot on the receptor, IL-1 inhibitors disrupt its activity.

IL-1 inhibitors generally aren't as effective as the other biologics for treating rheumatoid arthritis. But they may be helpful with other autoimmune inflammatory conditions, such as systemic JIA and periodic fever syndromes.

In addition, IL-1 inhibition may be beneficial for some people with acute gouty arthritis.

FDA-approved uses:
- Rheumatoid arthritis
- Systemic JIA
- Periodic fever syndromes
- Cryopyrin-associated periodic syndromes (CAPS)

How they're usually given:
- Subcutaneous injection

Benefits:
- Helps stall the disease process by targeting interleukin-1, another key player in the inflammatory cascade

Interleukin-1 inhibitors

Generic	Brand
anakinra	Kineret
canakinumab	Ilaris
rilonacept	Arcalyst

Risks:
- Local reaction at injection site
- Diarrhea
- Flu-like reactions
- Increased risk of serious infection

Precautions:
- Your healthcare team will monitor your white blood cell and platelet counts while you're on these drugs.
- This medication can increase your risk of serious infection, including tuberculosis and bacterial, viral and fungal infections.
- Contact your healthcare professional right away if you have a fever, don't feel well or experience unexplained weight loss, excessive sweating, coughing or difficulty breathing. These could be signs of infection.
- Receiving live virus vaccines isn't recommended while you're on medicines of this type.
- Anakinra is not recommended if you're pregnant or breastfeeding. Your healthcare team can suggest an alternative medication. The risks from other IL-1 inhibitors aren't known.

Interleukin-6 inhibitors

The cytokine interleukin-6 is capable of activating T cells, B cells and other immune cells. IL-6 inhibitors work by blocking the cytokine from binding to cell receptors. This medication can be given by an infusion through your blood or by a subcutaneous injection.

FDA-approved uses:
- Rheumatoid arthritis
- JIA
- Giant cell arteritis

How they're usually given:
- Subcutaneous injection, IV infusion

Benefits:
- Targets interleukin-6, disrupting the inflammatory process

Risks:
- Common cold symptoms
- Local reaction, such as a rash or swelling, at injection site
- Serious infections, including tuberculosis, bacterial sepsis and fungal infections
- Reactivation of dormant tuberculosis
- Allergic reaction, possibly severe, even leading to narrowed airways and difficulty breathing called anaphylaxis
- Tearing of the intestinal wall, known as bowel perforation, primarily if you have diverticulitis
- High cholesterol
- Blood cell deficiencies, resulting in bleeding and bruising more easily than normal, fatigue, or weakness
- Liver damage

Precautions:
- Prior to receiving an IL-6 inhibitor, you'll be screened for tuberculosis

Interleukin-6 inhibitors

Generic	Brand
sarilumab	Kevzara
tocilizumab	Actemra

and hepatitis B and C. If necessary, an infection will be treated before you start therapy.

- Your healthcare team will monitor you closely for signs of infection while you're taking this drug. Call your healthcare professional right away if you have a fever, don't feel well or experience unexplained weight loss, excessive sweating, coughing or difficulty breathing.
- While taking this medication, you'll be monitored regularly for changes in your blood cell counts and liver function.
- Receiving live virus vaccines isn't recommended while you're on this medicine.
- IL-6 inhibitors may not be appropriate in patients with underlying liver problems or a history of diverticulosis.
- The risks of using this during pregnancy and breastfeeding aren't known.

Interleukin-17 inhibitors

IL-17 inhibitors target the cytokine interleukin-17. The IL-17 pathway has a role in psoriasis, psoriatic arthritis and ankylosing spondylitis.

Interleukin-17 inhibitors

Generic	Brand
ixekizumab	Taltz
secukinumab	Cosentyx
bimekizumab	Bimzelx

FDA-approved uses:
- Psoriasis and psoriatic arthritis
- Ankylosing spondylitis

How they're usually given:
- Subcutaneous injection

Benefits:
- Inhibits IL-17, a key cytokine in inflammation

Risks:
- Local reaction at injection site
- Diarrhea
- Headache
- Upper respiratory tract infection
- Candida infection
- Uveitis
- Low number of neutrophils, a type of white blood cell
- May exacerbate inflammatory bowel disease activity
- May worsen depression
- May increase cholesterol

Precautions:
- You'll need to be screened for tuberculosis and hepatitis B and C. If necessary, an infection will be treated before you start therapy.
- Your healthcare team will monitor you closely for signs of infection while you're taking this drug. Call your healthcare professional right away if you have a fever, don't feel well or experience unexplained weight loss, excessive sweating, coughing or difficulty breathing.
- Receiving live virus vaccines isn't recommended while taking these medicines.

- IL-17 inhibitors may not be appropriate if you have chronic or recurring infections or a history of inflammatory bowel disease.
- Biologics can affect certain blood cells, so let your healthcare professional know if you experience bleeding, bruising, fatigue or weakness more easily than usual.
- These medications are not recommended if you're pregnant. Your healthcare team can suggest an alternative medication. The risks of using IL-17 inhibitors while breastfeeding aren't known.

IL-12/IL-23 inhibitor

The medication ustekinumab blocks both cytokines IL-12 and IL-23. It has been found to be effective in treating psoriasis and psoriatic arthritis. It can also be used to treat patients with Crohn's disease and ulcerative colitis, types of inflammatory bowel disease.

FDA-approved uses:
- Psoriasis
- Psoriatic arthritis
- Crohn's disease
- Ulcerative colitis

How it's usually given:
- Subcutaneous injection, IV infusion

IL-12/IL-23 inhibitor

Generic	Brand
ustekinumab	Stelara

Benefits:
- Blocks cytokines that aggravate psoriasis and psoriatic arthritis

Risks:
- Local reaction at injection site or infusion reaction
- Increased risk of infection
- Upper respiratory tract infections
- May increase risk of nonmelanoma skin cancer

Precautions:
- Prior to starting this medication, you'll be screened for tuberculosis and hepatitis B and C. If necessary, an infection will be treated before you start therapy.
- Your healthcare team will monitor you closely for signs of infection while you're taking this drug. Call your healthcare professional right away if you have a fever, don't feel well, or experience unexplained weight loss, excessive sweating, coughing or difficulty breathing.
- Receiving live virus vaccines isn't recommended while you're on an IL-12/IL-23 inhibitor.
- This drug may not be appropriate if you have chronic or recurring infections.
- This medication may damage the protective coating that surrounds nerve fibers in the brain and spinal cord.
- Biologics can affect certain blood cells, so let your care team know if you experience bleeding, bruising, fatigue or weakness more easily than usual.

- This medication is not recommended if you're pregnant. Your healthcare team can suggest an alternative. Ustekinumab may be safely used while breastfeeding, though it's important to discuss the risks and benefits beforehand.

IL-23 inhibitors

IL-23 inhibitors block this key cytokine found in the development of psoriasis and psoriatic arthritis.

FDA-approved uses:
- Psoriasis
- Psoriatic arthritis
- Crohn's disease
- Ulcerative colitis

How they're usually given:
- Subcutaneous injection

Benefits:
- Block the IL-23 cytokine, which is increased in psoriasis and psoriatic arthritis

Risks:
- Local reaction at injection site
- Increased risk of infection
- Upper respiratory tract infection
- Headache

IL-23 inhibitors

Generic	Brand
guselkumab	Tremfya
risankizumab	Skyrizi
tildrakizumab	Ilumya

Precautions:
- Prior to starting these medications, you'll be screened for tuberculosis and hepatitis B and C. If necessary, an infection will be treated before you start therapy.
- Your healthcare team will monitor you closely for signs of infection while you're taking this drug. Call your healthcare professional right away if you have a fever, don't feel well, or experience unexplained weight loss, excessive sweating, coughing or difficulty breathing.
- Receiving live virus vaccines isn't recommended while you're on these drugs.
- IL-23 inhibitors may not be appropriate if you have chronic or recurring infections.
- Biologics can affect certain blood cells, so let your healthcare team know if you experience bleeding, bruising, fatigue or weakness more easily than usual.
- The risks of using these during pregnancy and breastfeeding aren't known.

T cell inhibitor

The medication abatacept inhibits the action of T cells, which recognize invaders and trigger inflammation. The drug binds to the cells and blocks their signals.

T cell inhibitor

Generic	Brand
abatacept	Orencia

It's generally prescribed for people with moderate to severe rheumatoid arthritis that hasn't responded to other drugs.

Abatacept can slow damage to joints and improve physical function. It can be used with conventional DMARDs, but it shouldn't be taken with other cytokine inhibitors.

FDA-approved uses:
- Rheumatoid arthritis
- Juvenile idiopathic arthritis
- Psoriatic arthritis

How it's usually given:
- Subcutaneous injection, IV infusion

Benefits:
- Inhibits activation of T cells, blocking the perpetuation of inflammation

Risks:
- Headache
- Dizziness
- Nausea
- Upper respiratory infection
- Increased risk of infection
- May aggravate chronic obstructive pulmonary disease

Precautions:
- Prior to receiving abatacept, you'll be screened for tuberculosis and hepatitis B and C and treated, if necessary.
- Your healthcare team will monitor you closely for signs of infection while you're taking this drug. Call your healthcare professional right away if you have a fever, don't feel well, or experience unexplained weight loss, excessive sweating, coughing or difficulty breathing.
- Receiving live virus vaccines isn't recommended while you're taking this medication.
- Abatacept may not be appropriate if you have chronic or recurring infections or if you have a history of chronic obstructive pulmonary disease.
- This medication is not recommended if you're pregnant. Your healthcare team can suggest an alternative. Abatacept may be safely used while breastfeeding, though it's important to discuss the risks and benefits beforehand.

B cell inhibitor

B cells play an important role in sustaining the inflammation that's caused by rheumatoid arthritis. The drug rituximab is a genetically engineered protein that binds to B cells, causing them to self-destruct. Rituximab was first found to be effective in treating lymphoma, a type of cancer.

FDA-approved uses:
- Rheumatoid arthritis
- Vasculitis
- Lymphoma

How it's usually given:
- Intravenous infusion

B cell inhibitor

Generic	Brand
rituximab	Rituxan, others

Benefits:
- Targets and destroys immune system B cells
- Is usually reserved for severe disease that hasn't responded to other treatment
- Can be used in combination therapy with methotrexate

Risks:
- Infusion reactions
- Upper respiratory infection
- Urinary tract infection
- Fluid retention
- Rash, skin itching
- Nausea
- Diarrhea
- Infection of the nervous system

Precautions:
- Prior to receiving rituximab, you'll be screened for tuberculosis and hepatitis B and C and treated, if necessary.
- This medication can cause side effects for 24 hours after receiving the infusion.
- To minimize its side effects, your healthcare professional may give you a dose of a corticosteroid, acetaminophen or antihistamines.
- Receiving live virus vaccines isn't recommended while you're on this medication.
- This medication may damage the protective coating that surrounds nerve fibers in the brain and spinal cord.
- This drug lowers immunoglobulin levels.
- Your healthcare team will monitor you closely for signs of infection while you're taking this drug. Call

your healthcare professional right away if you have a fever, don't feel well, or experience unexplained weight loss, excessive sweating, coughing or difficulty breathing.
- A small number of people may develop antibodies to this medicine, but this effect is lessened when used with methotrexate.
- Avoid this drug during pregnancy, as it can affect the baby's developing immune system.

TARGETED DMARDS

While conventional DMARDs restrict your immune system broadly, targeted DMARDs block specific pathways inside immune cells. Targeted DMARDs are small molecules that affect cell communication mechanisms, such as kinase and phosphodiesterase pathways.

Kinase inhibitors

Kinase inhibitors are not true biologic medications, as they aren't proteins. Rather, they're small molecules that block the action of the enzyme Janus kinase, which is important in activating the immune system. This category of medica-

Kinase inhibitors

Generic	Brand
baricitinib	Olumiant
tofacitinib	Xeljanz
upadacitinib	Rinvoq

tion is approved for treating moderate to severe rheumatoid arthritis that hasn't responded well to methotrexate. An advantage of these drugs is that they can be taken by mouth.

FDA-approved uses:
- Rheumatoid arthritis
- Psoriatic arthritis
- Ulcerative colitis

How they're usually given:
- By mouth

Benefits:
- Inhibit the activation of Janus kinase (JAK), an enzyme that contributes to inflammation
- Used in adults who have moderate to severe rheumatoid arthritis who haven't responded well to methotrexate

Risks:
- Upper respiratory tract infections
- Headache
- Diarrhea
- Inflammation of the nose and upper throat
- Increased risk of serious infection
- Can increase cholesterol
- Increased risk of GI perforation if you have a history of diverticulitis
- Weight loss
- May increase hair growth
- Increased liver function on tests
- May increase the risk of non-melanoma skin cancer
- May increase the risk of interstitial lung disease

Precautions:
- A kinase inhibitor can be used in combination with methotrexate or other nonbiologic DMARDS, but it shouldn't be used in combination with biologics or strong immunosuppressive drugs, such as azathioprine or cyclosporine.
- Before starting this drug, you'll need to be tested for a latent tuberculosis infection and treated if necessary. Even if you test negative, you should be monitored for active tuberculosis while on this medication.
- While taking this medication, you'll be monitored regularly for changes in your blood cell counts, liver enzymes and blood cholesterol levels.
- This medication may not be appropriate if you have chronic or recurring infection or a history of diverticulosis.
- This drug may increase your risk of a blood clot.
- If you develop kidney disease, you may need to reduce the dose of this medication.
- The risks of using these during pregnancy and breastfeeding are unknown.

Phosphodiesterase 4 (PDE4) inhibitor

The drug apremilast helps to stem inflammatory responses by blocking the enzyme phosphodiesterase 4 (PDE4). It's used to treat psoriatic arthritis when conventional DMARDs haven't been effective. It's easy to take by mouth, and unlike biologics, this drug doesn't weaken

Phosphodiesterase 4 (PDE4) inhibitor

Generic	Brand
apremilast	Otezla

the immune system. If you have psoriatic arthritis and biologics are not an option for you, your healthcare team may suggest this medication.

FDA-approved uses:
• Psoriasis
• Psoriatic arthritis

How it's usually given:
• By mouth

Benefits:
• No effect on liver
• Does not increase infection risk

Risks:
• Depression
• Weight loss
• Diarrhea
• Nausea
• Headache
• Upper respiratory tract infection

Precautions:
• The dosage may need to be decreased if you have or develop kidney disease.
• This drug is not recommended if you're interested in getting pregnant.

11 Surgical treatments

If your joint pain from arthritis doesn't go away with other treatments, your healthcare team may recommend surgery to ease your symptoms. In certain cases, joint surgery can reduce pain and help you reach a more active and fulfilling life.

The primary goals of using surgery to treat arthritis are to relieve chronic pain, to slow or prevent cartilage damage, and to correct the joint's range of motion and stability. A surgical procedure aims to restore as much function to the joint as possible.

Some people choose surgery when they can no longer tolerate the pain and when other nonsurgical therapies they've tried, such as medications, exercise and weight loss, don't seem to help.

Other people need surgery because arthritis interferes with their family life, work or ability to maintain a home.

Deciding to have joint surgery involves careful consideration and planning with your healthcare professional. There are many different surgical procedures, and each offers different benefits and risks.

Before deciding on surgery, it's important to understand the possible outcomes and what each might mean for you. Is the surgery likely to completely resolve the pain? How long can you expect the improvement to last? How will the recovery time affect your routine? It's also important to be aware of any physical limitations that surgery may impose on the joint. For example, if you choose to go with a certain procedure, do you lose some flexibility in that joint? Are some movements restricted?

The outcome of surgery can be different for each person. It depends on several factors, including the strength of the bones, tendons and ligaments supporting your joints, your age, your weight, and your ability to participate in rehabilitation.

COMMON TYPES OF JOINT SURGERY

Different types of surgical procedures are used to treat the joints affected by arthritis and make them more functional. A surgeon will recommend certain procedures in order to address your specific needs. Depending on your age and overall health, your form of arthritis, and your specific joint problems, one or more of the following procedures may be recommended.

Debridement

Surgeons use this procedure to remove loose fragments of bone, cartilage or synovial membrane that cause joint pain, most often in the knees. The surgeon makes a small incision and inserts an arthroscope, a thin fiber-optic tube with a tiny camera. The camera lets the surgeon see inside the joint while other narrow tools cut or grind loose pieces as needed to suction out the fragments. The surgeon may make additional small incisions at different points around the joint to insert these instruments.

Debridement is often helpful to people in the early stages of osteoarthritis. The loose fragments can create the sensation of your knee joint "catching" or "locking up." Removing the loose pieces won't reverse the arthritis, but the procedure may help the joint move more smoothly and with less pain.

Synovectomy

Synovectomy (sin-o-VEK-tuh-me) removes some of the synovial tissue lining an inflamed joint. It is used especially when rheumatoid arthritis is the cause of inflammation. Removing this tissue can reduce pain and swelling and delay cartilage and bone destruction. Although it may provide pain relief, synovectomy is not a cure. Inflammation may recur as the synovium grows back over time.

Synovectomy is routinely performed on knees, fingers, wrists and elbows before significant cartilage erosion or deformity occurs. Some specialists also perform synovectomy on the elbow. Synovectomy can be done arthroscopically or as an open surgery. Arthroscopic surgery typically allows you to recover faster.

Cartilage transplantation

One form of this procedure is also known as autologous cartilage implantation (ACI). A small sample of cells is removed from the cartilage of the joint and cultivated in a lab. Six to eight weeks later, the lab-grown cartilage cells are inserted into a damaged joint as a tissue "scaffold" to help new cartilage grow.

Healthcare professionals use this procedure as a treatment for small areas of damaged cartilage — up to about 0.6 square inches. Transplantation for larger areas of damage has not yet been successful. To help advance this technique, scientists are working to identify substances that will stimulate healthy cartilage growth, called cartilage growth factors.

Osteotomy

During this procedure, a surgeon cuts and repositions bones near a damaged joint to help correct deformities and improve the malalignment causing the arthritis. These adjustments realign the joint and also help slow cartilage damage by distributing body weight more evenly across the joint. Osteotomy (os-tee-OT-uh-me) is most commonly used to correct curvature or bowing in the lower leg bones caused by osteoarthritis around the knee joint. It may be a good option for younger people wanting to avoid a joint replacement, particularly in the knee.

Resection

Surgeons sometimes remove all or part of a damaged bone when diseased joints make movement painful. Called resection — the full term is resection arthroplasty — this procedure may be used in the feet to make walking easier. It's also done to reduce pain in the wrists and hands. It's less commonly used in larger joints such as hips or knees, as it can result in limited mobility and function in these joints.

Joint replacement

When arthritis severely damages a joint, your healthcare team may recommend replacing it with an artificial joint. This joint replacement procedure is called arthroplasty (AHR-throe-plas-tee).

In the procedure, the surgeon removes certain parts of the damaged joint and replaces them with an implant made of high-density plastic, metal alloy or ceramic material. The implant is also called a prosthesis. Most of the major ligaments and tendons are left in place and rebalanced so that the joint straightens and bends well and is stable from side to side and front to back.

The hip and the knee are the most commonly replaced joints, but implants can also replace damaged bone and cartilage in other joints.

In some cases, the surgeon may choose to preserve more of the joint and replace only the most damaged part. In a knee joint, for example, damage may be limited to the inner or outer part of the knee or where the kneecap meets the thigh bone. Replacing only one part of the joint preserves more natural movement of the knee. A partial joint replacement may also allow for a faster recovery.

Joint fusion

Also called arthrodesis (ahr-throe-DEE-sis), joint fusion is used most often to reduce pain and improve stability in the spine, wrist, ankle, and the joints of the fingers and toes. During this procedure, surgeons remove a thin layer of tissue from the ends of two bones and bind them together, often using pins, rods or plates. Fresh bone cells then grow at the

SELECTING A SURGEON

If your decision is to have surgery, your primary care professional or rheumatologist can refer you to an orthopedic surgeon. Orthopedic surgeons perform operations involving joints, muscles and bones. Typically, you want someone with extensive experience in joint procedures.

It's important to have confidence in the orthopedic surgeon you choose. Board-certified surgeons have met extensive requirements for training and experience. Some surgeons have also completed additional training through a fellowship and focus their practice on the treatment of specific joints. An experienced orthopedic surgeon should be able to answer questions about the options available to you, the risks and benefits associated with each, and what to expect during your recovery.

Questions you may ask the surgeon include:
- How often have you performed this kind of surgery in the past?
- Are you board-certified and fellowship-trained?
- What are the short-term and long-term risks associated with this surgery?
- If the surgery involves implants, what type do you recommend?
- What kind of anesthesia will be used, and what are the risks?
- Should I expect a lot of pain, and what measures can I use to relieve it?
- How long is the recovery process, and what is involved?
- What outcome should I expect after this surgery?

Given the potential risks and costs associated with surgery, seeking a second opinion before proceeding may be sensible. You or a member of your healthcare team can initiate the process of getting a second opinion. Don't be afraid to ask about it.

juncture, fusing the two bones. Once healed, the fused joint can bear weight but has no flexibility.

Joint fusion is typically used when total joint replacement isn't possible. This may be the case after an infection or a failed joint replacement with significant bone loss.

Tendon and ligament repair

Surgeons can repair tendon tears to reduce pain, restore function and, in some cases, prevent tendon rupture. For example, you may need surgery if one of the tendons in the rotator cuff in your shoulder partially or fully tears. Other procedures can tighten or loosen tendons and ligaments. These are sometimes recommended to decrease pain, increase joint mobility or prepare a joint for total joint replacement. Surgeons may also perform procedures to relieve pressure on nerves that become pinched or irritated by tight ligaments.

CHOOSING THE RIGHT PROCEDURE

Your joints vary greatly in size, shape, design and function. When you see a surgeon about procedures to treat your joint pain, the surgeon will consider these differences and tailor your treatment accordingly.

This section explores how surgeons select procedures such as the ones described in the previous section to help relieve your arthritis symptoms in specific joints.

ANATOMY OF AN ARTIFICIAL JOINT

When the gradual deterioration of a joint occurs due to arthritis, implanting an artificial joint can help eliminate pain and restore near-normal function. The implants are also called prostheses.

Artificial joints are made of various metals, ceramics or plastic-like materials called polymers. Surgeons choose the implants best suited to your needs from a wide selection of sizes, shapes and constructions. At some medical centers, healthcare professionals may use computers to custom design the implants.

Traditionally, surgeons have secured joint implants to bones with a special cement. This method generally works well, but sometimes the cement eventually cracks, causing the implant to loosen. If loosening occurs, you may need additional procedures to reattach or replace the implant.

Uncemented implants are used more commonly now, especially in hip surgery. These implants have a porous surface that allows the bone to grow into them. This may improve durability. But uncemented implants may also loosen. On rare occasions, the bone fails to attach itself to the implant and the implant becomes fixed with scar tissue.

Over time, wear and tear from artificial joints creates debris. The tiny particles can cause inflammation that destroys the bone or soft tissue in the joint and may ultimately contribute to loosening of the implant. Typically, you'll be asked to schedule regular follow-ups every few years to monitor your joint's condition.

Hands and wrists

The ability to grasp a spoon, turn a doorknob or button a shirt is something you may take for granted until arthritis starts affecting your hands or wrists. It's no secret that arthritis pain can make these movements difficult, if not impossible.

The primary goals of hand or wrist procedures are the same for all joint surgeries — to improve function and reduce pain. Some procedures can also improve the appearance of finger joints deformed by arthritis. But surgery is rarely recommended for cosmetic reasons alone — unless the arthritis is greatly hurting your self-image and social interactions.

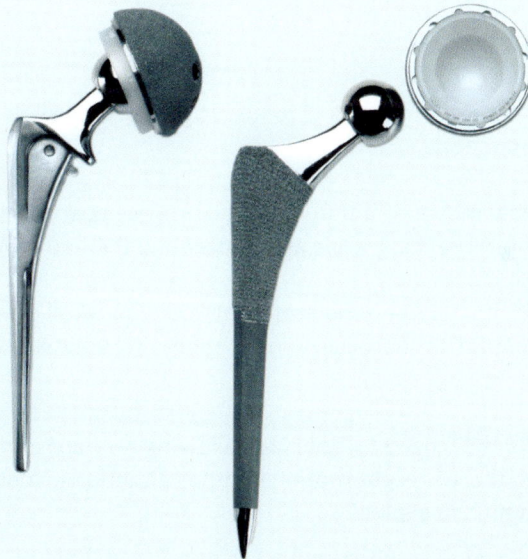

The components of an artificial hip implant are shown above, assembled (left) and apart (right). The implant on the right is cementless, with a surface on the long stem to which bone attaches itself. Typically, younger, active people with good bone quality are better candidates for cementless total hip arthroplasty. A cemented implant is preferred in people who have poor bone stock and in older people with lower activity levels. Regardless of the type of implant, recent studies show that 85% to 90% of total hip replacements are still successful 15 years after surgery.

Tendon and ligament adjustments

Sometimes rheumatoid arthritis causes tears in the tendons of the hand and wrist, and an operation is performed to repair the damage and prevent rupture of these tendons.

Other surgical procedures may be used to help tighten or loosen tendons and ligaments in the hand and wrist to decrease pain and increase your mobility and grip strength.

Synovectomy or resection

Removing inflamed tissue or damaged bone may help reduce pain in the wrists and fingers caused by rheumatoid arthritis.

Joint fusion

If you have severely damaged finger or wrist joints, fusing the joints together may relieve pain and improve stability. But fusing wrist joints also limits how you can move your hand.

YOUR BODY'S JOINTS

Your body has several different types of joints. Together they allow you to perform a variety of essential functions.

Fixed joints don't allow movement between bones. They absorb shock to help prevent the bones from breaking while also protecting the underlying tissue.

For example, fixed joints between the bony plates of your skull protect the sensitive brain tissue underneath. The sacroiliac joints connecting your spine and pelvis are another example.

Hinge joints work like the hinge in a doorway, allowing forward and backward movement, although there is slight motion in other directions. Your elbows, fingers, knees and toes contain hinge joints.

Pivot joints allow a rotating movement. The pivot joint in your neck allows your head to turn from side to side. Your elbow includes both hinge and pivot joints.

In ball-and-socket joints, the large round end of one bone fits snugly into a cup-shaped cavity of another bone. This allows movement in almost every direction, making swinging and rotation movements possible. Your shoulders and hips are ball-and-socket joints.

Joint replacement

Hand and wrist joint replacements are performed less often than hip and knee replacements are. This is partly because the joints are small and require precise repair of ligaments and tendons.

The hand is a complex structure with many moving parts. Other surgical procedures, such as joint fusion and tendon adjustment, can usually have good results, so surgeons often use joint replacement for only the most severely damaged hand and wrist joints. Some surgeons reserve knuckle replacement for older adults who tend to use their hands less, allowing the artificial knuckles to last longer.

If you have joint replacement surgery on a hand or wrist, your hand will be placed in a splint for 2 to 3 weeks while your muscles and other soft tissues heal. After

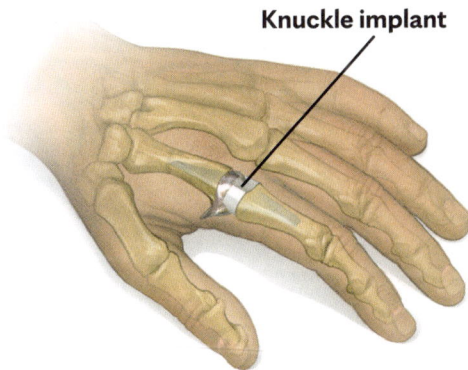

Knuckle implant

An artificial implant is shown in the knuckle of the index finger. The implant can reduce pain and restore motion in the knuckle joint and improve overall function of the hand.

that, you'll have physical therapy to retrain the tissues. Post-surgical therapy is essential in wrist or finger joint replacement because so much soft tissue reconstruction is involved.

Elbows

If medications and daily exercise aren't providing enough relief from arthritis pain in your elbow, you may consider other options. Several surgical procedures can reduce pain and increase the range of motion, including complete surgical replacement of your elbow joint.

Elbow surgery is generally performed in one of two ways. Open surgery refers to working on the joint through an incision in the arm — the more traditional method. Open surgery on the elbow is widely available, and surgeons have been doing it for years.

The other option is arthroscopic surgery, done through small incisions. It has a lower risk of infection and leaves less scarring. But the procedure requires special expertise to move a tiny camera and surgical tools within your elbow. If the joint has deteriorated from arthritis, arthroscopic elbow surgery may not be an option. And because this is a relatively specialized procedure, it may not be available at all medical centers.

The specific surgical procedure that's right for you will depend on several factors, including the type of arthritis you have and the condition of your elbow joint.

Synovectomy or resection

Removing inflamed tissue and, sometimes, damaged bone is usually the first choice of surgery for people in the early stages of rheumatoid arthritis. The procedure can help increase your elbow's range of motion and relieve pain. You and your healthcare team may consider synovectomy if you've tried medication and therapy for six months or more and you're still experiencing severe elbow pain.

The procedure can be open or done arthroscopically. Arthroscopic synovectomy is typically more thorough than the open option, because arthroscopy uses high-powered optics and small surgical

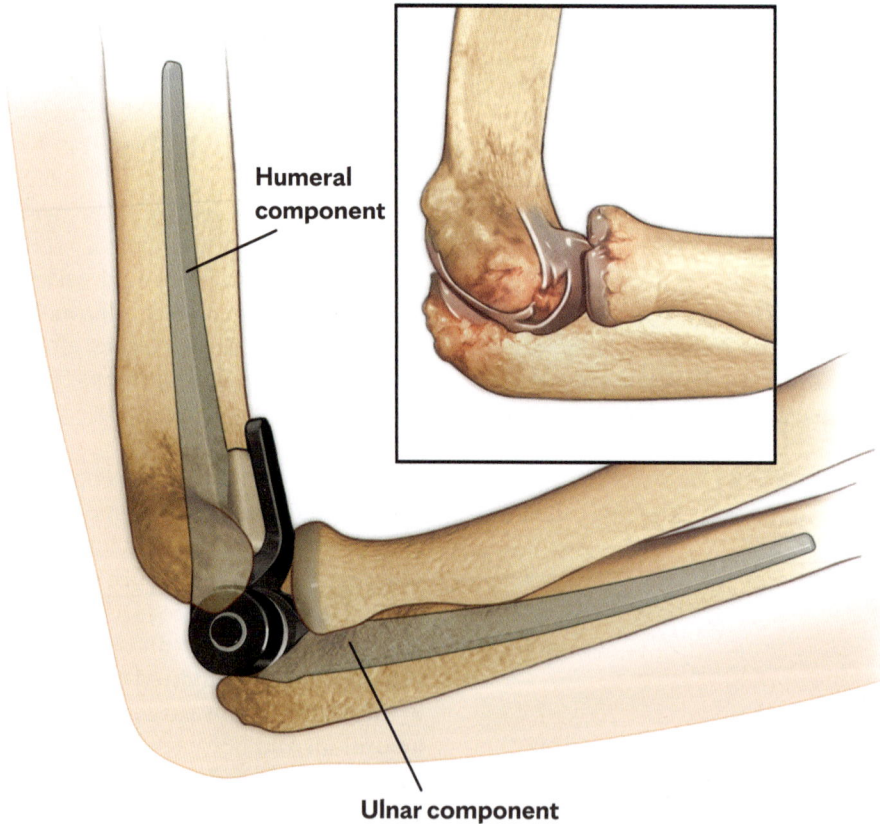

Humeral component

Ulnar component

Total elbow replacement may be recommended if arthritis has severely damaged the cartilage and bone (see inset). The components of the artificial joint are anchored with the help of long stems inserted into the humerus and ulna. Some implants permit movement in only one plane (hinge joint), while others permit rotation of the forearm (hinge and pivot joints), similar to a typical elbow joint.

instruments that allow your surgeon to access more of the joint.

The synovium in your joints eventually grows back, which means that your elbow pain could return. But a synovectomy can delay the need for more invasive surgical treatments, such as elbow replacement. Plus, medications can prevent the synovium from becoming inflamed again.

Debridement

For osteoarthritis, removing loose fragments is usually the first choice of surgery if medications and physical therapy fail to bring pain relief. Debridement can be performed either open or arthroscopically.

A more thorough form of debridement known as osteocapsular arthroplasty involves removing bone spurs, loose bone and cartilage, as well as performing a synovectomy and recontouring bones that have deteriorated due to arthritis. Osteocapsular arthroplasty can be an extremely successful procedure, relieving pain and improving range of motion. However, it's also relatively new and difficult to perform, so it may not be widely available.

Interpositional arthroplasty

In this open-surgery procedure, your surgeon removes bone spurs or loose fragments from the elbow joint. Your surgeon then separates your elbow and stitches a piece of skin tissue or tendon — usually taken from elsewhere in your body or from a donor — in place between the bones that make up the elbow joint. This tissue resurfaces the joint, keeping your bones from rubbing together to reduce pain.

This procedure is typically offered to younger or very active adults with severe arthritis of the elbow as a way to increase functionality and delay total joint replacement. Having total joint replacement carries limitations on activities and the amount of weight you can lift, which can be a difficult lifestyle change for some active people. However, neither surgery is a good fix for heavy laborers.

While interpositional arthroplasty may be the best choice for some people, pain relief and range of motion after the surgery can be unpredictable. Joint instability also is a significant risk. In addition, there's still a chance you may need to have replacement surgery later.

Joint replacement

If your arthritis causes severe elbow pain that doesn't respond to medication and limits your daily activities, you might be considered for total elbow replacement, also known as total elbow arthroplasty.

Replacing the entire joint is usually reserved for people with advanced arthritis that hasn't responded to nonsurgical treatments and less aggressive surgical options. It's generally done in adults ages 60 and older and isn't recommended for younger people unless other types of surgery have failed.

Replacing the diseased bone and tissue with an artificial joint can relieve pain and restore range of motion. During the procedure, your surgeon makes an incision in the back of the elbow and moves muscles and nerves out of the way. Then the surgeon removes diseased parts of the bones, reshapes the remaining bones and places the prosthetic joint in place. Elbow implants are typically secured partly with cement and partly with bone regrowth into certain uncemented parts of the implant.

As with any surgery, elbow replacement carries the risk of infection and bleeding. Also, mechanical problems with the new elbow joint, such as loosening or breakage, are more likely to occur than in other joints because of the tremendous stress that the elbow typically undergoes with use. Damage to the nerves in your elbow also is possible as a result of the operation.

While elbow replacement can increase range of motion and reduce pain, you'll have limitations on the new joint. After surgery, you shouldn't lift more than 1 or 2 pounds regularly, and lifting up to 10 pounds should only be done occasionally. Heavier lifting could damage the new joint or the bones holding it in place. These restrictions remain for the life of your new joint.

Shoulders

Doctors typically recommend daily exercise and medications as the first treatments for arthritis of the shoulder.

However, if you've tried these options and you still have pain and limited motion, it may be time to consider surgery. Joint replacement is the most common surgical procedure for shoulder arthritis, but you and your healthcare team may consider other procedures.

Synovectomy

If you have rheumatoid arthritis and the bones in your shoulder joint aren't damaged, a synovectomy might be all that's needed to restore motion and reduce pain. A synovectomy can be done as either open or arthroscopic surgery.

While it's true that the synovium can grow back and become inflamed again, medications can usually prevent that from happening. Most people with rheumatoid arthritis of the shoulder who have this procedure will have pain-free motion in the joint.

Joint fusion

When bone or cartilage damage in your shoulder is extensive, a more aggressive form of surgery may be needed. Joint fusion can reduce pain and offer long-term stability. But because the fusion immobilizes your joint, the procedure significantly reduces your ability to use the shoulder.

Joint fusion is less common today than it once was. You may be a candidate for this procedure if damage from arthritis makes it impossible for the muscles and tendons in your shoulder to hold an artificial joint securely in place, or if you've lost cartilage due to an infection of the shoulder joint.

Debridement

Osteocapsular arthroplasty is another surgical option for shoulder arthritis. During this arthroscopic procedure, your surgeon removes bone spurs and reshapes and smooths the joint surfaces of the shoulder. This makes it easier for the bones in your shoulder to move without friction and pain.

Joint replacement

Total shoulder replacement, also called arthroplasty, is the most common type of shoulder surgery for arthritis. It can increase the range of motion in your shoulder, making it easier to move your arm. It also improves strength and reduces pain in your shoulder.

During total shoulder replacement, your surgeon removes damaged parts of the bones that make up your shoulder joint, including the ball-shaped top of your humerus, or upper arm bone, and the

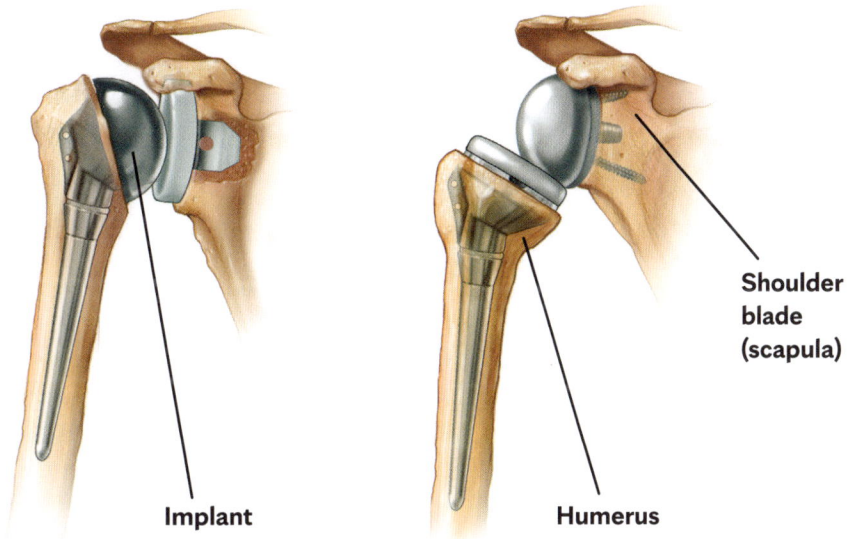

In total shoulder replacement (left), the ball component of the artificial joint is anchored to the humerus with the help of a long stem that's inserted into the bone, while the socket component is fixed to the shoulder blade. The implant replicates the structure and function of your natural shoulder joint. In reverse shoulder replacement (right), the implant design is reversed. The ball component is fixed to the shoulder blade, and the socket component is attached to the humerus.

glenoid cavity, or socket, of your shoulder blade. They're replaced with an artificial joint consisting of a metal ball and plastic socket. Your surgeon might also clean up the area around the joint by removing bone spurs and inflamed synovium.

Shoulder replacement can be associated with a longer rehabilitation period than other types of joint replacement. Learning to use your new joint and recovering its strength may take months, while regaining full function can take up to a year.

You'll need to diligently follow a prescribed set of exercises beginning the first day after surgery. Not sticking to the exercise regimen can lead to stiffness or instability in your new shoulder joint.

Shoulder replacement surgery is fairly safe and predictable, and most people are satisfied with their new shoulder joints. Like any surgery, though, it carries the risk of infection and bleeding, and complications can arise. A small number of artificial joints will eventually need to be replaced. The implant can loosen, requiring refitting. Sometimes the shoulder becomes weak and unstable, which may require another surgery.

Hemiarthroplasty

If the ball-shaped top of your humerus is damaged but the socket of your shoulder blade is still in good shape, your surgeon may recommend a version of joint replacement called hemiarthroplasty.

In this procedure, only the ball is replaced. The socket remains, although your surgeon may smooth it out. This procedure may also be considered if you have a tear in the muscles and tendons that support your shoulder, known as the rotator cuff, in addition to arthritis. A rotator cuff tear may make it difficult for your shoulder muscles to firmly hold a prosthetic socket in place, which would lead to early loosening of the artificial joint.

If you're younger and want to use your shoulder more vigorously than is possible with total joint replacement, your surgeon may recommend resurfacing hemiarthroplasty, which affixes a synthetic surface cap to the ball part of the joint. This procedure provides pain relief — although perhaps with less predictable results than with a total replacement — and avoids years of wear and tear on an artificial joint. The possibility of a total shoulder replacement remains open for a later time.

Reverse shoulder arthroplasty

As its name implies, a reverse shoulder arthroplasty swaps the ball and socket parts of the typical shoulder implant. A reverse prosthesis is placed so that the ball portion is attached to the shoulder blade and the socket portion is attached to the upper arm bone.

This procedure is most appropriate for people who have shoulder arthritis along with extensive tears of muscles and tendons in their rotator cuff, severely limiting motion. It may also be the best choice if you have a failed previous shoulder joint replacement and a weak rotator cuff. The reverse technique compensates for a lack of strength and support from the rotator cuff. It allows the deltoid, another muscle of the shoulder, to take over your shoulder's pulling function. This allows you to lift your arm again with relative ease.

Reverse shoulder arthroplasty is a newer procedure than traditional shoulder replacement. But for people who aren't otherwise good candidates for total shoulder arthroplasty, it has shown very promising results.

Hips

The daily demands on your hips are impressive: bearing your weight, walking, climbing stairs, bending and twisting. It's no wonder the hips are commonly affected by arthritis. When weight loss, medications, reduced activity and use of a cane fail to provide relief, your healthcare team may recommend hip surgery.

Osteotomy

This surgery, used to adjust and realign the bones of your hip joint, is occasionally used to help reduce hip pain, particularly in younger people without severe arthritis.

During this procedure, the surgeon makes a cut in the bone just below the joint to move healthier cartilage to the area that bears the most weight. This changes the joint alignment and helps distribute your body weight more evenly. For some people, it brings pain relief and improved function of the hip joint. In the best-case scenario, osteotomy may delay the need for total hip replacement for 10 years or even longer.

Joint fusion

Although less common today, fusing the bones of an arthritic hip joint is another surgical option. Fusion of the hip joint is generally reserved for people who aren't good candidates for hip replacement, including younger people. During this procedure, your surgeon joins the round upper end of your thigh bone, called the femur, and the socket in your pelvic bone, the acetabulum, eliminating all motion. This surgery changes the mechanics of how you walk, but it can provide good relief from joint pain for many years.

Joint replacement

Hip replacement surgery, also called total hip arthroplasty, is by far the most successful surgical procedure for treating advanced arthritis of the hip. It's also one of the most common joint replacement surgeries, with more than 370,000 done annually in the United States.

The implants for an artificial hip joint come in many shapes, styles and materials. Your surgeon will decide which joint is best suited for you. The implants, which mimic the natural design of your hip, fit together and function like a normal joint. They are biocompatible — meaning they're designed to be accepted by your body — and made to resist corrosion, degradation and wear.

Some artificial hip joints are held in place with bone cement. More commonly, the new joint is uncemented and held in place by new bone growth into a section of the prosthesis over time. No hard and fast rules dictate whether cemented or uncemented fixation should be used — it typically depends on the quality of the bone around the implant.

In general, uncemented fixation is used for people who have good bone quality. In certain cases, you may need to wait a few weeks for new bone growth to form before applying your full weight to the new joint. Cemented fixation is used for people with weakened health or weaker bones, such as from osteoporosis. A cemented joint can usually withstand your full weight immediately after surgery. For older adults, the surgeon may use a hybrid form of joint fixation, in which the socket is placed uncemented while the stem is cemented.

During the procedure, your thigh bone is separated from the socket on your pelvis. Working between the large hip muscles, your surgeon removes damaged bone and tissue and leaves the healthy bone intact. Next, an artificial socket is pressed into place on the pelvis. The top end of the thigh bone is

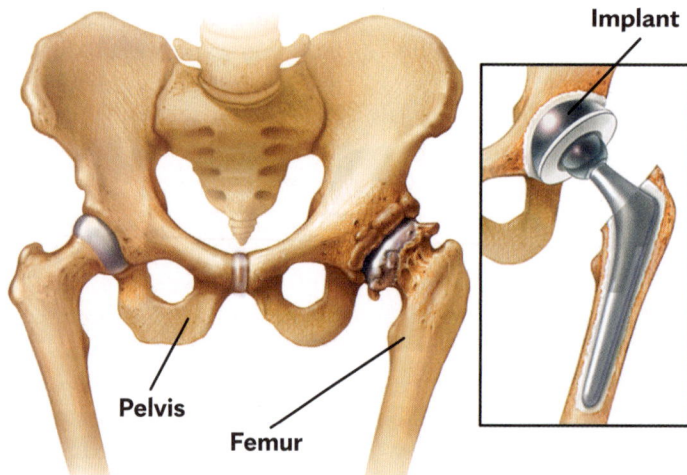

In this image, severe osteoarthritis has destroyed cartilage and bone in the left hip. In total hip replacement, the surgeon replaces the ball of the thigh bone, or femur, with an implant consisting of a metal ball attached to a metal stem that is inserted into the femur (see inset). A socket implant is also attached to your pelvic bone. The components may be cemented or uncemented, often depending on your bone quality.

hollowed out so that the stem of the ball implant can be inserted. The ball and the socket join to form a new hip joint. Before closing the incision, your surgeon checks the alignment and stability of the new joint.

Hip replacement surgery is successful more than 90% of the time. It usually allows pain-free movement for many years after the procedure. Still, don't expect to do things that you couldn't do before surgery. High-impact activities, such as running and playing basketball, may not be possible after a hip replacement. But with time, you may be able to swim, play golf, walk or ride a bike comfortably.

Hip replacement surgery is generally safe, but complications — sometimes serious ones — may occur. Most can be treated successfully. Rare complications may include blood clots, dislocation, infection, fracture, loosening or breakage of the prosthesis, change in leg length, or joint stiffening.

Hip replacement used to be an option primarily for older adults because implants would wear out. But improved technology has produced longer-lasting artificial joints available for more active people, including young adults. However, active people face the possibility of more surgery to replace worn-out artificial joints if they don't reduce their activity after a hip replacement.

Repeat surgery, also called revision surgery, is more difficult and often isn't as successful as the original procedure.

A newer surgical approach to hip replacement is minimally invasive, avoiding the need to detach or cut through muscles to reach the joint. This surgery is similar to traditional hip replacement but is performed with specially designed instruments inserted through a relatively small incision. It can still have the same complications, such as dislocated hips, bone fractures, and nerve and blood vessel injuries.

Because this technique is newer, the number of studies comparing outcomes with those of traditional hip replacement is limited. Some studies have shown that people undergoing minimally invasive hip replacement may have a faster, easier recovery. Other research has shown no difference in long-term outcomes compared to the more traditional approaches. However, longer follow-up is still needed to evaluate these less invasive techniques.

Resurfacing

In younger, more active people, some surgeons opt for a form of hip replacement that retains most of the ball of the hip joint, trimming only damaged portions and capping the ball with a smooth metal surface. The damaged socket on the pelvis is removed, just as with traditional hip replacement, and replaced with an artificial one.

An advantage of resurfacing is that the entire femoral head can be replaced at a later time, if necessary. This may be easier than correcting a total hip replacement if dislocation or implant failure occurs.

One risk of hip resurfacing is that the femoral neck — the narrow area just below the ball of the hip joint — might eventually fracture, requiring a full joint replacement. Hip resurfacing has fallen out of favor due to concerns over the metal debris generated from the metal-on-metal components used for resurfacing.

Knees

Surgery offers various options to relieve pain and restore mobility to an arthritic knee.

Debridement

This minimally invasive procedure is frequently used to remove cartilage tears or loose tissue fragments from around the knee joint. This may be a good option if you're young or middle-aged and the arthritis is a result of sports injuries. It's less effective for people with severe or long-term knee arthritis.

Synovectomy

If the cartilage isn't significantly damaged, removing inflamed tissue from around the knee joint can decrease pain and swelling in people with rheumatoid arthritis. It doesn't appear to slow the progress of arthritis. But in younger people, synovectomy may delay the need for total joint replacement.

Because the knee is a relatively large joint, surgeons typically perform the procedure with arthroscopy, which allows the surgeon to view inside the joint and remove diseased tissue with small instruments. An arthroscopic procedure requires a much smaller incision than a conventional operation does, so recovery is usually quicker.

Osteotomy

Healthcare professionals sometimes recommend surgery to realign the bone — a procedure called osteotomy. This is done to slow cartilage damage in the knee and relieve pain.

The act of trimming and repositioning the leg bones allows your body weight to be more evenly distributed across the knee joint, taking pressure off the arthritic area and moving it to intact cartilage. The process also corrects curvature or bowing in the lower leg bones caused by osteoarthritis. Surgeons typically recommend this procedure for younger, more active people with damage mostly on one side of the knee.

Joint fusion

Permanently fusing the parts of the knee together is an option for people who aren't candidates for knee replacement surgery — perhaps because of age, activity level, or weight or if an artificial knee becomes infected and can't be saved. Although fusion limits knee motion, it allows your leg to bear weight without pain.

EASING THE PAIN AFTER SURGERY

After joint replacement surgery, you may receive an anesthetic to numb the nerves surrounding the painful joint, in what is known as a peripheral nerve block. You'll get the medication through a catheter that's set up on the day of surgery and can remain in place for the first couple of days after surgery. It typically provides good pain relief. Some increase in pain is normal as the effect of the nerve block gradually wears off.

Another option is to inject a combination of pain-relieving medications into the joint and surrounding tissues at the time of surgery. Both techniques reduce or eliminate the side effects from opioid pain medications normally used in such cases. They have also reduced the recovery time after surgery.

When the nerve block is stopped, you'll be given oral pain medication. The medication helps ease discomfort but may not completely relieve the pain. Taking the medication before pain becomes significant is usually the most helpful, so tell your care team sooner rather than later if pain increases.

Express the level of pain you feel on a scale of 0 to 10, with 0 equal to no pain and 10 equal to the worst pain imaginable. Also tell your care team if you have any other discomfort or suspect that the pain medication is causing nausea or other symptoms. Cold packs can help reduce swelling and discomfort around the surgical incision.

Joint replacement

Knee replacement surgery, also called total knee arthroplasty, can help relieve pain and restore function in severely diseased knee joints. More than 600,000 knee replacement surgeries are performed in the United States each year. A wide variety of implant designs are available, depending on your age, size, activity level and overall health.

Most replacement procedures attempt to replicate your knee's natural ability to roll and glide as it bends. Although most people who undergo knee replacement are between the ages of 50 and 80, surgeons occasionally replace the knees of people who are younger. The active lifestyles of younger people may cause greater wear on an artificial knee, requiring the joint to be replaced again in the future.

During the surgery, your surgeon cuts away damaged bone and cartilage from the lower thigh bone, called the femur; the upper portion of the lower leg bone, the tibia; and the kneecap. Your knee is kept in a bent position so that all surfaces of the joint are fully exposed.

After making an incision, the muscles, kneecap and connective tissues are moved aside, and the damaged bone and cartilage are cut away. The ligaments are realigned to hold the joint together after the prosthesis is in place. Leg bones also may be realigned.

Your surgeon smooths the bones' rough edges and carefully measures the cut to ensure a good fit for your new prosthesis. The artificial joint is then put in place. Most implants are affixed with bone cement. Others are held in place by new

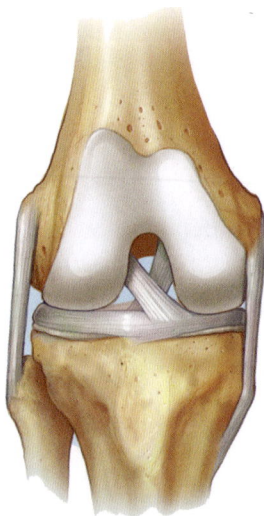

Total knee arthroplasty

Knee joint

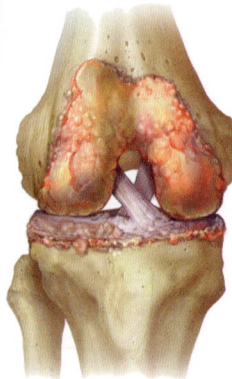

Knee with osteoarthritis

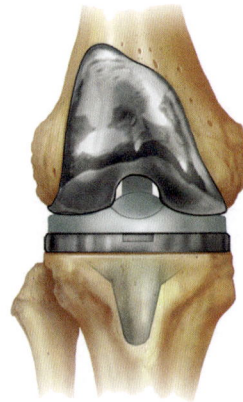

In total knee replacement, diseased bone and cartilage are removed from the end of the femur and a U-shaped component is attached. A T-shaped component is attached to the tibia, firmly anchored in the bone. The top of the T provides a resting place for the femoral component. A plastic spacer inserted between the two components functions as artificial cartilage by creating a smooth gliding surface. Some joints include another small component, a circular piece of plastic that attaches to your kneecap to replace damaged cartilage.

bone growth. Before closing the incision, the surgeon will bend and rotate the new joint, testing and balancing it to ensure proper function.

You probably won't forget that you have an artificial knee — your range of motion with a knee implant may never completely return to normal, or you might hear clicking sounds when you walk. Still, about 90% of people who have total knee replacement experience significant pain relief, improved mobility and better overall quality of life.

During the first weeks after surgery, physical activity will typically include a graduated walking program — first indoors, then outdoors — and knee-strengthening exercises that you learn from a physical therapist. You may also be advised to slowly resume other normal household activities, including walking up and down stairs.

Three to six weeks after surgery — depending on your doctor's assessment — you can typically resume most normal daily activities, such as shopping and light housekeeping. You can usually start driving in four to six weeks if you can bend your knee far enough to sit in a car and you have enough muscle control to properly operate the brakes and accelerator. As early as six weeks after surgery, you may start to notice the improvement in your knee, compared with how it felt before the joint replacement.

Being active after joint replacement is important for keeping your new artifi-

cial joint working smoothly. After recovery, you can enjoy low-impact activities such as walking, moderate hiking, swimming, golf and recreational biking. Some surgeons recommend avoiding high-impact activities such as running or jogging, contact or jumping sports, high-impact aerobics, skiing, and tennis. Also avoid repetitive lifting of objects over 50 pounds. The stress these activities place on the knee may increase the risk of early artificial joint failure.

Partial knee replacement

The knee joint includes three parts: the inside, or medial, compartment; the outside, or lateral, compartment; and the patellofemoral compartment, where the kneecap meets the femur.

If arthritis has affected only one part of your knee, your doctor may suggest an implant to replace just the damaged part. This is known as a unicompartmental knee arthroplasty. This procedure is less extensive than total replacement and usually allows for faster recovery. A partial replacement may also feel and move more like your natural knee.

To determine whether you're a candidate for the partial procedure, your surgeon must be certain that other parts of the joint are undamaged. Usually this can be determined by X-rays or MRI scans, but in some cases your surgeon may not make the decision until the time of surgery.

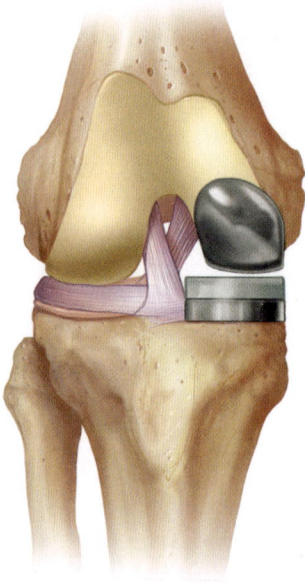

A partial knee replacement may be a good option for you if arthritis has affected only part of your knee joint. This surgery preserves the joint's healthy bone and tissues. Here, only the inside, or medial, compartment of the knee joint has been removed and replaced.

Minimally invasive surgery

In recent years, some surgeons have offered a procedure using a smaller incision. This may reduce trauma to muscles and tendons and result in a faster recovery and less scarring. Some early research has suggested that overall limb alignment may suffer when knee surgery is performed through smaller incisions, leading to complications. More research is still needed to know whether the procedure is as safe and effective as the conventional procedure in the long term.

WHAT ABOUT ARTHRITIS INVOLVING MULTIPLE JOINTS?

If you need more than one surgery to treat arthritis pain, you and your healthcare team can discuss which procedure should be performed first.

Surgery on the hips, knees, ankles and feet is usually done before surgery on the upper body joints. That's because using crutches after surgery on the lower extremities puts a lot of stress on the upper body.

When multiple lower body surgeries are required, hip surgery is typically performed before knee surgery to get the best possible knee alignment and pain relief. Ankle and foot surgeries are usually done before hip or knee replacement to provide stability for hip or knee rehabilitation.

When more than one surgery is needed on upper body joints, the order is controversial. Often, the more symptomatic joint is done first, but it's best to discuss the options with your surgeon.

Ankles and feet

The joints in your ankles and feet, like those in your hips and knees, help carry the weight of your body. Various procedures are used to relieve pain and stabilize these joints. Bone resection in the feet — for example, the removal of bunions, bone spurs or other bony growths — can make walking and standing less painful.

Debridement or osteotomy

The removal of cartilage and bone spurs, known as debridement, or the surgical realignment of the bone, known as osteotomy, can provide temporary relief from pain. These procedures may delay the need for more extensive surgery, perhaps for several years. They are most often performed arthroscopically. However, they can also be done as open surgery.

Synovectomy

For people with rheumatoid arthritis in the front of the foot, removing the inflamed synovial tissue in early stages of the disease may provide pain relief before the cartilage becomes badly eroded. After the procedure, your healthcare professional will likely recommend taking certain drugs to help control disease activity and reduce inflammation in your foot. (For more on medications, see Chapter 10.)

Joint fusion

If your symptoms are severe, the surgeon may recommend fusing the bones in your foot or ankle to improve stability and reduce pain, particularly if the condition has changed the shape of the joint, in what is called a caused deformity. Joint fusion is a standard treatment for arthritis of the ankle, although it can lead to changes in your gait. It may also eventually cause arthritic changes in other joints of your foot. The procedure may be a good option if you're younger and you want to resume more strenuous activities.

Joint replacement

Ankle joint and foot joint replacements are newer and evolving procedures that aren't widely used, partly because they lack a strong record of success. Early ankle implants often had complications, such as loosening, infection and persistent pain after the procedure.

Newer implant designs have reduced some of the problems and can provide good pain relief. And because implants allow the joint to move, unlike in a joint fusion, they don't risk causing arthritis in other parts of the foot. But more research is still needed to know how these newer ankle replacements perform over time and who the best candidates are. If an artificial joint fails, it may be difficult to find a different treatment that can be successful.

THINGS TO KNOW BEFORE SURGERY

Once your surgery is planned, you and your surgeon will determine when you can be admitted to the hospital. It's also good to arrange meals and other assistance ahead of time to help you cope with changes in your activity level during recovery. (See "Plan ahead for recovery" on pages 176-177.)

Before surgery, your healthcare team will want to know your medical history and do a physical exam. People with arthritis need special considerations before surgery because of certain risks related to the disease:

Cardiovascular risk

People with arthritis have a greater risk of heart disease. A preoperative cardiac stress test may be recommended to check whether you're at risk of a heart attack or another heart problem during or after surgery.

Anesthesia concerns

Your surgeon will discuss the risks of anesthesia with you before surgery. Arthritis in the neck or jaw, known as the cervical spine and temporomandibular joint, respectively, may increase the risk of problems with your airway while under anesthesia. If you have subluxation — severe shifting — of the cervical spine, the risk of spinal cord injury is higher. In addition, having limited range of motion in your joints may make positioning your body for surgery difficult. X-rays may be needed before the surgery to assess these concerns.

Infection risk

While taking your medical history and doing a physical exam, your healthcare team will assess your risk of infection. You may be checked for dental cavities; open, crater-like wounds especially around the feet, known as skin ulcerations; and signs or symptoms of a urinary tract infection. Your nutrition level also may be assessed since you're more likely to develop an infection if you're malnourished. As prevention, your care team may prescribe preoperative antibiotics.

Disease activity and medication use

Before you have elective surgery, your rheumatologist should evaluate your level of disease activity and identify major organ involvement that may impact the surgery. Ideally, you should have surgery during periods when the disease is well controlled and you have a successful medication regimen. Your healthcare team will review your medications with you and explain any changes that may need to occur before, during and after surgery. They will assess the risks and benefits of changing any drug or dosage in your specific situation.

- **Steroids.** Some corticosteroids may increase the risk of surgical site infection, skin tearing, fracture, gastrointestinal hemorrhage or ulcer. Most physicians will taper the steroid dose to the lowest dose possible prior to surgery to reduce these risks. One study found that among people who had hip or knee replacements, those taking more than 15 milligrams of prednisone daily had a 20-fold increase in the risk of postoperative infection.

- *Nonsteroidal anti-inflammatory drugs (NSAIDs).* These medications are typically stopped about a week before surgery to minimize the risk of bleeding. Acetaminophen (Tylenol, others) can usually be substituted for pain control, if necessary.
- *Disease-modifying antirheumatic drugs (DMARDs).* In the past, DMARDs such as methotrexate were often stopped before surgery to minimize the risk of infection. But newer research suggests that in most cases, you can safely continue taking these medications leading up to joint surgery. If you have a high risk of infection — say, due to uncontrolled diabetes or lung or liver disease — or a weakened immune system, your healthcare team may recommend skipping a few doses of the DMARD before and after surgery. Some professionals still recommend stopping medications such as leflunomide, sulfasalazine and azathioprine for a brief time before surgery.
- *Biologics.* These medications are still not as well studied regarding the safety of taking them near the time of surgery. Because of this, you may need to stop taking them at least one cycle before the procedure to minimize the risk of infection. Your surgeon may want to balance the risk of infection or wound complication against the risk of a disease flare-up if you stop taking your medications. If you do discontinue a medication, you can usually start it again one or two weeks after surgery.

Potential risks and complications

Joint surgeries can greatly improve your quality of life. Still, every surgery carries a risk of complications. Your medical team will monitor you closely during and after surgery to reduce the chance of infection, a blood clot in the lung, blood loss or a heart attack. Other rare complications may include injury of a nerve or blood vessel, a joint dislocation, bone loss, and even death.

Infection

The location of an artificial joint implant is susceptible to infection, even in the long term. Bacteria can travel through your bloodstream and infect the site years after the procedure. Let your healthcare team know immediately if you notice warning signs such as a fever over 100 F, shaking, chills, incision drainage, and increasing redness, tenderness, swelling and pain around the artificial joint.

If you take a course of antibiotics and they fail to clear up the infection, you will likely need surgery to either clean the artificial joint or remove the infected joint and replace it with a new joint.

To reduce the risk of implant infection, your healthcare professional may recommend antibiotics each time you have certain dental procedures, such as tooth extraction or periodontal work, as well as urological procedures and bowel surgery. Bacteria may also enter your bloodstream through cuts, scrapes and skin ulcers.

PLAN AHEAD FOR RECOVERY

Expect your recovery from surgery to take some time. It may be several months before you can resume all your normal activities. To make things easier on yourself, plan for your return home after surgery before you go to the hospital:

- Talk with your surgeon about how long you can expect to stay in the hospital after surgery. Some people now go home the same day after total hip or knee replacement surgery. Most people stay one or two nights, while some may need to stay longer. Certain other surgeries are outpatient procedures, meaning that most people can plan to go home the same day.
- The best option after you've been discharged is to go directly home. Another option is to go to a loved one's home. Ask someone to accompany you as you leave the hospital, as you may not be able to drive right away.
- Ask someone — a family member, friend or neighbor — to assist you for the first week or two at home. Or you may arrange for a temporary caregiver from a home health-care agency or a short stay at a step-down care facility during this time. You shouldn't be alone for more than three or four hours at a time during this period.
- Your caregiver must be able to help you with activities around the house, such as getting dressed, using the bathroom, preparing meals and doing laundry.
- Leave your home clean and tidy before you go to surgery so that you won't need to clean much during your recovery.
- Move throw rugs, cords and other tripping hazards and clutter out of walkways.
- If possible, rearrange your bedroom with extra space around the bed to allow room to get in and out while using a walker or crutches. If your bedroom is up or down a flight

Blood clots

Dangerous blood clots may form in a vein of the leg (deep vein thrombosis) or lung (pulmonary embolus) after surgery. Blood thinners are commonly prescribed, especially after hip and knee replacement, to help reduce the risk of developing a clot. During your hospital stay, you'll be encouraged to move your foot and ankle, which increases blood flow to your leg muscles and helps prevent swelling and blood clots. You may also need to wear support hose or compression boots to further protect against swelling and clotting.

Blood loss

Joint surgeries may require a blood transfusion. The vast majority of people who receive transfusions have no adverse reactions. The use of a person's own blood (autologous transfusion), while popular in the past, is now rare.

of stairs, you may need to have your bed temporarily moved to a room on the main level of your home.

- Be sure to get instructions on how best to lie down and sit up in bed (see the illustration on page 299).
- Consider installing safety bars or a secure handrail in your shower or bath and arrange for a toilet-seat riser with arms if you have a low toilet. Try using a stable bench or chair in your shower.
- Make sure the handrails along your stairways are secure.
- Rearrange your kitchen so that you can easily reach utensils, tableware and food without bending, stretching or lifting.
- Stock up on food supplies. Prepare some meals in advance and freeze them for use after you return home.
- Set up one location as a "recovery center" where you'll spend most of your time. Make sure to have a sturdy armchair with a firm seat cushion and back — not a recliner. Gather the things you might want to have within easy reach: remote controls, telephone or cell phone, laptop computer or tablet, chargers, books, music player, tissues, medicine, and a pitcher of water.
- Ask your mail carrier to deliver to your door, if possible.
- If you wish, request a visit from your clergyperson or spiritual adviser while you recover.
- Consider placing a clean plastic trash bag on the car seat to make it easier to turn and adjust your body once you're seated in the vehicle.
- If you're interested in getting assistance from a home healthcare agency or public health nurse while you recover from surgery, arrange it beforehand. Your healthcare team may be able to help you with referrals and arrangements.

Analysis of people who used their own blood versus donated blood shows no difference in terms of side effects or reactions.

Certain methods now commonly used can lower the likelihood that you'll need a blood transfusion. These include medications given during surgery and blood collection devices used during the procedure that quickly infuse lost blood back into your body. The method used will depend on the results of blood tests taken before your surgery and the anticipated blood loss.

Loosening of artificial joints

Implants may loosen, dislocate or wear out. However, improved designs and surgical techniques have helped replacement joints last longer. On rare occasions, certain movements or an injury can dislocate an implanted artificial hip joint.

Hospital stay

The length of your hospital stay after surgery will depend on many factors, including the type of joint operation you've had, your age and your overall health. It also depends on whether you experience any complications after surgery.

After the procedure, the surgical care team will monitor your vital signs, alertness, and pain or comfort level and adjust your medications accordingly. Your surgeon may prescribe an antibiotic to prevent infection and a blood thinner medication called an anticoagulant to reduce the risk of blood clots.

Procedures that use only small incisions and local anesthesia, such as arthroscopic debridement or synovectomy, frequently do not require an overnight stay in the hospital. Joint replacement surgery is also increasingly being done on an outpatient basis in younger healthy patients.

Physical therapy begins almost immediately after most joint procedures. Even though you might need assistance at first, you can expect to be up and out of your hospital bed several times daily. A physical therapist will help you practice the best ways to dress, sit down in a chair, get out of bed, use the toilet and climb stairs. Remarkably, most people leave the hospital within two to three days after total joint replacement — if not sooner.

Rehabilitation

Exercise and rest are both important elements of recovery from joint surgery. It's absolutely essential that you follow the activity guidelines that your surgeon or physical therapist prescribes.

If you don't do the exercises, you can end up with a stiff, painful joint. But appropriate rest also is important. If you have rheumatoid arthritis in other joints, putting extra stress on them during the recovery period, while you're protecting the operated joint, may cause a flare-up.

Physical therapists can help you learn the proper way to move and protect a new or altered joint. Exercise can improve joint motion, strengthen the muscles around your joint, reduce pain and improve mobility. You may need to learn how to use assistive devices such as a walker, cane or crutches for support while the surgical site heals.

Occupational therapists can help you become more independent in daily activities. They may work with you on getting dressed, preparing food and bathing. They can also help you learn to use assistive devices such as dressing aids, grab bars, raised toilet seats and bath benches. The goal of rehabilitation is for you to become as independent as possible in your daily living.

Depending on your age, physical condition and home situation, your surgeon may recommend a short stay in a skilled nursing facility or rehabilitation center to

DISEASE-SPECIFIC ISSUES

Some forms of arthritis involve greater risk of certain complications during or after surgery. These include:

- *Sjögren's syndrome.* This condition causes dry eyes and mouth. During surgery, your care team may use lubricating gel and artificial tears to keep your corneas from becoming dry and scratched.
- *Rheumatoid arthritis.* People with rheumatoid arthritis have an increased risk of problems of the neck, known as the cervical spine, or jaw. Special cervical spine X-rays may be necessary before surgery, and your anesthesiologist may need to use a flexible tube for intubation. In addition, people with rheumatoid arthritis may have low white blood cell counts and have an increased risk of infection, especially if they are taking arthritis medication that weakens the immune system.
- *Juvenile idiopathic arthritis (JIA).* Children with JIA may have disturbances in bone growth after surgery. Joint replacement is usually delayed until their bones are done growing. Intubation — for help with breathing during surgery — may be difficult for children with disease activity in the cervical spine and jaw.
- *Ankylosing spondylitis.* People with this form of arthritis have an increased risk of heart disease and problems with the aortic valve. They also are at risk of lung disease, and changes in their upper back can affect breathing motion. Positioning and intubation for surgery also may be difficult. After surgery, the disease may cause extra bone to form at the surgical site. This can cause pain and limit motion.
- *Psoriatic arthritis.* The risk of a skin flare may be higher at the time of surgery, due to the stopping of medication and the stress of the procedure.
- *Connective tissue diseases.* Diseases of this type, which include lupus and scleroderma, may affect multiple organs and can increase the risk of infection, blood clots and anemia, as well as heart, kidney and lung disease.

allow you to focus fully on recovery before returning home.

Recovery at home

To recover more quickly, you'll likely need to continue doing the recommended exercises at home. Your surgeon and physical therapist can help you determine when you'll be able to resume your favorite activities. They can also identify positions or movements to avoid that may damage your joint.

If your surgery involved any joint below your waist — the weight-bearing joints — you'll probably need to use a walker, cane or crutches for a time after returning home. If you have difficulty getting around, your healthcare team may recommend in-home visits by a physical or occupational therapist.

Joint infection may still be a risk after you leave the hospital. Make sure to contact your healthcare professional if you develop a fever, if your incision opens or if you notice an increase of pain, tenderness, swelling, redness, warmth or fluid draining near the surgical site. Also watch for signs of circulation problems, such as increased swelling, pain or tenderness in your limbs.

During the first few weeks at home after getting a new weight-bearing joint, you'll typically have a graduated walking program. You'll start slowly and then build activity as you become more fit and accustomed to the artificial joint. You'll also continue strengthening exercises. You may be advised to slowly resume other normal household activities, including walking up and down stairs.

Three to eight weeks after a joint replacement — depending on the procedure you had and on your healthcare professional's assessment — you generally can resume most normal daily activities, such as shopping and light housekeeping. Driving is generally possible in 4 to 8 weeks after hip or knee replacement. You'll need to be able to bend your knee far enough to sit in a car and have enough muscle control to operate the brakes and accelerator.

NEW LEASE ON LIFE

Full recovery from a joint operation may take only a few weeks for certain tendon, ligament or cartilage procedures. Some types of joint fusion, osteotomy or joint replacements can require several months to a year of recovery before your bones fully heal and you regain maximum strength, stability and mobility.

Many people have less pain and swelling, as well as easier movement, in just days after the procedure. Your age, overall physical health and commitment to rehabilitation can all play a role in how quickly you recover. Follow-up visits with your healthcare team also are important.

Although recovering from joint surgery takes time, the outcome gives many people a new lease on life. Many years after surgery, most recipients of an artificial hip or knee are still able to move around comfortably. You may need to permanently avoid vigorous, high-impact activities, even after successful joint replacement and dedicated rehabilitation and care. Nevertheless, if you and your healthcare team decide it's time, joint surgery can lead you to an active, fulfilling future.

12 Pain management

Sharp. Throbbing. Nagging. Stiff. Burning. Achy. Agonizing. There may be millions of ways to talk about arthritis pain — one for each person who has arthritis.

No matter how you describe the sensation, joint pain can keep you from doing the things you would like to do. Treatment can help fix what's making your joint hurt. But meanwhile, you may have to deal with the discomfort.

Your approach to treating pain may be as individualistic as the symptoms you're experiencing. The use of medications to reduce inflammation and relieve pain is a major element of most treatment plans (see Chapter 10).

Some approaches focus on building a lifestyle that minimizes pain. You can learn better posture and body mechanics and use special devices to help with daily tasks (see Chapter 18).

You can also work at strengthening your muscles, tendons and ligaments to stabilize your damaged joints (see Chapter 15). In addition, losing weight may lessen the stress on joints (see Chapter 16). And building a positive attitude that helps keep pain in perspective can be valuable as well (see Chapter 17).

In many ways, this entire book is about the defining characteristic of arthritis — pain. There are many ways to understand it and to deal with it.

This chapter focuses on common approaches to pain management. The first section explains the cycle of pain. The section directly following reviews simple treatments for acute pain, the term for short-term pain. Many of these can be performed at home. The last section discusses professional treatment of pain aside from medications.

THE PAIN CYCLE

To best understand pain management, it is important to understand the cycle of pain. Pain starts when an area of the body is stimulated or experiences discomfort. Pain is influenced by many factors, including your activity level, your physical condition, the amount of swelling or inflammation in your joints, your tolerance of pain, and your state of mind. Physical discomfort can trigger feelings of frustration, anxiety or sadness. These feelings can also intensify your perception of pain. As pain worsens, you may start avoiding activities that you previously enjoyed. This can lead to decreased physical activity, weakening of the muscles, increased sadness and fatigue. The cycle then repeats, resulting in more pain.

Understanding your physical limits is essential for pain management because it helps prevent further injury. When you push your body beyond what it can handle, especially when you have chronic pain, you risk exacerbating your condition. For example, you might agree to help your friend move even though you have arthritis in your knees and hands. You may push through the pain lifting heavy boxes, but these repetitive motions can significantly increase your pain after the work is done and even cause a flare-up in your arthritis.

Knowing your limits and working on "not overdoing it" will go a long way in promoting healing and maintaining your physical function without further aggravating your pain.

The best way to disrupt the pain cycle is to address both the physical and emotional aspects of pain. Below we describe a variety of techniques to treat pain. Pain management works best when using multiple modalities.

TREATING ACUTE PAIN

Acute arthritis pain comes on quickly and lasts a short time, but it completely disrupts your day. It's severe pain that prevents you from working in the kitchen, typing on a keyboard or climbing a flight of stairs.

You can use either cold or heat to help relieve pain. It may be a matter of trial and error to find which temperature — or combination of temperatures — works best. Before using cold or heat, make sure your skin is dry and free of cuts and sores. Use a towel to protect the skin from direct contact with cold or heat, especially in areas where bone is close to the skin surface.

Cold

Cold is especially good for pain from arthritis flare-ups, as well as overuse injuries. Cold has a numbing effect on the painful area, dulling the sensation. It decreases muscle spasms and may reduce swelling and inflammation. Applying cold is typically recommended in the initial days of a flare-up. However, don't use cold if you have poor circulation or numbness in your skin.

Ice packs

You can pick up ice packs at many drugstores, department stores and pharmacies. Instant ice packs may be helpful if you don't have easy access to freezer gel packs. They're simple to use — squeezing the pack will activate its contents.

Before using an ice pack, make sure to wrap it in a thin towel so that the cold surface doesn't touch your skin directly. This will also help the pack stay cold longer.

You may apply cold several times a day for 15 to 20 minutes at a time. Regularly check that skin color is normal where you apply it. Losing color in your skin may mean that you're starting to get frostbite. Stop immediately if this happens.

Helpful hint: To make your own ice pack, combine ⅓ cup of rubbing alcohol with ⅔ cup of water. Seal the mixture inside a freezer bag. Put this bag inside another freezer bag, seal it and chill the pack in a freezer. It's ready to use when it's slushy. You can refreeze the contents after use. A bag of frozen vegetables, such as corn or peas, also can work. Just take care not to eat the frozen vegetables if they have been defrosted and frozen again.

Ice massage

This method also applies cold to your skin. Wrap an ice cube or a small block of ice in cloth and hold it comfortably in your hand. Use a circular motion to move the ice in and around your painful joint for 5 to 7 minutes. Apply mild pressure and remember to keep the ice moving when it's in direct contact with your skin.

Remember to watch for color changes in your skin. If you notice your skin losing its underlying natural tone, stop immediately. If your skin becomes numb during the massage, stop the treatment.

Helpful hint: Make a block of ice by freezing water in a paper cup. Peel back part of the cup to expose enough ice for a massage. Wrap the sides of the cup in a towel to protect your hands.

HOT AND COLD PACKS

A reusable gel-filled pack is perhaps the safest and most convenient commercially available product for applying either heat or cold to an affected joint. It's inexpensive and is found in most pharmacies.

You typically heat the pack in hot water or a microwave oven or chill the pack in a freezer. The heat or cold dissipates as the pack is used, so it's generally safe to apply it for 20 to 30 minutes at a time. You can also use it to treat minor muscle sprains and strains and minor tendinitis. Be sure to follow the product manufacturer's instructions.

Heat

Heat helps relax muscles and soothes painful joints. It also encourages blood flow to the affected area. Heat is especially good for easing stiffness and getting muscles limber.

If you have poor circulation or numbness in the area, don't apply high heat — you won't know if you're getting burned. In addition, don't apply heat after acute trauma or over an area that is swollen. It could increase the swelling and pain even more.

Hot packs and heating pads

Drape a towel or cloth over the painful area. Place a hot pack on top of the towel. Cover the pack with another layer or two of towels to keep it hot. Add or remove towels above or below to vary the heat. You may add extra layers over your skin in spots where bones sit close to the skin. Apply the heat for 20 to 30 minutes.

Check your skin every 15 minutes. If you see red and white blotches, stop treatment immediately. Continuing to heat the area could cause a burn or blister.

To protect your skin from burning, don't lie on a hot pack or heating pad or apply pressure during treatment.

Helpful hint: Make your own heat pack by placing a wet washcloth in a freezer bag and heating it in the microwave for one minute. Wrap the hot pack in a towel and place it near the affected joint. You can also fill a cotton tube sock with rice or another grain (other than popcorn), knot the open end, and warm it in the microwave.

Baths, showers and hot tubs

One of the easiest and most effective ways to apply heat to a painful joint is to take a 15-minute hot shower or bath. A standard bathtub can be just as effective as a hot tub.

In a very warm bath or shower, remember to use extra caution — and the grab bars — when entering or leaving the stall. You could become lightheaded or even faint, causing a fall.

Helpful hint: Placing clothes in the dryer for a few minutes before dressing can help ease morning stiffness. Or turn on an electric blanket for a few minutes before getting out of bed.

Heat lamps

You can also warm a painful joint using an infrared heat lamp with a reflector heat bulb, or clamp lamps or incubator lights equipped with low-cost incandescent bulbs. Incandescent lights release most of their energy as heat, and the heat can significantly increase blood circulation in the affected area.

Position the heat source approximately 18 to 20 inches from your skin. Then apply the heat for 20 to 30 minutes. You can decrease the intensity of the heat by moving the lamp farther away. Direct the lamp at the skin from the side rather than from above.

Helpful hint: Use an alarm clock or timer while you're using the heat lamp to make sure the heat doesn't stay on too long. Or ask someone to wake you if you think you might fall asleep.

Contrast baths

Contrast baths are helpful to many people with rheumatoid arthritis or osteoarthritis of the hands and feet. Alternating between warm and cold water may provide more relief than a hot or cold bath alone.

Start with two large pans. Fill one pan with warm water (approximately 97 to 104 F) and the other one with cool water (approximately 55 to 61 F). Place your joint in the warm water first for 10 minutes and then in the cool water for one minute. Cycle back to the warm water for four minutes and then to the cool water for one minute.

Repeat this process for half an hour. Always end with your hands or feet in the warm water. If pans aren't available, twin sinks work just as well for soaking your hands.

Helpful hint: Because you're immersing your skin directly into the baths, use water that is warm, not hot, and cool, not icy.

Topical treatments

There are multiple topical options in the form of creams or patches to manage pain. Topical options should never be used on broken, irritated, or infected skin. Some people may also experience photosensitivity or an increased likelihood of skin burning when exposed to the rays of the sun while using topical solutions. If you are allergic to an oral formulation of a topical cream or patch, you should not use the cream or patch, as you will likely have the same allergic reaction.

Topical nonsteroidal anti-inflammatory drugs (NSAIDs) come in gels, creams and patches. These medications can help reduce inflammation and relieve pain, especially in arthritis.

Topical NSAIDs should be used with caution, as they can be absorbed by the body. If you have underlying ulcers of the stomach or a history of bleeding from your gastrointestinal tract, you should not use topical NSAIDs, as they can exacerbate these issues. Asthma can be triggered by NSAIDs. If you have an allergy to NSAIDs, like ibuprofen, you should not use the topical form. It is uncommon, but topical NSAIDs can interact with other medications such as blood thinners, also known as anticoagulants, or blood pressure medications. You should talk to your healthcare professional before using topical NSAIDs.

Capsaicin cream, which is made from chili peppers, can help reduce pain by decreasing certain chemicals in your body that pass on pain signals. Capsaicin cream does have a burning sensation, and some may find this uncomfortable. Wash your hands thoroughly after use of this cream and take great care not to touch your eyes or mouth as accidental transfer could cause significant irritation.

Menthol or camphor cream has ingredients that create a cooling or warming sensation. Certain essential oils such as

DESCRIBING PAIN

It's not hard to recognize pain when you experience it. It's more difficult to describe what you're feeling to your healthcare team. And yet the details you provide at a medical visit may be extremely valuable in diagnosing and treating a condition such as arthritis or in helping you manage its symptoms.

In fact, it's hard to be objective when you're describing pain. Your personal experience of pain is influenced, in part, by your physical and emotional health and your mood, all of which may change from day to day. Pain tolerance varies greatly, and the pain that you brush off as "nothing" one day may feel unbearable on another.

Your healthcare team may use a numerical rating scale, which allows you to verbally rate pain on a scale of 0 to 10, with 0 representing no pain and 10 representing the worst pain imaginable. When you're talking to your healthcare team, the following questions also may help you describe your symptoms better:
- Where is the pain located? Does it remain in that place or does it tend to spread to other areas?
- When and how did the pain start? Were you doing any activities that you normally don't do? Did you have any illness before the pain started?
- Is the pain continuous or intermittent? If intermittent, how long does the discomfort last?
- Does the pain feel mild, moderate or severe?
- What is the quality of the pain? For example, does it feel throbbing, dull, sharp or burning?
- Are there associated symptoms? For example, is there weakness, headache, or numbness and tingling along with the pain?
- Does the pain change when you do certain activities or movements? Does it affect your ability to perform simple tasks?
- Does the pain keep you from sleeping, or does it awaken you from sleep?
- Have you tried anything to manage the pain?

eucalyptus or peppermint can have similar effects. These sensations can decrease pain by distracting the brain from discomfort. Like capsaicin cream, menthol or camphor cream can also cause a burning sensation.

Lidocaine patches or gels, which provide a numbing effect to the applied area, are often used for nerve pain. If you have a heart condition such as arrhythmia, you should be cautious when using lidocaine patches. Patches or gels should be used as prescribed, generally only once every 12 hours. Excessive or prolonged application can lead to systemic absorption, which can be toxic.

Cannabidiol (CBD) cream and oil are derived from cannabis but do not contain THC, the psychoactive part of marijuana that can result in dependency. Topical CBD interacts with the part of the body's system involved in controlling pain and inflammation. Using CBD cream can reduce inflammation and is helpful in conditions with more localized pain such as arthritis.

The regulation and understanding of CBD products continue to evolve with time. Some products may contain higher or lower amounts than advertised. Although CBD creams tend to be more localized, it is also possible to absorb them systemically. This could result in drowsiness, dry mouth or changes in appetite, though these side effects are more often seen with oral CBD products compared to topical.

CBD goes through the liver, using a mechanism similar to many commonly prescribed medications. Blood thinners, antiplatelet drugs (such as clopidogrel), anti-seizure medications, benzodiazepines (such as alprazolam), antidepressants, antipsychotics, beta-blockers (such as metoprolol), calcium channel blockers (such as amlodipine), immunosuppressants and chemotherapy drugs may interact with CBD.

PROFESSIONAL HELP FOR PAIN

Various healthcare professionals may bring a broad range of experience and expertise to your pain management team. Your family physician or rheumatologist may prescribe medication to help control your discomfort, along with exercises and other therapies. But your treatment may also include seeing a physical therapist, occupational therapist, physiatrist, psychiatrist, psychologist or perhaps even a specialist of integrative medicine, such as an acupuncturist. These professionals may use different methods and techniques to help you manage your pain.

Devices to control pain

Orthotics is a medical specialty dealing with supportive devices for the body. The devices may control the function of a joint, assist or restrict its movement, and reduce pressure on the joint. Many products, including insoles, splints and braces, can be used to help relieve arthritis pain.

Foot orthotics

If you've lost foot or ankle support due to the deterioration of a joint, usually as a result of rheumatoid arthritis, it can lead to strain on the associated knee or hip. Foot orthotic devices, including heel cups, arch supports and molded boots, can help stabilize arthritic joints, thus reducing stress on other joints and helping relieve pain.

Shoe insoles

Special insoles placed inside your shoes may provide pain relief due to osteo-arthritis of the knee. The healthcare professional may recommend a medial-wedge insole or a lateral-wedge insole, depending on how it alters knee function. When using insoles, it's important to wear appropriate footwear with cushioning that properly supports your weight-bearing joints and your back.

Knee braces

Braces are used on the lower limbs to decrease weight-bearing pressure and provide stability. Knee braces are helpful to some individuals with osteoarthritis. They may help reduce pain and increase knee mobility.

Therapies to control pain

Healthcare professionals may prescribe the following to help you reduce or manage pain. Some of these fall under the heading of integrative medicine. A full discussion of various integrative medicine treatments used for treating arthritis pain can be found in Chapter 13.

Physical exercise

Exercise is perhaps your best defense against pain. Your healthcare professional may have you work with a physical therapist to develop an exercise program that maximizes your range of motion. Exercise can also strengthen the muscles around your painful joints. (For more on exercise, see Chapter 15.)

Massage

Massage can improve blood circulation, help you relax, and reduce pain and swelling. Some therapists are specially trained in massage techniques for people with arthritis.

During massage, heed the warnings of pain. If you're giving yourself a massage or a family member is massaging you, remember to stop as soon as it starts to hurt. If the joint itself is swollen or painful, avoid massaging it and instead massage adjacent muscles.

Try warming or cooling the area before massage. Use a lotion or massage oil to help hands glide smoothly over the skin.

Helpful hint: If you're using massage oil or lotion on the affected area, wash it off before heat treatment to avoid burns.

Specialized heat treatments

Unlike more simplified home heat treatments, a physical therapist may use specialized techniques or equipment to provide pain relief.

One of these treatments may involve soaking sore joints, particularly in the hands, in a warm paraffin bath. With instruction from the therapist, you may be able to use warm paraffin at home.

For deeper penetration, the therapist may use ultrasound or shortwave diathermy, which applies an electromagnetic current at higher frequencies to generate heat. This procedure requires careful monitoring because it may worsen some forms of arthritis.

Steroid injections

Steroid medications are prescribed to reduce pain and inflammation in joints. Your healthcare professional may inject cortisone directly into an acutely inflamed joint — for example, a knee, a hip or an ankle — to ease discomfort. (For more on joint injections, see Chapter 14.)

Nerve block

Your doctor may use an anesthetic injection to deaden the nerves in a targeted area of your body that's experiencing pain, interrupting the pain signals to the brain. The relief is temporary, but the treatment provides a welcome respite from chronic arthritic pain.

Transcutaneous electrical nerve stimulation (TENS)

This therapy is used to treat targeted areas of your body that are experiencing pain. Electrodes placed on your skin near the painful areas deliver mild, painless electric pulses to nearby nerve pathways. The strength of the pulses may be adjusted as needed to control pain.

TENS is thought to work in several ways. The stimulation may overpower pain signals in nerve pathways, reducing the pain messages that reach your brain. TENS treatment may also trigger a release of endorphins, which are chemicals in your body with painkilling effects similar to those of morphine.

TENS generally works best for acute pain from a pinched nerve. Studies show that TENS has mixed results in treating chronic pain, but it does give relief for some people with arthritis. Most often, TENS is used in combination with exercise and other pain treatments.

Similar to TENS, a treatment called percutaneous electrical nerve stimulation (PENS) delivers electric pulses to the nerve pathways. But instead of delivering the current through electrodes, PENS uses needles that penetrate your skin to just below the surface. These needles are very thin, like those used in acupuncture. Most people feel some sensation, but not pain, when the needles are inserted.

Behavioral approaches to control pain

Pain and trauma are often closely linked. Trauma can be physical (an injury to the body) or emotional or psychological (a distressing life event). The body and the mind are deeply interconnected, and emotional or psychological distress can be expressed physically in the form of pain.

Traumatic events in childhood, often referred to as adverse childhood experiences, can have a more lasting impact on physical and mental health by changing the way the brain develops and processes stress and pain. Addressing underlying trauma can be an important step to getting to the bottom of pain.

Self-coping strategies

Positive thinking can be vital in coping with chronic pain. Being positive doesn't mean you're trying to ignore the hurt. It means that you're approaching your condition in a positive, productive manner, looking for ways to make the best happen, not the worst. To manage pain, you must pace yourself. Pacing is the act of breaking down activities into manageable chunks and taking regular breaks to prevent overexertion. (For self-coping strategies such as mindfulness meditation, see Chapter 17.)

You may reach a point at which you need extra support to cope with arthritis symptoms. That's when professionals may be able to help you.

Cognitive behavioral therapy

With cognitive behavioral therapy, you work with a counselor in a structured way to become more aware of inaccurate or negative thinking. The therapy allows you to view challenging situations clearly and respond to them in more effective ways.

The goals for treating arthritis will likely include identifying and modifying your negative reactions to pain. And you'll learn how to change behavior in ways that help you better manage life despite the pain.

Cognitive behavioral therapy is generally focused on specific problems and uses a goal-oriented approach. It requires you to become more aware of your thoughts, emotions and beliefs about your condition. It also helps you recognize habits in everyday life that may be contributing to the problem.

Related treatments

In addition to behavioral approaches to managing pain, you may learn other ways to build support.

Biofeedback

Your body has automatic involuntary reactions to stress and pain: changes in muscle tension, skin temperature, blood pressure and heart rate. The goals of biofeedback are to teach you to recognize these reactions and to learn to modify them.

During a session with a therapist, you're attached to monitors that track your physiologic systems — heart, respiration, muscle tension, skin temperature and brain activity. The therapist, with the help of this output, can teach you to control involuntary reactions that trigger the stress symptoms.

Relaxation training

You can learn to relax your body and mind with a variety of techniques, including progressive muscle relaxation, deep breathing, guided imagery and meditation. (For more on these techniques, see Chapter 13.)

With the help of an instructor, you can learn how to take short breaks whenever you're feeling overwhelmed by stress or pain as a way of helping you concentrate and relax. Eventually, you will learn to relax on your own, without taking cues from someone else.

The ideal location for relaxation is a quiet room where you can rest comfortably on a bed, in a reclining chair or even on the floor. You should feel at ease, not cramped or confined.

You may enjoy audiovisual resources to help you focus, for example, softly playing a recording of ocean waves or forest sounds. Soft lighting that's easy on the eyes is often preferable.

The goal of relaxation strategy is to reduce tension buildup in your body. You can employ the strategy throughout the day, whenever you feel stress or pain building up. In this way you may prevent the tension from getting worse and successfully complete activities in your daily life.

Chronic pain centers

If your arthritis pain is severe, your healthcare professional may recommend visiting a chronic pain center. In this setting, you may undergo outpatient treatment from a team of pain specialists. The program may last from several days to several weeks.

The center may be useful if you're not getting any respite from chronic pain, and the pain treatments you're using, such as medications, injections and surgery, don't seem to be working. An interdisciplinary approach to pain relief at these centers is essential because it's unlikely that any one technique will work to control pain.

The team of professionals at these centers can help treat pain and associated conditions such as depression. They may also help you deal with potential consequences of arthritis, such as family disruption and loss of income.

13 Holistic and integrative medicine

Conventional medicine has much to offer in helping you manage your arthritis. But standard arthritis medicines may not "cure" arthritis or completely control your symptoms. You may still have good days and not-so-good days.

In addition, some conventional arthritis treatments carry the risk of unwanted and even serious side effects, especially after long-term use. For these reasons and others, many people with arthritis turn to holistic and integrative medicine.

Holistic healthcare considers the whole person — mind, body and spirit. The focus isn't just on a specific part, such as the joints, but on how that part fits in with the rest of the body, and how the rest of the body impacts that part.

Integrative medicine can be a key part of holistic care. In the medical field, integrative medicine is the practice of using

proven complementary treatments alongside conventional treatments to achieve optimal health and healing of the whole person. Integrative treatments don't replace conventional medicine. Instead, they complement existing treatments with the goal of improving outcomes. You may also know these treatments by other names, such as complementary medicine or alternative medicine.

More than a third of adults in the United States use some kind of integrative medicine as part of their healthcare. Supplements, meditation, chiropractic care, yoga and massage are all examples.

Pain is a powerful motivator in the hunt for new treatments that may provide relief. In fact, research shows that chronic pain is the top reason people try integrative medicine. Integrative therapies can effectively treat many types of pain, including back pain, neck pain, and arthritis and joint pain.

This chapter will help you learn about integrative therapies that may enhance your treatment plan. You'll find background information as well as tips on using these treatments wisely. Use the information here to guide you when you talk with your arthritis care team about options for your care.

CHOOSING AN INTEGRATIVE THERAPY

One of the key differences between integrative therapies and conventional medicine is testing. Conventional medicine, particularly in the United States, is designed around clinical trials that rigorously test the medicines on thousands of people.

When a medicine or therapy is approved by the U.S. Food and Drug Administration, it means that regulators are fairly certain that the drug is safe and effective for most people who are meant to take it and who take it as instructed.

Many integrative therapies — such as massage therapy, herbal supplements and meditation — have been used for a thousand years or more. But these therapies didn't start out in a lab or in a study. Instead, they were found by trial and error. Scientific research has more recently shown evidence for some of these methods. But overall, they're still used today because many people find them helpful.

This means that scientists are playing catch-up in their efforts to test many of these therapies on a large scale. Researchers are still learning how they work and making sure they're truly safe and effective. Evidence is still emerging, so it's important to use common sense when considering integrative therapies.

Discuss your options

Many people who use integrative therapies often don't talk about them with their healthcare team. They assume that medical professionals either won't be interested or will be opposed to the treatments. But not telling your healthcare team about all the therapies you're using, whether traditional or nontraditional, can be dangerous.

For example, just because an integrative therapy is said to be "natural" doesn't mean it's safe to use. Some dietary supplements and herbs touted as being natural can cause problems with the conventional medications you may be taking.

If you're thinking about trying an integrative therapy, talk about it with your care team first. Many healthcare professionals see the value of integrative practices and can help you blend them into your treatment plan.

Your healthcare professional may not know enough about a particular therapy to endorse it, but they may be able to show you studies on its risks and

WHAT'S IN A NAME?

The terms used to describe healthcare methods that fall outside of mainstream medicine have shifted over the last several decades.

In the early 1990s, many of these methods were labeled as "unconventional" or "alternative." Later, they were referred to as complementary and alternative medicine (CAM), an umbrella term that's still used today. It includes a diverse range of systems, practices and products that aren't typically part of conventional practice.

There's an important distinction to be made:
- Complementary therapies are treatments used in conjunction with conventional medicine. For example, you may practice tai chi along with taking standard pain medication to relieve pain.
- Alternative therapies are used in place of conventional medicine. An example of this is seeing a homeopath or naturopath instead of a conventionally trained healthcare professional.

Among the general public, this distinction isn't always clear. Many people use the term *alternative medicine* as a catchall phrase for all health practices that aren't typically part of mainstream medicine.

Today, medicine has shifted in focus toward prevention and whole-body wellness, and healthcare professionals are integrating unconventional therapies into their practices.

Therapies that were once called "alternative" or "complementary" may now be described as integrative. As the term suggests, integrative medicine refers to using natural or holistic practices as a complement to conventional medicine. Integrative therapies are used alongside conventional medicine to optimize health through nutrition, exercise, stress management and social connection.

This is done by combining the best of today's high-tech tests and procedures with the best of nontraditional practice and principles of holistic care. This approach can help soothe stress, reduce pain and anxiety, maintain strength and flexibility, and promote a sense of well-being.

benefits or give you resources that can help you evaluate your options.

Regardless of what your healthcare team thinks about integrative medicine, it's important that they know what you're doing. That will allow you to get the best possible care and avoid dangerous interactions.

Assess the risks and benefits

Some integrative therapies pose very little risk while offering wonderful benefits. For example, meditation and relaxed breathing are unlikely to cause harm. They're easy to learn, you can do them anywhere at any time, and they can help you to relax and reduce stress.

On the flip side, buying an herbal supplement that's touted as an arthritis cure may be risky. Supplements are complex mixtures of compounds found in nature. While there are many reputable supplement manufacturers in the United States, dietary supplements in general aren't regulated with the same strict oversight as are prescription drugs. Your product may have varying or unknown amounts of the active ingredient.

Even though stronger regulations have been in place in the United States since 2010, herbal products of poor or unreliable quality can still reach store shelves. This may cause your healthcare team to be skeptical about taking them. Keep in mind that any potential benefits may be offset by the risks. So think critically and use reputable sources and providers.

Finding a provider

When you're looking for someone who practices the type of integrative therapy you're interested in, choose someone in the same way you would choose a new physician. Look at their qualifications and experience. Ask for a referral from a trusted healthcare professional or a friend or family member who has had the treatment you're considering. Many universities and teaching hospitals, including Mayo Clinic, now have integrative health programs that offer a holistic, evidence-based approach to healthcare.

If you're evaluating a licensed practitioner, check with your local and state medical boards for information on credentials and whether any complaints have been filed against the individual.

You can also contact well-established professional organizations, such as the American Academy of Medical Acupuncture, for the names of certified practitioners in your area. Keep in mind, though, that for many integrative therapies, there are no licensure or certification standards.

Consider treatment cost

The integrative treatment you're considering may not be covered by your health insurance plan. Check with your insurance company first. If you have to pay for it out of pocket, find out how much it will cost. If possible, get it in writing before you start treatment.

WHAT MAKES A GOOD STUDY?

When doing research on treatments for arthritis, here are two types of studies you may find.

Randomized controlled trial
A randomized controlled trial is basic to most medical research. It's designed to evaluate a new medication or other form of treatment. In this type of study, participants are usually divided into two groups. One group gets the treatment being studied. The other group is the control group. People in the control group get standard treatment, no treatment or an inactive substance called a placebo. Participants are placed in these groups randomly. This helps ensure both groups will be similar.

Double-blind study
In this type of trial, neither the researchers nor the participants know who's getting the active treatment and who's getting the placebo. With this approach, the results are objective. Still, because people can vary so much, many healthcare professionals prefer to see whether the results of later trials can confirm the results of a particular study. Only then are a study's results considered to be conclusive, in many cases.

Keep your mind open and stay objective

Look at integrative therapies objectively. Stay open to possibilities, but take a close look at any treatment you're considering.

FORMS OF INTEGRATIVE THERAPY

Many different forms of integrative medicine can ease symptoms and help you cope with arthritis. Each type of therapy may work in a different way to improve your physical and emotional health and your quality of life.

This section outlines five common types of integrative medicine:
- Mind-body medicine
- Herbs and other dietary supplements
- Energy therapies
- Hands-on therapies
- Alternative medical and healing systems

In each section, you'll learn about the therapies that are used the most and have been shown to be the most helpful.

MIND-BODY MEDICINE

People have long believed that your state of mind can influence your physical body and your health. More recently, research using imaging techniques such as functional MRI has confirmed this. Mind-body techniques that promote relaxation can be helpful for people with arthritis. They can help ease tension, which may also help reduce pain and improve physical functioning. Mind-body techniques usually get the green light for use from medical professionals.

You can learn to do most of these techniques yourself. Many are inexpensive or free. To get the full benefit, practice them regularly.

Aromatherapy

This ancient form of healing uses essential oils from flowers, herbs and trees to promote health and well-being. Practitioners believe that when these oils are massaged into the skin or inhaled, they help treat symptoms, including arthritis pain and inflammation.

Originally popular in Europe, aromatherapy is increasingly being used in the United States. Aromatherapy treatments are found in stores that sell natural health products.

More study is needed to say for sure if the plant oils used in aromatherapy are of benefit to health and well-being. Limited

BIOFEEDBACK AND NEUROFEEDBACK

Biofeedback is a type of mind-body therapy that helps you learn how to control your body's functions, such as your responses to pain. During a biofeedback session, a trained therapist applies electrodes and electronic sensors to your body. The sensors monitor your physical response — including your heart rate, breathing patterns, body temperature and muscle activity. The sensors then feed the information back to you via sound and visual cues. With this feedback, you can learn how to control your body's responses and enter into a relaxed state. The goal is to learn to control them on your own.

Some research has looked at whether biofeedback can help in managing arthritis pain. So far, studies have not shown a clear benefit, but more high-quality research is needed.

Neurofeedback is a type of biofeedback that focuses on brain activity. Sensors, usually attached to a headband or cap, are placed on the scalp. A connected app gives you real-time feedback, such as identifying an active or a calm brain state, and the app may offer guided meditation or breathing exercises. Training the brain with neurofeedback has been shown to help with stress management. While further studies are needed, some research suggests it also could help in managing pain conditions such as fibromyalgia.

research has been done on the use of aromatherapy for arthritis.

Guided imagery

Imagery is a thought process that invokes the senses — you use it to see in your mind's eye. Guided imagery, also called visualization, has been used by different cultures through the ages as a healing tool.

With guided imagery, you close your eyes to the outside world and create a soothing mental picture that helps your mind promote healing. In your mind's eye, for example, you might see yourself lying on a beach on a warm summer day listening to gentle waves lapping on the shore.

When you imagine the beach, your brain is activated almost as if you were actually feeling the sand beneath your toes. The message your brain receives is relayed to other parts of your body that control your heart rate and blood pressure. With repeated practice, your relaxed state during guided imagery may help relieve pain, fatigue and other symptoms. In turn, this may reduce your need for medications.

Hypnosis

Hypnosis is often portrayed humorously on TV and in films, but it can be an effective health treatment. Hypnosis induces a state of deep relaxation that helps you concentrate and makes you more open to the power of suggestion.

For instance, if you're open to a suggestion to relax, you may respond less to the world around you. You can use hypnosis to help manage pain — or at least shift your attention away from it. Several studies have found that hypnosis can be useful in pain management, although they haven't focused specifically on its use with arthritis. Research shows that hypnosis works better for some adults than others.

Scientists don't understand exactly how hypnosis works. It appears to alter brain wave patterns in much the same way that other relaxation techniques do. It seems to influence the nerve impulses, hormones and chemicals that affect how your brain communicates with your body.

Meditation

Meditation has been around for thousands of years. It can help you enter a deep, restful state that reduces your body's stress response.

There are many paths to meditation. In general, when you're meditating, you're paying attention to the present moment, not on past concerns or future anxieties. You focus on your breathing or on a mantra — a simple sound or phrase repeated over and over.

During meditation, you suspend the flow of emotions and thoughts that normally fill your mind. This helps you achieve a deep mental calmness and state of relaxation. It may also help you control

GET STARTED WITH RELAXATION TECHNIQUES

You can master simple relaxation techniques with a little practice. Use this approach whenever you feel increasing stress, pain or muscle tension.

Relaxed breathing
Stress or pain typically causes rapid, shallow breathing. This kind of breathing helps your body respond to stress by boosting your heart rate and causing you to sweat. By controlling your breathing, the effects of stress will become less intense, and you'll be able to keep the effects of stress from spiraling out of control.

Here's how to use relaxed breathing in times of stress:
• *Inhale.* With your mouth closed and your shoulders relaxed, inhale deeply by slowly pushing your stomach out as you count to six. Allow the air to fill your diaphragm, the muscle under your rib cage.
• *Exhale.* Release the air through your mouth as you slowly count to six.
• *Repeat.* Complete this cycle 3 to 5 times.

Progressive muscle relaxation
The goal of progressive muscle relaxation is to reduce muscle tension. First, find a quiet place where you'll be free from interruption. Loosen tight clothing and remove your glasses or contacts if you like. Find a comfortable position — seated or lying down.

Starting with your feet and working up through your body to your neck and head, tense each muscle group for at least five seconds and then relax the muscles for up to 30 seconds. Repeat before moving to the next muscle group. Areas to concentrate on include your feet, legs, stomach, back, chest, hands, arms, shoulders, neck and face. Each session should last about 10 minutes.

As you learn to relax, you'll start to notice when stress causes your muscles to tense up. You'll also start to notice other physical changes that stress causes in your body. Knowing how stress makes you feel will help you make a conscious effort to relax whenever you feel stress building. And remember, relaxation is a skill. As with any skill, you'll get better with practice.

how you respond to challenging and stressful situations.

Today, many people meditate for spiritual reasons, but meditation may have health benefits, too. Meditating regularly can slow your brain waves, boost your mood and decrease your muscle tension, blood pressure and heart rate. It can also lessen your body's response to the chemicals it produces when you're stressed by pain.

Meditation is often practiced on its own. Some people start with simply sitting quietly and paying attention to their breathing. Meditation can be combined with other therapies, such as yoga and tai chi. You can even meditate while walking or jogging.

Yoga and tai chi

Yoga and tai chi are efficient, low-impact activities that can help you maintain both physical fitness and mental clarity. With regular practice, you can gradually increase your strength and flexibility while enhancing the connection of your mind, body and spirit.

Yoga combines breathing exercises, physical postures, meditation and other techniques that originated in India more than 5,000 years ago.

There are many different styles of yoga. Hatha is one of the most common forms. It involves different body postures that are held for various lengths of time and done in a sequence.

In the United States, yoga has become increasingly popular as a fitness activity. Don't be intimidated, though, if what comes to mind are "power yoga" and "hot yoga" classes featuring strength-intensive moves. Many forms of yoga can benefit your strength and flexibility with gentler movements. In a class, you also can ask the instructor to suggest modified poses to accommodate joint pain or a limited range of motion.

Tai chi is an ancient Chinese tradition that combines rhythmic movements,

REST AND REPAIR

For many people, the brain is frequently being triggered into the "fight or flight" response by modern stressors throughout the day. However, very few of the triggering events require the stress hormones that are released (cortisol, epinephrine, norepinephrine and others). Because we do not "use" the stress hormones, they may have negative effects, including hurting our immune function, increasing inflammation, impairing sleep, hurting cognitive function and affecting the heart. Mind body practice works to enhance our "rest and repair" response such that when we do experience stressors, we are less likely to release the stress hormones and therefore avoid the negative impact of chronic stress.

breathing techniques and focused attention. A self-paced series of postures is performed in a slow, graceful manner. Each body position flows into the next as one continuous movement.

Yoga and tai chi may improve quality of life and relieve pain from osteoarthritis. In part, these practices help by improving how well you move and enhancing your strength, flexibility and balance. Studies have shown that tai chi can improve range of motion in people with rheumatoid arthritis. Both yoga and tai chi promote relaxation and help reduce stress, which often goes hand in hand with chronic pain.

Some postures may strain your lower back and joints, so be careful. Don't push to perform a pose that feels uncomfortable. It's best to work with a yoga or tai chi instructor who knows about your health condition and can help you make adjustments if needed.

HERBS AND OTHER DIETARY SUPPLEMENTS

Herbs and dietary supplements make up the broadest category of integrative therapies. This category encompasses a range of ingredients found in nature, including herbs, vitamins, minerals, amino acids, animal extracts and enzymes.

Herbs and dietary supplements are the most commonly used form of integrative medicine in the United States. About 1 in 5 adults use some type of natural product.

Herbal treatments have been in use for thousands of years. Many of today's conventional medicines, including digoxin, which is used for congestive heart failure, and quinine, used for malaria, were once considered folk medicines. Scientists continue to discover new medicines derived from plants and herbs.

Many herbal preparations are marketed as alternative pain relievers and inflammation fighters for arthritis. As experts learn more about how to treat pain and other symptoms of arthritis, researchers are also working to improve evidence-based knowledge about these herbal treatments.

But it's hard to apply traditional scientific research to dietary supplements. Many products are complex mixtures of natural ingredients that often can't be tested in the same manner as conventional medications, in which one compound is tested for one disease. Different brands of the same herb may have varying amounts of the active ingredient in them.

In addition, research hasn't established guidelines around how much of a supplement to take and what side effects supplements may cause. So it's important to talk to your healthcare team before taking any herbs or dietary supplements.

Best bets

If you're interested in adding an integrative medicine supplement to your arthritis treatment, you may want to look at the following products. While everyone responds differently to treatments, research has shown these to be generally safe and sometimes helpful.

Glucosamine and chondroitin

Glucosamine and chondroitin are natural compounds found in cartilage, the tough, pliable tissue that cushions joints. Glucosamine supplements are made from the outer skeletons of shellfish. Chondroitin supplements are made from sources such as shark cartilage. The two compounds are often used together. Taken separately or together, these supplements are the second-most used of all natural products, after fish oil.

There have been dozens of clinical trials on glucosamine for osteoarthritis — most often for osteoarthritis of the knee. Unfortunately, these studies have yielded mixed results.

In a two-year study from the National Institutes of Health known as the Glucosamine/ Chondroitin Arthritis Intervention Trial (GAIT), glucosamine and chondroitin were used to treat more than 1,500 people with osteoarthritis of the knee. Results suggested that glucosamine sulfate, when used with chondroitin, helped a small group of people with moderate to severe knee pain. But the researchers couldn't say for sure if it was helpful for overall pain relief.

More research is also needed to say how effective these supplements are in treating rheumatoid arthritis. Early research suggests that glucosamine and chondroitin may lessen pain, but they don't seem to lessen inflammation or help with painful and swollen joints.

Glucosamine and chondroitin appear to be safe, with few side effects. However, if you're allergic to shellfish, you should avoid them. And be cautious if you take a blood thinner, such as warfarin, because glucosamine may increase the risk of bleeding.

A NOTE ON DIET

You may have read about specific diets that help with arthritis symptoms. Some of them involve removing wheat, bacon, pork, milk, rye bread, beef or coffee from your diet. But there's no proof that these strategies help relieve symptoms.

Research suggests that following a Mediterranean diet benefits rheumatoid arthritis. The diet focuses on eating whole grains, fruits and vegetables and limiting saturated fats, sodium and processed foods. (For more on healthful eating and arthritis, see Chapter 16.)

Gout is the one type of arthritis that does require a specific diet, because certain foods can contribute to the excess uric acid in the body. (For more on eating to help manage gout symptoms, see pages 260-261.)

Like many supplements, glucosamine can take longer than most prescription drugs to be effective. So, you may want to use a supplement for 4 to 6 weeks or even longer before deciding if it is helpful or not. Keep track of your pain levels and the side effects to see if the treatment is working for you.

Glucosamine may take up to eight weeks to become most effective.

Gamma-linolenic acid (GLA)

Gamma-linolenic acid is an omega-6 fatty acid. It's necessary for good health, but it isn't produced in the body. Your body obtains GLA from the breakdown of certain foods during digestion. GLA supplements are typically made from borage, black currant and evening primrose.

Once in your body, GLA is converted into compounds with anti-inflammatory properties. There's some proof that it may moderately reduce pain, joint tenderness and morning stiffness from rheumatoid arthritis.

Borage seed oil is available in liquid or capsule form, as are oils made from black currant seeds and the evening primrose plant. These oils may cause mild stomach upset.

S-adenosyl-L-methionine (SAMe)

S-adenosyl-L-methionine is a dietary supplement that has gained attention as a treatment for osteoarthritis. It's a man-made version of a compound that occurs naturally in the body. Pronounced "sam-E," this supplement is thought to repair, stimulate growth in and increase the thickness of cartilage. In Europe, SAMe is available as a prescription medication for arthritis and depression.

SAMe has been studied in several clinical trials. It appears to relieve pain from osteoarthritis as well as NSAIDs do, but with fewer side effects. And it can improve how well your joints work. You may need to take SAMe for more than a month before you see significant relief from your symptoms.

Side effects are uncommon and may include minor nausea or stomach upset. SAMe may lessen the effects of a drug used to treat Parkinson's disease. It may also interact with drugs and supplements used to increase levels of serotonin in the body, such as antidepressants. SAMe may also worsen symptoms of mania in people with bipolar disorder.

Fish oil

Cold-water fish such as salmon, mackerel, herring, sardines and trout are high in polyunsaturated fats called omega-3 fatty acids. These fatty acids play an important role in many bodily functions and can help reduce inflammation. Eating at least two servings of fish a week has many health benefits.

For people with arthritis, taking a supplement of the oil derived from fatty fish may also be helpful. Fish oils are high in two specific fatty acids, eicosapentaenoic acid (EPA) and docosahexaenoic acid (DHA), that play a role in the anti-inflammatory process.

Fish oil has been shown to improve pain, tender joints, morning stiffness and other symptoms in people with rheumatoid arthritis. In addition, fish oil supplements may protect against developing heart disease, which is more likely in people with rheumatoid arthritis.

Fish oil supplements may also allow some people with rheumatoid arthritis to reduce their use of anti-inflammatory drugs. Taking a low dose of fish oil daily may also improve pain and function for people with osteoarthritis.

Fish oil is sold as a supplement in liquid, capsule or pill form. Side effects are usually mild and may include a fishy aftertaste, bad-smelling sweat, head-ache, heartburn, nausea and diarrhea. Fish oil supplements may cause problems with drugs that affect how the blood clots.

Ginger

Ginger is an aromatic spice native to Asia. The product you buy in the grocery store is the underground stem of the plant. It's also available as a powder, tablet, extract, tincture and oil.

Some studies have found that ginger can modestly reduce pain associated with arthritis. Researchers believe that com-pounds in ginger have anti-inflammatory effects. Research is ongoing.

In low doses, ginger causes few side effects. In some people, it may cause mild stomach discomfort, heartburn, diarrhea and gas. It may interact with blood thinners, and people with gallstone disease should use ginger with caution.

Vitamins

Vitamin C, vitamin E and beta carotene, which contain antioxidants, have been studied as possible treatments of arthritis because they may help prevent cell damage that leads to joint pain and further progression of the disease. Dietary sources include fruits and vegetables, which are important parts of a healthy diet in general. Should you take vitamin supplements as well? More studies are needed to answer this question.

So far, some research indicates that vitamin C may make it less likely that your osteoarthritis will get worse. Taking vitamin E along with standard care for rheumatoid arthritis seems to help with pain, but not with inflammation. Vitamin E doesn't seem to help with the pain and stiffness of osteoarthritis.

Vitamin D, best known for its bone-protecting properties, is sometimes taken to treat and prevent arthritis. Some research shows that low levels of vitamin D are common in people with rheumatoid arthritis. However, there is no clear evidence that deficiency of this vitamin increases the risk of developing rheumatoid arthritis, and taking vitamin D supplements doesn't seem to reduce pain from this type of arthritis. There are indications that vitamin D may help with pain and function in people who have osteoarthritis and don't get enough of the vitamin in their diets.

Vitamin B-3 is made up of niacin and niacinamide. Preliminary studies suggest that niacinamide — found in meat, fish, milk, eggs, green vegetables and cereals — may be useful in treating osteoarthritis. But more research is needed before a recommendation can be made about taking vitamin B-3 supplements.

Avocado-soybean unsaponifiables

This supplement is a mixture of avocado and soybean oils. It's widely used in Europe to treat knee and hip osteoarthritis. It acts as an anti-inflammatory, and some studies have shown it can slow or even prevent joint damage. Some research shows that it may improve pain and help you move more easily, but more research is needed.

Capsaicin

This topical cream made from chili peppers is widely used for pain relief. The product is generally considered safe for use but can cause unpleasant effects such as a burning sensation on the skin. Some experts recommend this cream for hand osteoarthritis but not for some cases of osteoarthritis of the knee.

Turmeric

Turmeric contains the chemical curcumin, a yellow pigment that makes for a popular fabric dye. It's a popular spice in Indian and Asian dishes. Studies suggest that its anti-inflammatory qualities may help treat osteoarthritis. Specifically, turmeric may reduce pain and make it easier to move. It may also help lessen joint swelling and morning stiffness in rheumatoid arthritis.

When it's taken by mouth or applied to the skin, it's generally considered safe. Because turmeric may slow blood clotting, it should be avoided if you take blood thinners.

Devil's claw

Devil's claw is widely marketed as a remedy for osteoarthritis. It's been used extensively in Europe, and indications are increasing that it can lessen arthritis pain.

The plant may have some anti-inflammatory, pain-relieving and antioxidant properties. Studies have shown that it reduces pain from osteoarthritis, especially hip and knee pain. Unfortunately, it doesn't appear that devil's claw can help with symptoms of rheumatoid arthritis.

The side effects of devil's claw appear to be minimal, the most common being diarrhea and stomach upset. It may also cause problems with drugs used to treat and prevent blood clots and some medications used to treat high blood pressure.

More evidence needed

A number of other herbs and supplements on the market may also have therapeutic effects. But more research is needed to better understand how the possible benefits balance any risks.

Marijuana

Now that a number of states have legalized marijuana for medical use, healthcare professionals are often asked about using it. It may be available in the form of a pill, oil, oral solution and spray, or whole plant material. Studies show that marijuana may help treat symptoms of a variety of conditions, including chronic pain. However, the evidence for this use is limited, particularly for pain from rheumatic disease.

Some evidence suggests that a specific mouth spray containing a certain marijuana extract may help with sleep and morning pain in rheumatoid arthritis. It doesn't seem to help joint stiffness in the morning or make pain less intense, though.

Safety concerns and side effects are two more reasons that marijuana generally isn't recommended for treating pain. The side effects of medical marijuana can include dizziness, slower reaction times, increased heart rate and, in rare cases, psychosis. It has additional risks when used with other medications.

Experts in rheumatology and pain management offer this advice for using medical marijuana to treat arthritis symptoms:

- Don't smoke it. Inhaling it through a vaporizer or ingesting it brings fewer health risks.
- Know the levels of active ingredients and choose an application with low tetrahydrocannabinol (THC) content, up to 9%, and high cannabidiol (CBD) content.
- Start with a low dose.
- Don't drive or operate heavy machinery for 24 hours after taking it. It can impair reaction time.
- Avoid cannabis if you're under 25 years old, as the brain is still maturing until this age. Marijuana can negatively affect brain development.
- Consider using medical marijuana only when your symptoms flare, and follow up with your healthcare team regularly to monitor its effects.

Bovine cartilage

Cartilage that comes from cow tissue is thought to have anti-inflammatory effects. Some researchers think it can spur growth of new cartilage in people with osteoarthritis. Injections of bovine cartilage given under the skin seem to help ease symptoms of both osteoarthritis and rheumatoid arthritis.

Cat's claw

Cat's claw is made from a woody vine from the tropical rainforests of Central and South America. Its name comes from the hooked thorns that run along the vine's surface. The herb comes in tablet or capsule form and is sold as tea.

Cat's claw inhibits two substances that trigger inflammation. For osteoarthritis, this supplement may relieve knee pain. For rheumatoid arthritis, it may have a modest effect on reducing joint pain and swelling.

More study on the benefits and risks of cat's claw is needed. The supplement may lower your blood pressure, so if you take drugs to lower high blood pressure, talk to your healthcare team before taking cat's claw.

Dimethyl sulfoxide (DMSO) and methyl-sulfonylmethane (MSM)

These related supplements are used for many conditions, including osteoarthritis.

RISK OF DRUG INTERACTIONS WITH CBD

Cannabidiol (CBD) is one of the components of marijuana, known for having anti-inflammatory effects without psychoactive effects that make you "high." CBD oil is on the rise as an integrative therapy for a number of conditions, including arthritis. But because of the ways that certain medications and CBD work in the body, they may interact if you use both. This could make each less effective or increase the risk of adverse effects.

The following medications may interact with CBD:
- Certain antidepressants, including amitriptyline, citalopram (Celexa), fluoxetine (Prozac), mirtazapine (Remeron), paroxetine (Paxil) and sertraline (Zoloft)
- Gabapentin (Neurontin)
- Certain NSAIDs, including celecoxib (Celebrex) and naproxen (Naprosyn)
- Steroids, including prednisone, prednisolone and hydrocortisone
- Pregabalin (Lyrica)
- Tofacitinib (Xeljanz)
- Tramadol (Ultram)

Some other arthritis medications appear less likely to interact with CBD. These include certain conventional DMARDs, such as hydroxychloroquine, methotrexate and sulfasalazine, and biologic DMARDs, such as abatacept, adalimumab, anakinra, baricitinib, etanercept, infliximab, rituximab and tocilizumab.

Research in this area is still early and ongoing. In addition, some emerging reports show high liver enzyme levels after CBD use. Talk with your healthcare team about the risks of using CBD or other marijuana components as part of your treatment. (For more on topical use of CBD, see page 187.)

Some research shows that used alone or with glucosamine, MSM may lessen symptoms of pain and swelling and improve how well your joints work. But not enough research has been done to indicate if these supplements are helpful for osteoarthritis.

Selenium

Some studies suggest that selenium, a trace mineral with antioxidant properties, may decrease joint pain and inflammation. Other research, however, has failed to show a benefit. More research is needed.

Willow bark

Willow bark contains salicin, an ingredient similar to the active ingredient in aspirin. Yet there's no strong evidence that willow bark can help treat osteoporosis or rheumatoid arthritis. This supplement should not be taken with blood thinners.

ENERGY THERAPIES

Energy therapies center on the belief that illness results from a blockage or disturbance of the free flow of energy through your body. According to this theory, rebalancing your energy fields can restore health and allow healing to occur. Of all the energy-based therapies, the best known and most well studied is acupuncture.

Acupuncture

Originating in China more than 2,500 years ago, acupuncture is one of the oldest forms of medicine in the world. The system is based on a belief that the body contains a vital life energy that runs along pathways within the body. Imbalances in energy flow are thought to cause illness.

The energy pathways, called meridians, are accessible at approximately 400 different locations, or points, on the body. Practitioners of acupuncture attempt to rebalance energy flow by inserting extremely fine needles into these points.

During a typical acupuncture session, the practitioner inserts disposable, sterilized stainless steel needles into the skin. The practitioner may manipulate the needles manually or by electrical stimulation or heat.

A typical acupuncture visit may last from 15 to 60 minutes. Therapy usually involves a series of weekly or biweekly treatments. It's common to have several treatments, which can get expensive if acupuncture isn't covered by your insurance.

Scientists don't fully understand how or why acupuncture works. It's possible that it may work, in part, by stimulating your body's painkilling chemicals, called endorphins. When performed properly by a trained practitioner, it has proved to be safe and effective for various pain-related conditions, including lower back pain, headaches and fibromyalgia.

In a study on acupuncture for osteoarthritis of the knee, people were randomly assigned to get one of three treatments: acupuncture, sham acupuncture or a self-help program. People receiving acupuncture saw a significant decrease in pain and were able to move more easily compared with people in the other groups.

Researchers suggest that acupuncture can complement standard care for knee osteoarthritis. Other studies on the use of acupuncture for arthritis have varied in quality, but most have shown some benefit.

Acupuncture may be particularly appealing to people who can't tolerate side effects from long-term use of NSAIDs, as well as those with moderate to severe pain who don't want to or can't undergo surgery.

Dry needling

Dry needling is a type of therapy often used by physical therapists for intramuscular stimulation. It's also known as trigger point therapy. A needle is inserted directly into tender areas, or trigger points, to try to break up scar tissue and calcifications. The idea behind dry needling is that irritating the surface of the bone may increase muscle relaxation and stimulate faster healing. However, it's not clear how it works, and more study of its use in treating arthritis is needed. In contrast to acupuncture, dry needling is strictly based on Western medicine principles and research.

Magnetic therapy

Many people wear magnets based on the idea that they can help reduce arthritis pain. Static magnets are placed in shoe insoles, headbands and bracelets. They aren't very strong. Electromagnets, on the other hand, are made to be magnetic with the help of electrical current. Devices with these types of magnets are used for health purposes, but it's not clear if they can relieve the pain of rheumatoid arthritis or osteoarthritis much, if at all. Magnets can disrupt implantable defibrillators and pacemakers and shouldn't be used during pregnancy.

Copper bracelets

Some people wear copper bracelets to ease arthritis pain. The practice is based on the thought that your body may not be getting enough copper from your diet, so you might absorb some from the bracelet. However, researchers who have studied their use for both osteoarthritis and rheumatoid arthritis have found that they bring no relief.

Cryotherapy

Imagine walking into something that looks like a sauna, but instead of feeling a pleasant relaxing warmth, the chamber is cooled to minus 148 degrees F or below. The concept is similar to applying ice to an injury to prevent or decrease inflammatory processes that cause swelling. In a cryotherapy chamber, you wear minimal clothing, gloves, a woolen headband covering the ears, a nose and mouth mask, and dry shoes and socks to reduce the risk of cold-related injury. The blasts of freezing air last 2 to 3 minutes.

Evidence is still lacking on the safety and effectiveness of cryotherapy chambers, but some studies suggest benefits for use in sports medicine and in the treatment of inflammatory conditions such as rheumatoid arthritis.

One study found that cryotherapy improved mobility and reduced the intensity of pain in people with rheumatoid arthritis. Other research has recorded a measurable decrease in specific inflammatory markers after the therapy.

Infrared saunas

An infrared sauna is a type of sauna that uses light to make heat. This type of sauna heats your body directly without warming the air around you. Generally, people like saunas because they cause reactions like those caused by moderate exercise, such as vigorous sweating and an increased heart rate. An infrared sauna gives these results at lower temperatures than does a regular sauna.

Many studies have looked at using infrared saunas in the treatment of long-lasting health problems, including arthritis, and found some proof that saunas may help. But larger and more exact studies are needed to prove these results. Meanwhile, no harmful effects have been reported with infrared saunas. So if you're thinking of trying a sauna to relax, an infrared sauna might be an option.

HANDS-ON THERAPIES

Also called manual therapies, this popular group of treatments involves the movement or manipulation of one or more parts of the body. These therapies may relax the tissues surrounding joints, improving blood circulation and joint mobility.

Chiropractic manipulation

A chiropractor may gently manipulate your soft tissues to stop muscle spasms and relieve tenderness. Chiropractors focus on the relationship between the structure and function of joints. If the structure of a joint is not right, then it can't work as it was designed. The American College of Rheumatology (ACR) supports chiropractic therapy for lower back pain. However, due to lack of research support and with potential to harm, the ACR recommends against chiropractic care in management of rheumatoid arthritis.

Massage

You might think of a massage as a luxury limited to exotic spas and upscale health clubs. But massage can be an excellent way to ease arthritis pain and stiffness. During a massage, a therapist uses their fingers, hands, and fists to knead, stroke and manipulate your body's soft tissues

— skin, muscles and tendons. There are many types of massage, and the practice is done in health clubs, salons, massage studios and hospitals.

According to one small study, massage helped lessen pain and increase grip strength in people with rheumatoid arthritis in the arms and shoulders. It may also help people with osteoarthritis in the knee.

Massage can help loosen tight muscles, improve flexibility and reduce stress. Studies show that it can temporarily relieve pain. But if you have painful, swollen joints from rheumatoid arthritis, massaging the area directly may worsen your pain. Any pain that's more than momentary discomfort could mean something is wrong. If you feel uncomfortable, speak up.

Prolotherapy

Prolotherapy is a natural therapy that reduces pain by relying on the body's ability to repair itself. A local irritant, such as dextrose solution, is injected into the soft tissue of a painful joint. The goal is to cause an inflammatory response that kick-starts the body's healing response. This, in turn, strengthens and repairs damaged tissues.

Prolotherapy has been used in many parts of the body, such as the back, knees, shoulders, and various joints and ligaments. Several shots at the site of the injury are usually needed for it to be helpful. Medical professionals who

support using prolotherapy believe that it may help with some chronic musculoskeletal injuries, but how well it works overall is still not known. Irritation at the site of the injections may occur.

ALTERNATIVE MEDICAL AND HEALING SYSTEMS

These complete medical systems are distinct from traditional Western medicine. They typically emphasize the whole person — mind, body and spirit — in treating and preventing disease. The systems are based on customs that may date back thousands of years. Traditional Asian, Native American, African, Tibetan and South American practices fall into this category.

These approaches are based on beliefs that the mind and body have a powerful connection and that the body has the power to heal itself. Alternative systems are individualized; no two people with similar symptoms get the same treatment. For example, you may take a different amount of herbs than someone else.

Ayurveda

Ayurveda dates back thousands of years to ancient India. The aim of ayurvedic medicine is to promote health rather than fight disease. This is done through an emphasis on harmony in body, mind and spirit. Treatment may include fasting, breathing exercises, massage, herbs, meditation and yoga.

Few scientific studies have examined the use of ayurveda in treating arthritis. The existing research has focused on the use of herbal medicine, not other aspects of ayurveda. Some studies have shown that various herbal mixtures may help with osteoarthritis and rheumatoid arthritis. Ayurvedic herbs may help reduce pain and stiffness, but better-designed research is needed to confirm these findings.

Homeopathy

Homeopathy was developed in Germany in the late 18th century. Today it's practiced around the globe. Homeopathy is based on two principles — the law of similars and the law of infinitesimals.

The law of similars maintains that a disease can be cured with a substance that produces similar symptoms in healthy people. According to the law of infinitesimals, the substances used to treat disease are most effective when they're highly diluted to the point that none of the original substance remains. Most homeopathic treatments are highly diluted forms of natural substances, such as plants and minerals.

Some researchers have tried to learn how homeopathic medicines might work. Since the active ingredients in the preparations are so diluted, most scientists are skeptical about their efficacy. A few studies have focused on the use of homeopathy for arthritis. Some indicate that these treatments may improve pain, stiffness, grip strength and other symp-

toms of rheumatoid arthritis. But for osteoarthritis, no studies have found it to be any more effective than conventional treatment.

Because homeopathic medicine mainly involves diluted substances, the risk to your health is likely to be minimal. A bigger concern may be the time and money you spend on something that may not work, while forgoing proven conventional treatment.

EVALUATING INTEGRATIVE THERAPIES

It's easy to become frustrated by the limitations of conventional medicine on treating arthritis. What's the point of using it if it's not going to cure you, right? You may believe that trying an unproven treatment is better than doing nothing at all.

In fact, you may encounter wonderful opportunities to improve your health with integrative therapies. Unfortunately, their practice also attracts a few unscrupulous or fraudulent businesses and practitioners who are ready to prey on people desperate for a cure at any cost.

So, it's important to protect yourself. If you opt to try an integrative approach, your safest bet is to separate the help from the hype. But finding out how effective and safe a therapy is can be hard because many haven't been studied as extensively as mainstream medicine has.

Conventional medicine practiced by most doctors is grounded in the scientific method, which relies on experimentation and established research practices. Before a new therapy is widely accepted, scientists typically publish study results in reputable journals that are reviewed by experts who aren't associated with the study or sale of the product.

Throughout the process, researchers attempt to identify the health benefits and risks of the therapy. They also try to sort effective treatments from the ineffective ones that are enhanced by the placebo effect. The placebo effect happens when someone feels better simply due to receiving treatment of any kind, whether it's a sugar pill or a real medication.

The cyclic nature of rheumatoid arthritis can make it hard to say how effective a treatment is. Because flares and remissions can occur suddenly and for no clear reason, you may be tempted to think that the treatment you just tried is what's making you feel better. This type of "coincidental cure" can be misleading and make a treatment appear more effective than it is.

The symptoms in osteoarthritis also may vary for reasons that are unclear. Changes may occur after a joint is used more strenuously than usual. Or you may see no recognizable cause at all. All these normal variations make it hard to say whether any therapy is working.

With this in mind, it's important to look carefully at a therapy before you try it. Here are some steps to take as you get started:

- *Gather information.* Find out what's known about the safety and effectiveness of any integrative therapy you're considering. Check scientific studies to determine the advantages and disadvantages, risks, side effects, expected results and length of treatment. The National Center for Complementary and Integrative Health (https://nccih.nih.gov) is an excellent resource.
- *Consider the source.* When looking for facts, rely on reputable sources, such as well-known medical schools or healthcare institutions, government agencies, and professional associations or organizations, such as the Arthritis Foundation.
- *Use the internet wisely.* When using the internet for research, look for a site featuring an editorial board or medical advisory board involved with developing its information. Check the dates posted on the site. Outdated information can be wrong and dangerous. Look for a site that regularly updates its information.
- *Know when to be suspicious.* Think twice about any product or practitioner that promises cures, makes claims that sound too good to be true or encourages you to give up conventional treatments. Be wary of terms such as quick cure, miracle cure, new discovery or secret formula. If a cure for arthritis or another disease had been discovered, it would be widely reported and prescribed. Also be suspicious of claims that a product cures a wide range of unrelated diseases, for example cancer, arthritis and AIDS.

In general, when it comes to using a nontraditional practice, try to steer a middle course between uncritical acceptance and outright rejection of the therapy. Stay open to various treatments but evaluate them carefully.

The list of what's considered integrative is ever-changing. Every day, new approaches to healthcare emerge, and what were once fringe therapies become part of mainstream practice. Indeed, many hospitals, healthcare professionals and health insurers are integrating a variety of nontraditional treatments into their services — with good reason.

Talk to your healthcare team about the best natural therapies and your treatment plan. If they are uncomfortable with these practices, ask for a referral to a pharmacist or specialist who can help.

14 Injections

When arthritis causes persistent joint pain, medications and other methods of pain management sometimes aren't enough to bring relief. What if other treatments haven't helped — or helped enough — but surgery still isn't recommended for your circumstances? Joint injections may be another option.

Injecting different substances into the joints can treat arthritis pain in a number of ways. Corticosteroid shots may be able to bring quick and targeted pain relief. Other types of injections can help replace natural lubrication in a joint or can work to boost your body's own ability to heal damaged tissues. Researchers are continuing to explore newer treatments such as stem cell therapy to see how these may help provide joint relief.

This chapter will explore several types of joint injections your healthcare professional may recommend.

CORTICOSTEROIDS

Corticosteroid shots are injections that may help relieve pain and inflammation in a specific area of your body. These shots use a synthetic form of cortisone, a hormone naturally made in your body. Cortisone reduces inflammation by blocking inflammatory molecules.

Cortisone shots are most commonly injected into joints such as the ankle, elbow, hip, knee, shoulder, spine and wrist. Even the small joints in your hands and feet may benefit. The injections usually contain the corticosteroid medication and a local anesthetic. Often you can receive a cortisone shot at your healthcare professional's office.

Cortisone shots are commonly used for several musculoskeletal pains, including osteoarthritis, inflammatory arthritis such as rheumatoid arthritis, bursitis, plantar fasciitis, tendinitis, trigger points, ganglion cysts and carpal tunnel syndrome.

As with any medication, cortisone shots carry a risk of certain complications. These are somewhat different from the side effects of corticosteroids taken by mouth, because the medication is concentrated in one area instead of circulating throughout your body. The risk increases with larger doses and repeated use. Side effects can include:

- Joint infection
- Nerve damage
- Thinning of skin and soft tissue around the injection site
- Temporary flare of pain and inflammation in the joint
- Tendon weakening or rupture
- Thinning of nearby bone (osteoporosis)
- Whitening or lightening of the skin around the injection site
- Death of nearby bone (osteonecrosis)
- Temporary increase in blood sugar

There's concern that repeated cortisone shots might cause the cartilage within a joint to deteriorate. So medical professionals typically limit the number of cortisone shots into a joint. In general, you shouldn't get cortisone injections more often than every 12 weeks and usually not more than three or four times a year.

Receiving the shot

If you take blood thinners, you might need to stop taking them for several days before your cortisone shot to reduce the risk of bleeding or bruising. This is especially true with spine injections, where bleeding can be more serious. Some dietary supplements also have a blood-thinning effect, which may increase your risk of bruising. Ask your healthcare professional what medications and supplements you should avoid before your cortisone shot.

When you go in for the shot, the area being injected will need to be easily accessible to your healthcare team. Tank tops or sports bras give easier access for shoulder injections, and wearing shorts is convenient for knee injections. Your healthcare professional may ask you to change into a gown if the clothing you are wearing makes getting to the site of

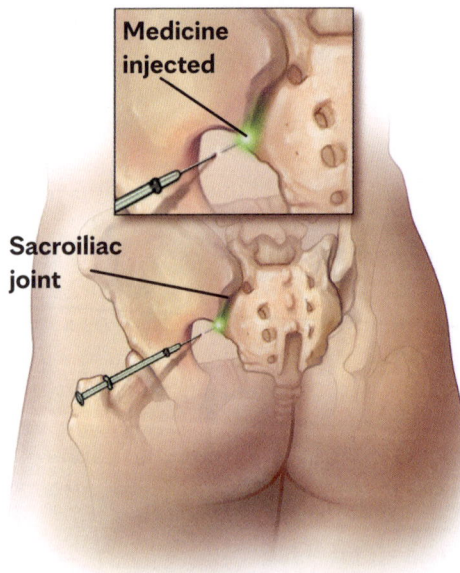

A cortisone shot in the sacroiliac joint may help relieve pain and inflammation in the lower back and pelvis.

injection difficult. You'll then be positioned so that the needle can easily be inserted. The area around the injection site is cleaned, and your healthcare team may also apply an anesthetic spray to numb the area. In some cases, your healthcare professional may use ultrasound or a type of X-ray called fluoroscopy to watch the needle's progress inside your body — to make sure it's placed in the right spot.

You'll likely feel some pressure when the needle is inserted. Let your healthcare team know if you are experiencing a lot of discomfort. The medication is then released into the injection site. Typically, an anesthetic in the cortisone shot provides immediate pain relief, while a corticosteroid medication relieves pain and inflammation over time. Pay attention to your pain relief right after the injection, since a response to the injection, even for a short period of time, lets your care team know that your pain is coming from the joint that was injected.

Some people experience redness and a feeling of warmth in the chest and face after receiving a cortisone shot. The shot also may temporarily increase blood sugar levels in people who have diabetes. If you take insulin, you'll need to pay close attention to your blood sugar level for the first few days after your shot.

Your healthcare team might ask that you take certain steps after the shot to minimize the risk of complications, including:
- Protect the injection area for a day or two. For instance, if you received a cortisone shot in your shoulder, avoid heavy lifting. If you received a cortisone shot in your knee, stay off your feet as much as you can.
- Apply ice to the injection site as needed to relieve pain. Don't use heating pads.
- Watch for signs of infection, including increasing pain, redness and swelling that lasts more than 48 hours.
- It may be recommended not to use a bathtub, hot tub or whirlpool for two days. It's OK to take a shower the day you receive your injection.

The results of cortisone shots typically depend on the reason for treatment. Cortisone shots commonly cause a temporary flare in pain and inflammation for up to 48 hours after the injection. After that, your pain and inflammation in the affected joint should decrease, and the relief can last up to several months. Any increase in pain, redness or swelling around the joint that was injected that does not improve after several days should be reported to your healthcare team.

HYALURONIC ACID

Hyaluronic acid, also called hyaluronan, is a natural substance found in joint fluid. It works by acting like a lubricant and shock absorber and helps the joint work properly. In people with osteoarthritis, natural hyaluronic acid molecules in the joints break down, and their lubricating effect is reduced. This can result in more rapid wearing down of the joints and in pain.

Scientists have discovered other sources for hyaluronan — most commonly, the red combs of roosters. They have discovered ways to extract and purify hyaluronan into a gel for clinical use. Animal-free products also are available. Treatment with this type of shot is commonly referred to as viscosupplementation. So far, the FDA has approved hyaluronan injections only for osteoarthritis of the knee and not for other joints, such as the shoulder or hip.

Injection of this compound into a knee joint affected by arthritis may help improve lubrication of the joint. For many people it can improve mobility and reduce pain, although the effect is usually modest. The injection may work by helping your body to produce more hyaluronic acid and preserve cells in your cartilage. It may also help reduce pain signals and limit your body's inflammatory response. However, more research is needed to prove whether it slows progression of the disease.

This type of injection may be recommended for people with osteoarthritis who are not getting relief from physical therapy and pain medications. It may also be a good option for people who can't take nonsteroidal anti-inflammatory drugs (NSAIDs) or other pain relievers. Usually, people might receive hyaluronic acid injections after trying a steroid shot first.

Receiving the shot

Hyaluronic acid can be given as a single shot or in a series of injections, depending on your healthcare team's preference. If the decision is to use a series of shots, you'll receive one a week for 3 to 5 weeks. You'll see your healthcare team for each one to make sure the injection is given safely and in the right location, as with cortisone shots. And similarly, it's best to avoid putting heavy stress on your knee for a day or two after the shot.

It may take several weeks to notice relief from symptoms. While cortisone shots work faster, relief from hyaluronic acid injections may last longer — up to six months or more.

As with any joint injection, there's a small risk of infection with this treatment. Occasionally, you may have muscle pain, stiffness or swelling in the joint for a day or two. If these symptoms persist, you should contact your healthcare team. But the risk of side effects is low, even with multiple courses of treatment. For many people, hyaluronic acid shots can safely provide better joint function and more manageable pain that may help delay knee surgery for months or years.

WHAT IS REGENERATIVE MEDICINE?

Regenerative medicine deals with the process of engineering or replacing human cells and tissues to help your body function normally. There is growing interest in regenerative medicine, such as stem cell therapy, for people with arthritis and other musculoskeletal issues.

Your body has the ability to heal itself from certain injuries or conditions. For

IS REGENERATIVE MEDICINE THE RIGHT TREATMENT FOR YOU?

Regenerative medicine therapy is a promising area of research and treatment for a wide range of conditions. But it's important to understand that this therapy doesn't work for everyone with joint pain. It's often one of the last treatments tried.

Some studies have shown that regenerative medicine may be helpful for musculo-skeletal and spine conditions. However, the FDA has not yet approved regenerative medicine as a treatment for these uses. In addition, these therapies have possible side effects and complications. Talk to your healthcare professional or a regenerative medicine specialist if you have questions.

You'll also want to talk with your care team about any medications you're already taking and how they may affect regenerative therapy. Corticosteroids can interfere with platelet and stem cell function. They also can affect how well you heal, so you may need to stop taking them several weeks before a stem cell procedure. You may need to stop blood-thinning medications and NSAIDs as well.

Finally, these treatments usually aren't covered by insurance plans, and they can be very expensive. If you have questions about the cost and how to pay for this, ask a member of your care team.

example, think about a paper cut. Within a day or so, most people get a scab at the site of the cut. That scab is the body working to heal the skin and the tissue beneath it. Regenerative medicine relies on the body's ability to heal itself. The goal is to replace or restore human cells, tissues or organs that aren't functioning or healthy to allow the joint to function normally again.

Regenerative medicine is still a relatively new type of treatment, with ongoing research. So far it has been used to treat a variety of musculoskeletal injuries and conditions, such as Achilles tendinosis,

rotator cuff injuries and tennis elbow. Muscle and ligament sprains, plantar fasciitis, degenerative disk disease and arthritis have also been treated by these experimental therapies. Studies are continuing to explore how different types of regenerative medicine may help people with arthritis pain.

Two regenerative therapies are used more commonly to treat joint pain: platelet-rich plasma (PRP) and stem cells from bone marrow aspirate concentrate (BMAC). These innovative procedures are mini-mally invasive, use local anesthesia and don't require a hospital stay.

PLATELET-RICH PLASMA (PRP) THERAPY

In recent years, there has been some enthusiasm that injecting whole blood, or more specifically, plasma, which is the liquid component of your blood, into painful tissues may help with healing and reducing pain. This treatment aims to take advantage of the blood's natural healing properties to repair damaged cartilage, tendons, ligaments, muscles or even bone. Plasma includes platelets, proteins and growth factors. Although not well understood, these growth factors may increase blood flow, provide healing and decrease inflammation.

How does PRP work?

When you're bleeding, your body quickly sends platelets to the injured area. Platelets act like "first responder" cells that form a clot to help stop the bleeding. Platelets contain several factors that are released when the platelet is activated due to tissue injury. These factors help healing by attracting other healing cells, forming a tissue scaffold for healthy tissue to grow into and help increase blood flow to the area by forming new blood vessels.

When PRP is injected into a diseased or injured area affected by arthritis, it works primarily as a natural anti-inflammatory to help decrease the pain caused by arthritis. PRP also has the potential to use the body's natural healing processes to help heal the

damage of arthritis. Multiple studies are evaluating PRP injections into painful areas of the body for treatment of different musculoskeletal conditions such as tendon injuries, plantar fasciitis and osteoarthritis. PRP has been proven to be an effective anti-inflammatory, but its role in healing cartilage remains to be determined.

How is PRP made?

Blood has different components, including:
- Red blood cells: cells that carry oxygen to the body
- White blood cells: cells that work to fight infection

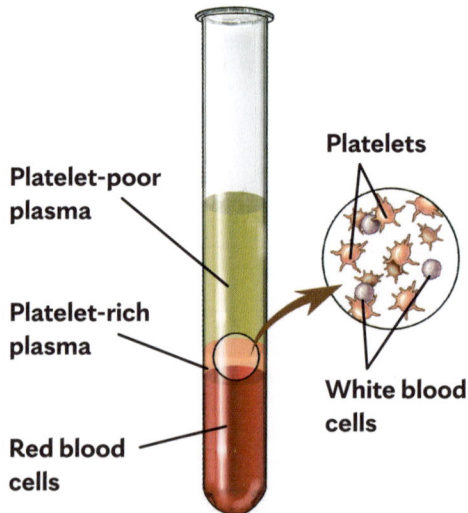

A blood sample is spun in a centrifuge to separate platelet-rich plasma (PRP) for use.

- Platelets: cells that help blood to clot and help the body heal from injury
- Plasma: the colorless, fluid part of blood

The first step in creating PRP is to draw blood from a vein and place it into a machine called a centrifuge. The centrifuge spins the blood at high speeds, separating the platelets from the other blood cells in 30 minutes or so.

The PRP layer is then injected into the arthritic joint, painful tendon degeneration or ligament tears to allow your body to regenerate tissue.

Is PRP effective?

PRP therapy acts very differently from cortisone injections, which simply decrease inflammation and have no healing capabilities. The anti-inflammatory properties of PRP tend to lead to long-standing pain relief compared to cortisone. This is because it potentially helps the damaged or worn-out tissue start to regenerate.

Recent research studies have looked at this treatment, with mixed results. Some people have experienced reduced pain with PRP injections in conditions such as tennis elbow, rotator cuff disease and osteoarthritis. Studies suggest that PRP may provide similar or better relief than hyaluronic acid shots for knee arthritis, and PRP therapy may have a longer-lasting effect. But not all PRP is created equal. There are different preparation and delivery techniques, which can lead to different results.

The FDA hasn't officially endorsed PRP as a treatment for musculoskeletal conditions. But physicians are able to provide this treatment off-label for people who've exhausted other options. Still, more high-quality, controlled clinical studies are needed to determine the best candidates and the most effective techniques before this becomes a more common therapy for joint pain.

STEM CELL THERAPY

Stem cells are cells with the potential of developing into many different cell types. In the body, they can divide and form more stem cells or become specialized cells with a more specific function, such as blood cells, red cells, heart muscle cells or bone cells. No other cell in the body has the natural ability to generate into different types of cells depending on the needs of the body.

In regenerative medicine, researchers and healthcare professionals are studying whether stem cells may be used to generate healthy cells and replace diseased cells. If stem cells can be guided to become specific cells that regenerate and repair diseased cells in people, this process could help with a wide range of diseases.

Stem cells are powerful cells. They can:
- Copy or replicate themselves
- Ooze or secrete anti-inflammatory proteins

- Turn into different types of cells, such as cartilage, bone and tendon

When you are sick or injured, stem cells help tissue heal and regenerate. They also help control any nearby inflammation.

Your bone marrow — the tissue inside your bones — has stem cells and many other cells that help in healing. Blood cells are made in bone marrow. Cells found in bone marrow can be used to treat damaged tissue, improve function and help control pain.

Stem cells are obtained from a concentrated form of bone marrow called bone marrow aspirate concentrate (BMAC). Compared with typical bone marrow, BMAC has more regenerative cells, including stem cells. It also has platelets and growth factors like those found in PRP.

BMAC has been injected into injured joints, tendons, ligaments, muscles, intervertebral disks and other areas.

How is BMAC made?

Bone marrow is most commonly taken from the back of your pelvic bone. While you lie on your side or your stomach, a

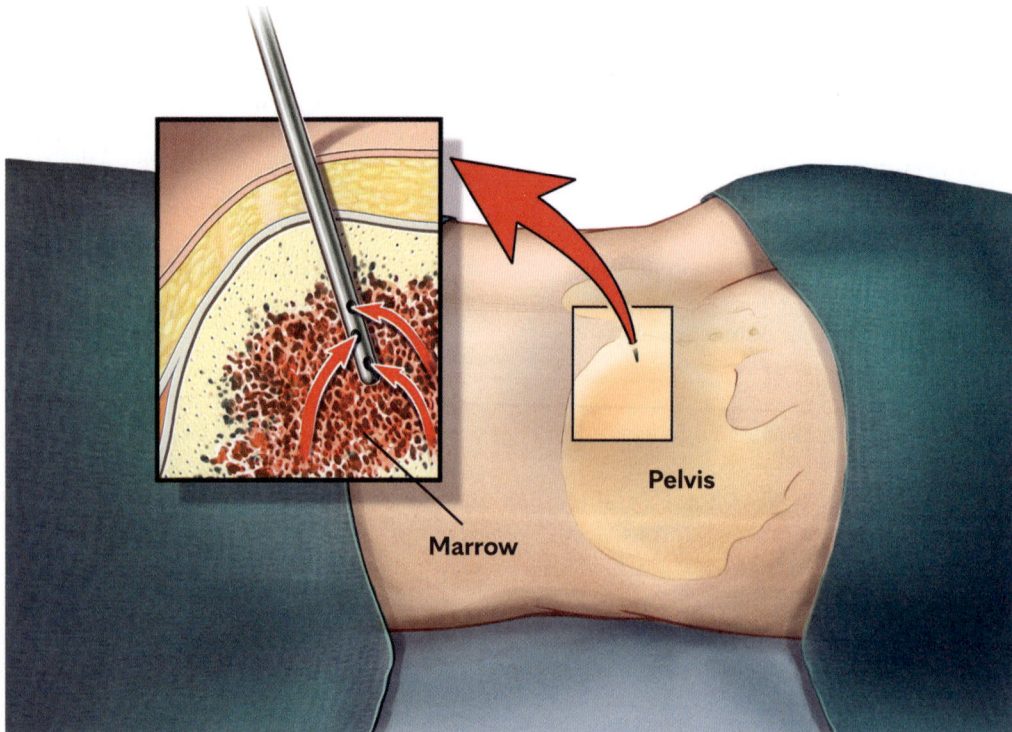

Bone marrow is removed from the pelvis.

member of your healthcare team will locate your pelvic bone with the help of an ultrasound machine or an instrument called a fluoroscope. Your skin will be cleaned, and you'll receive an anesthetic to numb the tissue down to the bone. A special needle is guided into the bone, and the marrow is withdrawn.

The bone marrow is placed in the centrifuge. Spinning the marrow removes much of the fluid and unwanted components, concentrating the bone marrow cells. The result is BMAC.

This process usually takes 30 to 60 minutes, depending on how much marrow was drawn from your bone.

Your healthcare team then uses ultrasound or fluoroscopy to identify the part of your joint to receive the stem cells, and the BMAC is injected into the target area. In all, it takes about two hours to make and inject BMAC.

Promising, but not yet proven

Unfortunately, the excitement surrounding emerging stem cell therapy has led some patients and healthcare professionals to overlook the lack of scientific evidence to support its use at this time. Stem cell therapies currently in use outside clinical studies do not contain pure stem cells. Instead, they include a variety of cells, of which only a very small percentage are stem cells. It is possible that many of these treatments do not contain enough stem cells to be of help.

In addition, many stem cell therapies are now marketed directly to patients. To meet the growing interest, some clinics offer these injections without proper assurance of the contents or quality. Some forms of mislabeled stem cell therapies do not contain any living stem cells. Such practices are cause for concern. While the risks with joint injections are low, misleading treatments used in other parts of the body may cause harm to people looking for relief. They can also delay the scientific progress needed to turn stem cell therapies into cures.

What the research into stem cells and arthritis shows is that there are opportunities for stem cell treatment to be used as injection therapy. It may be used alone or in addition to joint surgery procedures. Successful stem cell therapies thus far have resulted mostly in pain relief and improvement in function or quality of life. Only a few limited early studies have demonstrated improvement in new cartilage or bone formation needed to cure arthritis. Exactly how that cartilage regrowth occurs, or even how pain relief is achieved, is still unknown. That means if you have a stem cell procedure, it will be used to treat only the symptoms of arthritis. This therapy can't yet cure the disease entirely. At this point it is unlikely that someone who needs a total joint replacement will be able to avoid the procedure by using stem cells. The stem cells are simply treating the pain, not correcting the arthritis.

As with other types of regenerative medicine, stem cell treatment for arthritis also isn't covered by most insurance companies. You'll likely pay out of pocket for it, which can be expensive.

Stem cell therapy for joint pain appears to be a fairly safe treatment option. If evidence of its effectiveness continues to grow, it may possibly be used more widely for arthritis in the future. Meanwhile, until the scientific evidence provides proof of its promise, it remains an experimental option that you and your healthcare team might discuss if you haven't been able to manage your joint pain with other treatments.

15 Staying active

Your joints are stiff, swollen and achy. Sometimes it hurts when you stand, get up from a chair or climb stairs. Won't exercise just aggravate these symptoms and make you feel worse?

In fact, it's just the opposite. The idea that you should rest your joints when you have arthritis is outdated. Today, it's clear that movement is good medicine for osteoarthritis, rheumatoid arthritis and many other types of rheumatic disease. Physical activity is not only safe — it can also reduce pain and stiffness while improving your overall health, mood and quality of life.

In addition, physical activity can help fend off the natural loss of joint strength and range of motion that comes with arthritis. Being active helps you perform everyday tasks and maintain your independence. There's no reason not to be as physically active as your abilities and symptoms allow. Exercising at least 30 minutes on most days of the week is recommended.

If that's far more activity than you're used to, you're not alone. Many people don't meet this benchmark — with or without arthritis. But studies show that people affected by arthritis are typically less active than people without joint conditions.

The best plan for arthritis includes aerobic activity, as well as muscle-strengthening exercises, flexibility exercises and balance exercises. If you're already doing some of these things, keep it up. Or, if that sounds overwhelming, just start slowly — every bit helps. Use the tips in this chapter to build up your current activity level, whatever it may be.

BENEFITS OF EXERCISE

Being active has benefits for everyone. It improves sleep, concentration, energy and mood. Regular exercise can also help control blood pressure and cholesterol and may reduce your risk of many conditions, including heart disease, stroke, diabetes and depression. There are additional benefits for arthritis. Regular physical activity can help do all of the following:

Relieve pain and stiffness and increase energy

Regular exercise can triumph over two of the most common problems of arthritis — pain and lack of energy. Studies show that moderate-intensity aerobic and muscle-strengthening exercises can reduce pain and morning stiffness. Exercise improves your balance and boosts your endurance. It may also reduce inflammation.

Protect your bones and joints

Within a relatively short period of time, regular exercise can strengthen the muscles surrounding your joints. This helps stabilize weakened joints and increases flexibility. Stronger muscles may even help compensate for cartilage loss and can improve your range of motion.

Over the long term, exercise can help slow bone loss that leads to osteoporosis, a condition that causes bones to become weak and brittle and susceptible to fractures. Physical activity helps you maintain bone density and offset bone loss that happens naturally as you age. Exercise also helps improve your posture and balance.

Control your weight

Combined with healthy food choices, regular exercise can help you lose weight or maintain a healthy weight. Keeping off extra weight has many health benefits, and it's important for your joints. Excess weight adds stress to your weight-bearing joints, which can aggravate pain, stiffness and inflammation.

Reduce or delay disability

Regular exercise helps you gain strength and agility that can improve your ability to do everyday activities, such as carrying grocery bags and climbing stairs. Keeping up better function helps you maintain your independence and quality of life.

Exercise may also improve some of the workplace limitations that go hand in hand with arthritis. In one study of people with arthritis in the workplace, participants in a six-week walking program saw significant improvements in many aspects of their jobs. They reported less trouble concentrating, crouching or bending, working in awkward positions, moving objects, and standing for long periods of time.

Improve your mood

People with arthritis are at higher risk of anxiety and depression. Getting regular physical activity can help to reduce these mood disorders, relieve stress and improve your overall well-being.

You don't have to expend hours of hard work and sweat to get these health benefits. Any activity is better than no activity. And the more active you can be, the more it can help you.

GETTING STARTED

If you haven't been active for a while, starting an exercise program may be a challenge. You may feel some pain and stiffness at the beginning. You may be worried about hurting yourself. Or you just may not have much confidence.

Luckily, you don't need a lot of equipment to be active, and you don't have to log a lot of hours at the gym if that's not your thing. Your healthcare team can help design a simple program that caters to your needs, interests and capabilities.

Be patient with yourself. Your first few exercise outings may not be easy, but try to stick with it. For many people with arthritis, it takes 6 to 8 weeks to establish a routine and to see the health benefits. With the following guidelines, you'll be on your way.

Talk to your healthcare team

Before you begin or change an exercise routine, discuss your plans with your healthcare team. They can recommend specific exercises and precautions based on your abilities and symptoms. Your healthcare team may also suggest that you meet with a physical therapist or an occupational therapist. These profession-

als are trained to help people find ways to move effectively. A therapist who is experienced at working with people who have arthritis may be very helpful. They can show you how to modify exercises to make them work better for you.

Gather your equipment

Choose activities that are fun for you, and select the appropriate equipment. If you're planning to exercise on land (as opposed to in the pool), the most important piece of equipment is a comfortable, supportive pair of athletic shoes that are appropriate for the exercise you choose. Look for shoes with plenty of room in the toe box, especially if you have joint deformities such as bunions or hammertoes. Then check the sole. You want a thick, supportive sole for shock absorption. Some people with arthritis get a better fit with shoe inserts. Be sure to replace your shoes before they wear down and cause foot pain. This often occurs after walking or running approximately 500 miles.

Depending on what activities you enjoy, you may also benefit from specialized equipment, for example, a recumbent bike or special handles for golf clubs. You don't need to spend a lot of money on fancy equipment, though. Walking is free, and it's one of the best exercises for arthritis.

Exercise at the best time of day

Generally speaking, exercise whenever it's best for you. Try to loosen up with gentle exercises first thing in the morning. It's usually best to avoid exercising right after you eat. Also, keep in mind that exercising 5 to 6 hours before bedtime may help you sleep better and feel less stiff in the morning.

Start slow and focus on mechanics

Some people with arthritis are glad if they can take a step or two. Maybe you can easily walk several miles. Start wherever you are and build up gradually. Your goals will be different from those of someone else with arthritis.

If you haven't been physically active for a while, begin with 5 or 10 minutes of walking at a time. As you become more fit, increase the frequency, duration and intensity of your walks. Build slowly and gradually, allowing enough time for your body to adjust to each new level before adding more. Because of your arthritis, it may take you three or four weeks to adjust. Walking in a pool may help you build endurance, as the water relieves some of the pressure on your weight-bearing joints.

Keep your goals manageable. Perhaps you can walk only a minute each day at first. But if you add a minute each week, you'll be walking nearly an hour each day after a year. Doing several short sessions of activity throughout the day, such as three 10-minute walks, can have similar benefits to a longer exercise session.

Remember that body mechanics and positioning during exercise are very important. Poor positioning or body mechanics can make joints more painful or cause swelling. Some positions may be stressful to certain joints. Your doctor or physical therapist can show you how to adapt standard exercises so that they are comfortable for you.

Modify, modify, modify

Arthritis symptoms will tend to vary from day to day. On some days, you'll feel great — as if you could keep walking or swimming forever. On other days, you may feel like ditching your regular workout because you feel more pain and stiffness and have less energy due to fatigue.

On those tough days, try to modify your activity and stay as active as possible. It can be difficult to resume your routine after days of inactivity. So it's better to modify your plans than skip them entirely. For example:

- If you don't feel up to a 30-minute walk, try to accumulate 30 minutes of walking in shorter stints throughout the day.
- If it's painful to walk on a hard surface, try riding a bicycle or walking in a swimming pool.
- If you skip your walk, you can still do your flexibility exercises.
- Remember, any activity is better than no activity.

Know when to slow down

It's important to listen to your body carefully when you have arthritis. You'll

INCREASING YOUR ACTIVITY LEVEL

Start with less intense activity and get accustomed to it before attempting more intense exercise. To build up, increase your exercise in this order.

Frequency: The number of days you exercise a week

Duration: The length of each activity session

Intensity: How hard you're working

When you're ready, interval training is a good way to add intensity to your workout. This technique involves alternating short bursts of higher-intensity activity with periods of lower-intensity activity. For example, you might alternate walking quickly with walking at a leisurely pace. If you're a swimmer, try alternating a couple of fast laps with a couple of slow laps. Start with just one or two higher-intensity intervals per session, each lasting only 30 seconds. Gradually build up to 3 to 5 higher-intensity intervals per session on nonconsecutive days. You can also gradually increase the length of the higher-intensity intervals to 1 to 2 minutes each.

Interval training is an especially effective way to build your cardiovascular fitness. And by adding bursts of higher-intensity activity, you can reap the benefits of exercise in less time.

learn by trial and error how much exercise is too much. Pay attention to how you feel before and after each session. Do you feel the same or better? How about two hours — or two days — later?

It's normal to feel some new aches and pains in your joints and surrounding muscles during and after exercise, especially during the first 4 to 6 weeks of starting a new exercise program. However, if you have increased pain in the joints affected by arthritis or you experience new pain that lasts for two hours or more after you exercise, you may need to slow down a little and adjust your routine.

You can start by taking care of your acute symptoms. That may involve a little rest and taking an over-the-counter pain reliever as needed.

The next time you exercise, break up the activity into smaller segments or reduce the intensity or number of repetitions. Also think about your mechanics. Are you performing an activity in a way that aggravates your condition?

To minimize pain, make sure you're using good equipment and good posture. Try changing your activity to lower the impact on your joints.

Be sure to do a proper warm-up and cooldown every time you exercise. You can warm up your muscles with a warm shower or bath, heat packs, or massage to reduce stiffness before exercising. Just don't apply heat to an already inflamed joint.

At the end of each session, finish with slow, easy movements. After exercise, it may help to apply either heat or cold to affected joints for 10 to 15 minutes.

If you're not regularly taking an anti-inflammatory medication and heat and cold don't relieve your pain, you can try taking aspirin, ibuprofen (Advil, Motrin IB, others) or acetaminophen (Tylenol, others) one hour before exercise. These can help limit swelling and reduce pain. Just avoid mixing medications or over-medicating. You don't want to mask pain that warns you to stop.

If you're already treating arthritis pain with daily medications and you can't exercise without pain, you may need the help of a physical therapist. They can help develop an exercise plan that is best for you.

If exercise brings on a sharp cramp or muscle pain, gently rub and stretch the muscle until the pain subsides. Don't exercise joints that are tender, injured or severely inflamed.

Most people with arthritis can exercise safely. You don't have to give up on exercise at the first sign of discomfort. Adjust your routine and backtrack as needed. But stay focused on your goal of regular activity.

YOUR WEEKLY WORKOUT

To get relief from your symptoms and maintain strength and range of motion in your affected joints, you'll need to develop a well-rounded exercise program.

WHEN TO CALL YOUR HEALTHCARE TEAM

Introduce new activities gradually, and pay attention to warning signs. Call your healthcare team if you experience:
- Pain that is sharp, stabbing or constant
- Pain that causes you to limp
- Pain that persists for a few days despite rest, medication, or hot or cold packs
- Joints that are extremely swollen, red or "hot"

Seek emergency medical attention if you experience:
- Chest pain
- Severe shortness of breath
- Faintness, dizziness
- Nausea
- Discoloration in your arms or legs

Your starting point may be nothing more than a walk around the block, but eventually you should try to include the following components in your weekly routine:

Aerobic exercise Work up to at least 30 minutes on most days (150 minutes of moderate-intensity aerobic exercise every week).

Strength training and balance exercises Aim for at least three days a week, taking care not to work the same muscle group two days in a row.

Mobility exercises Stretch for 15 minutes every day.

Even if you can't always meet these activity goals, it's important to be as active as you can. And it's OK if you have to change your activity levels from week to week, depending on your arthritis symptoms.

Aerobic exercise

When you're doing aerobic activity, you're repeatedly moving large muscles in your arms, legs and hips. You breathe faster and deeper, which maximizes the amount of oxygen in your blood. Your heart beats faster, which increases blood flow to your muscles.

For the greatest health benefits, the U.S. Department of Health and Human Services recommends that most adults get at least 150 minutes a week of moderate-intensity aerobic activity, or 75

minutes a week of vigorous activity. Aim for either goal — or an equivalent combination of moderate and vigorous activity — if your arthritis allows. If not, be as active as you can. Especially if you're older, it's important to know your limits for safe activity.

Regular aerobic activity provides both short-term and long-term benefits for arthritis. It can reduce pain and joint tenderness while improving aerobic capacity and mobility. Aerobic activity is also important for burning calories and controlling your weight.

Studies investigating the benefits of various types of aerobic activity, such as walking, running, cycling, aquatics and aerobic dance, have declared no clear winner for arthritis symptoms, so choose the activities you like best.

Focus on joint-friendly activities that don't twist or pound your joints. Some people with arthritis are able to tolerate high-impact activities, such as running, basketball, tennis or aerobics. But these activities may aggravate your symptoms. If you're just getting started, stick with activities that are easy on the joints, such as walking, bicycling, water exercise or dancing. Elliptical machines and stationary bikes may also be good choices if they're available.

Whatever activity you choose, always allow time to warm up with some gentle range-of-motion exercises. Begin with a slow, steady rhythm. Don't jerk or bounce. Maintain good posture while you exercise.

As comfortably as you can, work up to a pace that gets your heart pumping a little harder and makes your breathing a little faster but still allows you to carry on a conversation. For the last 5 to 10 minutes, slow down and let your muscles and heart rate return to normal.

To meet the recommended aerobic activity goals, be creative about how and when to exercise. Walk on a treadmill or use an exercise bike while watching TV. Walk with a friend or your family after dinner. Schedule exercise into your day as you would an important appointment.

Although sustained, continuous exercise may provide the greatest benefit, you don't need to do all your exercises at one time. Break up the activity into smaller sessions if you need to.

As mentioned earlier in this chapter, begin any aerobic exercise program gradually, slowly increasing the intensity and length of your workouts. Try to build up to at least 30 minutes of aerobic activity five or more days a week, adding a minute or two at a time.

If you're comfortable with your level of activity and want an additional challenge, gradually increase to 45 or 60 minutes five days a week. This level of activity provides additional health benefits.

It may help to use an exercise journal, a smartphone app or an activity tracker such as a watch to help you log your progress.

Strength training and balance exercises

Another component of your program is to do muscle-strengthening and balance exercises 2 to 3 days a week. Always warm up first, with 5 to 10 minutes of stretching or gentle aerobic exercise. Be sure not to work the same group of muscles two days in a row so that the muscles have time to recover.

Choose a mix of activities that build strength and balance. Some activities — such as yoga and squats — are good for both. Other activities are more targeted at one area of fitness than at another.

Strength training exercises

As muscles become stronger, they provide better joint support. Strong muscles can also take some of the pressure off painful joints and contribute to better overall joint function. People with arthritis who do regular strength training exercises report less pain and stiffness and better quality of life.

Strength training is often done with free weights or weight machines. But strength training can also be done in your living room using inexpensive, lightweight resistance tubing, your body weight, or even canned goods from your pantry. Isometric exercises, which involve no movement, can be especially beneficial for people with arthritis. In the pool, the water can provide resistance for strength training. Talk to your healthcare team about the strength exercises that are best suited for your joints and symptoms.

MIX AND MATCH FOR BETTER HEALTH

Try to be active for at least 30 minutes on most days. Even three separate 10-minute bursts of activity can add up to a lot of calories burned. Bits of activity lasting less than 10 minutes can help improve your health, too — anything is better than nothing!

Activity	Calories burned in 10 minutes of activity*
Ballroom dancing, slow	37
Basketball game	97
Bicycling (less than 10 mph, leisurely pace)	48
Bowling	37
Elliptical trainer, moderate effort	61
Fishing	43
Gardening	46
Golfing (carrying clubs)	52
Jogging (5 mph)	100
Light housework, such as sweeping	28
Swimming laps, slow crawl	71
Swimming, treading water	43
Walking (2 mph, strolling)	34
Walking for exercise (3.5 mph, brisk pace)	52
Yoga (hatha)	30

*Calories are based on a 160-pound person. If you weigh less than 160 pounds, you need to spend more time to burn the same number of calories. If you weigh more than 160 pounds, the calories burned would be somewhat more. Adapted from Ainsworth, BE, et al., 2011 compendium of physical activities: A second update of codes and MET values, *Medicine and Science in Sports & Exercise,* 2011; doi:10.1249/MSS.0b013e31821ece12.

Balance exercises

Tai chi, yoga, Pilates, backward walking, side stepping and standing on one foot are good examples of balance exercises, also called body awareness exercises. These activities can improve your posture, balance, sense of joint position, core strength and coordination. Some also provide stress relief and relaxation.

Balance exercises are particularly important if you are worried about falling or if your age, medical history or arthritis symptoms increase your risk. If you have knee arthritis, the condition may cause muscle weakness that can increase your risk of falling.

Many group classes include some balance exercises. Or you can do balance exercises at home — even while brushing your teeth! For example, you can do the hip exercise on page 237 at your bathroom sink.

Mobility exercises

Mobility exercises are at the core of a good exercise program for arthritis. These stretching and range-of-motion exercises counteract the stiffness that arthritis causes in your joints and spine.

Performing these exercises daily can help maintain or improve your flexibility in the affected joints and surrounding muscles. In turn, this helps reduce your risk of injury and improve joint function, which makes daily activities and other forms of exercise easier.

Pick a regular time to do mobility exercises at least once a day — for some people, doing them in the evening reduces morning stiffness the next day. You'll need 5 to 10 repetitions of each mobility exercise once or twice a day to maintain your range of motion and flexibility.

If you're trying to increase range of motion and flexibility in a joint that has lost motion or is tight, you may need more repetitions or more daily sessions. Talk to your healthcare professional or physical therapist if you need help.

EVERY MOVE COUNTS

Take advantage of opportunities to get up and move around throughout the day — normal daily activities add up. You get health benefits from taking out the trash, cleaning, shopping, vacuuming, making the bed and mowing the lawn. But consider these activities a supplement to, not a substitute for, your regular exercises. And don't forget to balance these tasks with rest.

You can boost your exercise total by increasing physical activity in your routine daily tasks. Park your car farther away from your destination and walk a little farther. Or walk your dog farther than just around the block.

EXERCISE GUIDE

You may benefit from some of the exercises illustrated on the following pages. Your healthcare team can help identify the best set of exercises for your arthritis.

Exercises for strength and balance

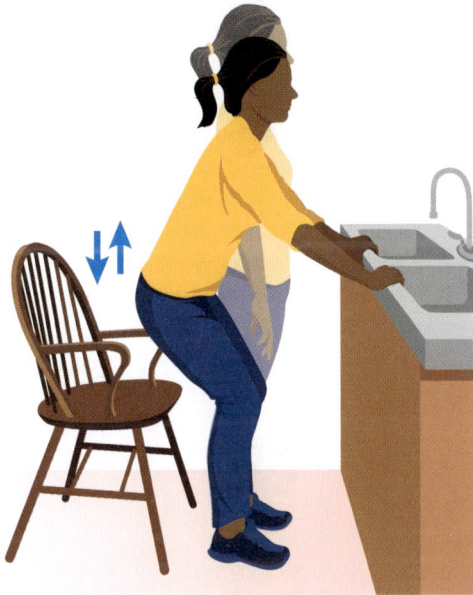

Squats

Stand with a sturdy chair behind you. Hold onto a counter for support. Breathe out as you sit back and squat down as far as you can comfortably go. Keep your knees in line with your toes, making sure they don't fall forward. Hold the position for five seconds. Inhale as you return to standing. Relax and repeat. As you build strength, hold the squat for longer or squat down farther.

Sit-to-stand

Sit in a sturdy chair that has arms. Keeping your spine straight, raise yourself up off the chair without using your arms or hands to assist you. Keep your knees over your toes during the motion. Relax and repeat. If your legs are weak, you may need to push your body up using your arms or hands for assistance. Skip this exercise if it causes pain to your hands, wrists or elbows.

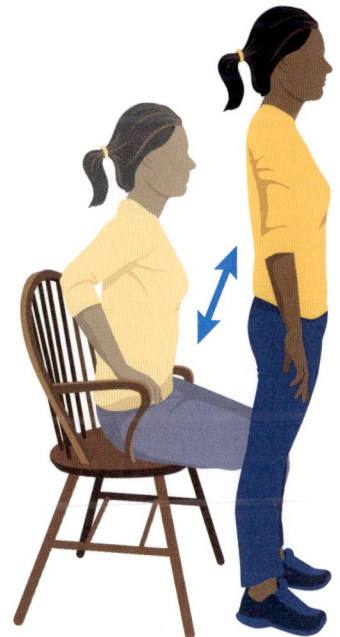

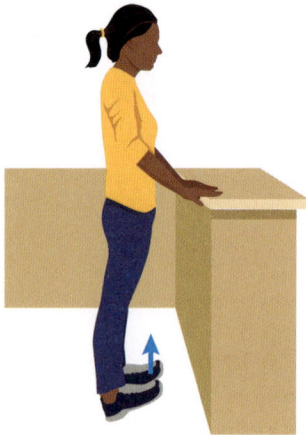

Toe lift

Stand with your feet as wide as your hips. Hold onto a counter for support. Keeping your heels firmly planted, lift your toes as high as you can. Lower your toes and repeat.

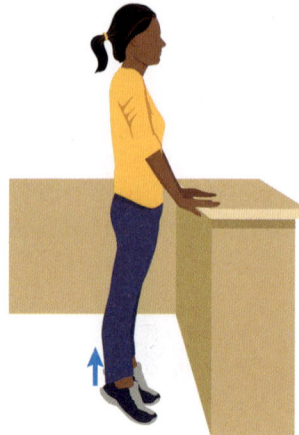

Heel lift

Stand with your feet as wide as your hips. Hold onto a counter for support. Keeping your toes firmly planted, lift your heels as high as you can. Lower your heels and repeat.

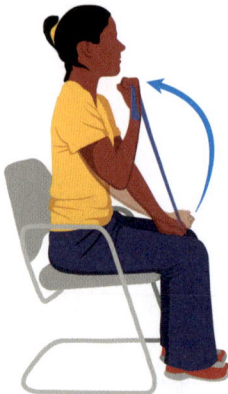

Biceps strengthening

Sit in a chair with a length of resistance tubing. Grasp one end of the tubing in each hand and place your hands on your knees, with palms up and arms straight. Pull upward with one arm. Slowly return to the starting position and repeat with the other arm.

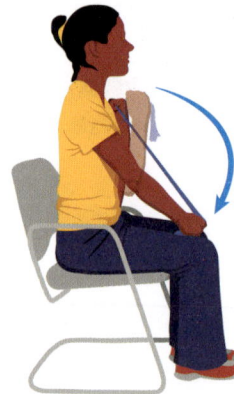

Triceps strengthening

Grasp one end of the resistance tubing in each hand at shoulder height, with thumbs up and elbows bent. Straighten one arm toward your knee, keeping your elbow at your side. Slowly return to the starting position and repeat with the other arm. Stand with your feet as wide as your hips.

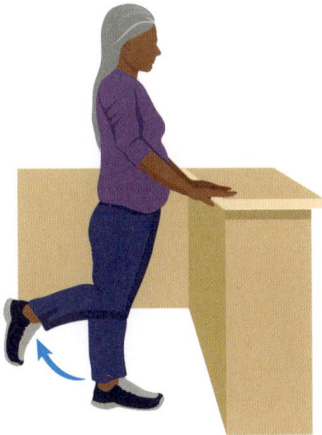

Knee bend

You may want to hold onto a counter for support. Slowly bend one knee, bringing your heel up toward your buttocks, and hold for a few seconds. Return to the starting position and repeat with the other knee. To help improve balance, stand in place for progressively longer periods of time with your knee bent.

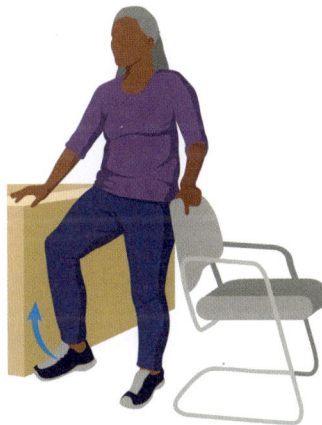

Standing march

Stand between a counter and a sturdy chair. Hold onto the counter and chair for support, if needed. Keep your spine straight and slowly march in place, lifting your feet as high as you can.

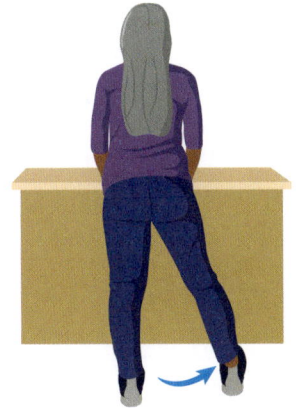

Hip swing

Stand with your feet shoulder-width apart. You may hold onto a counter for support. Slowly swing one foot off the floor to the side, as far as you can, and hold. Keep your spine neutral and do not allow it to bend, twist or rotate during the hip-swing motion. Return to the starting position and repeat with the other foot. To work on balance, remove one hand from the counter.

Exercises for mobility

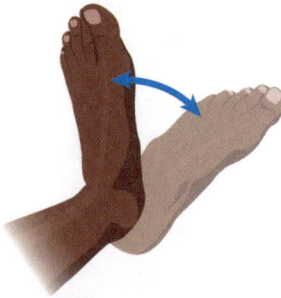

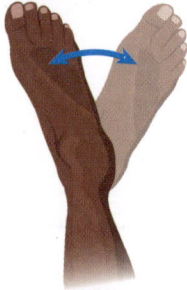

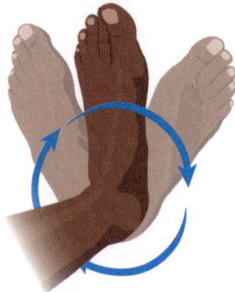

Ankle rotations

Sit or lie down with your legs out in front of you and your heels on the floor. Bring the toes of one foot toward you, then push them away from you (top). Move your toes to one side and then to the other side (middle). Move your foot in a circle in one direction, then the other direction (bottom). Repeat with the other foot.

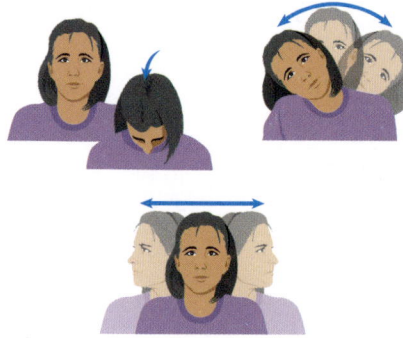

Neck stretch

Tilt your chin forward and down to your chest. Next, tilt your ear toward one shoulder and then the other, without raising your shoulders. Finally, keeping your neck, shoulders and spine straight, turn your face side to side.

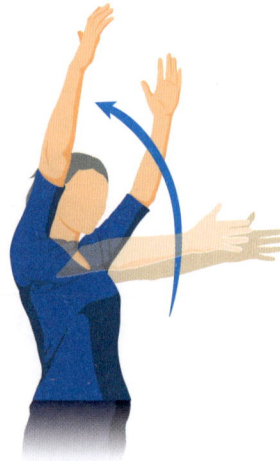

Overhead arm raise

Stand with your arms straight out at chest height. Gently raise your arms over your head. Lower them back to the starting position. Relax and repeat. For a variation, start with your arms out to the sides, palms facing forward.

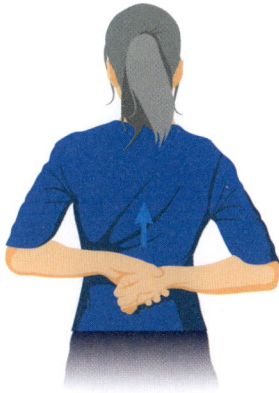

Behind-the-back stretch

Grasp your wrist behind your back. Gently pull your arm up until you feel a stretch in your shoulders. Relax and repeat. Switch arms.

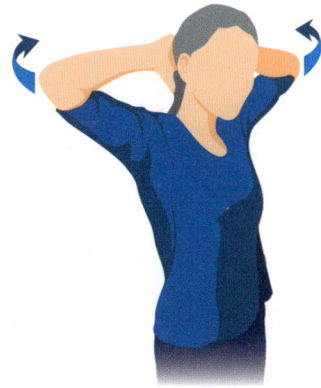

Shoulder blade squeeze

Place your hands on the back of your head. Pinch your shoulder blades together by moving your elbows back. Hold briefly. Relax and repeat.

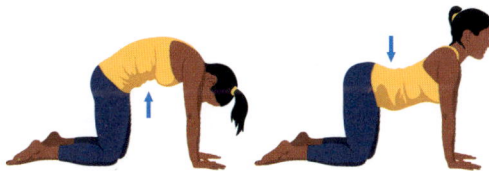

Cat stretch

Get on your hands and knees. Arch your back away from the floor and then let it sag toward the floor. Focus on your middle to lower back, where the motion should be taking place. Don't arch your head back too far. Relax and repeat. If you have hand or wrist arthritis, you may not be able to tolerate this position.

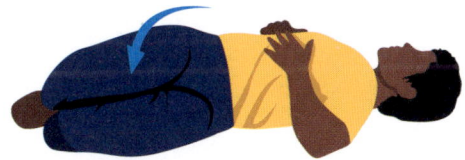

Lumbar rotation

Lie on your back, with knees bent and feet on the floor. Gently roll your knees to the left, all the way to the floor if you can. Hold this position for a few deep breaths. Return to the starting position. Then roll to the right. Repeat.
Lie on your back, with your knees bent and

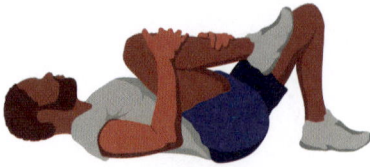

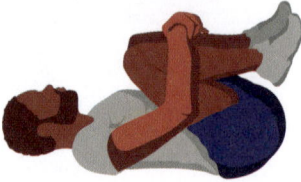

Lower back stretch

Pelvic tilt

your feet on the floor. Keeping your lower back on the floor, lift your right knee and hug it toward your chest, using your hands (top). Hold this position for a few deep breaths. Repeat with the left knee. Then hug both knees (bottom). If knee pain is aggravated by this exercise, place your hands behind the knee joints when pulling your knees toward your chest.

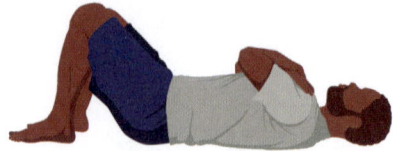

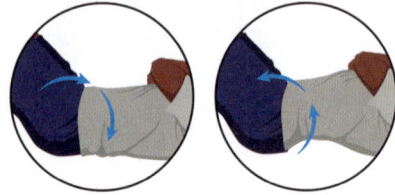

Lie on a firm, flat surface with your knees bent. Tighten your abdominal muscles to flatten the small of your back against the surface (lower left). Release tension in your abdominal muscles to arch the small of your back (lower right). Slowly return to the starting position.

Hand exercises

Arthritis is a cause of pain and deformity in the many small joints of your hands and fingers. Daily exercises can help maintain your strength, mobility and range of motion in these joints.

Knuckle bend

Hold your hand straight with your fingers close together. Bend the end and middle joints of your fingers. Keep your knuckles straight. Slowly return your hand to the starting position. Repeat multiple times, then switch hands.

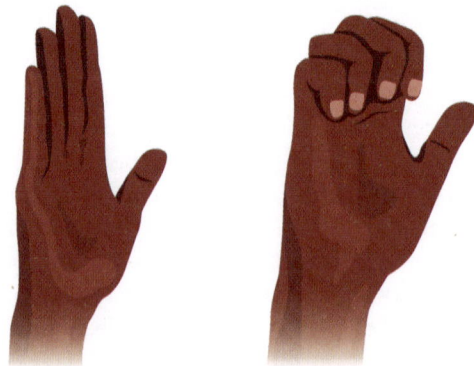

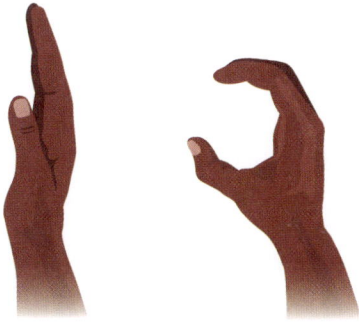

Thumb stabilization

Hold your hand straight with your fingers close together. Gently curve your fingers into a C shape. Slowly return your hand to the starting position. Repeat and switch hands.

Thumb stretch

Hold your hand in a relaxed position with your fingers straight. Bend your thumb across your palm, touching the tip to the base of your smallest finger. If you can't make your thumb touch, stretch it as far as you can. Return your thumb to the starting position. Repeat and switch hands.

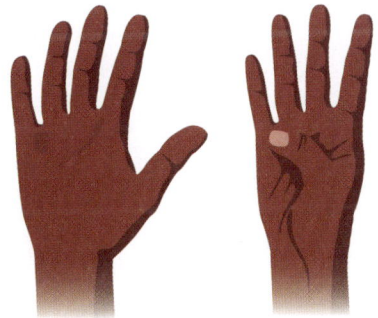

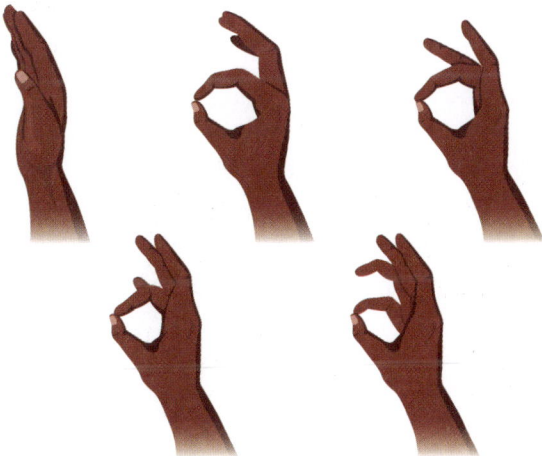

Fingertip touch

Hold your fingers straight and close together. Slowly form an O shape by touching your thumb to your index finger. Then follow with your middle, ring and smallest fingers. Repeat this exercise and switch hands.

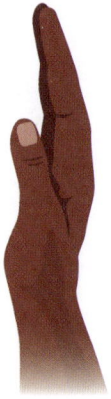

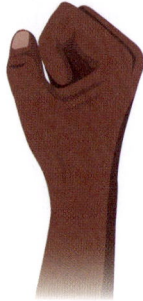

Closed fist

Hold your fingers straight and close together with the side of your wrist and hand resting on a table-top. Close your fingers into a gentle fist, wrapping your thumb around the outside of your fingers. Don't squeeze. Slowly return your hand to the starting position. Repeat and switch hands.

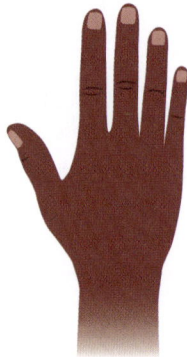

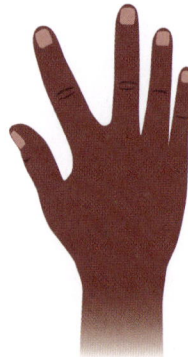

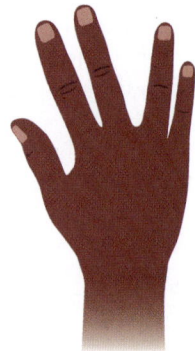

Finger walk

Rest your hand on a tabletop with your palm facing down. Move your thumb away from your fingers. Beginning with your index finger, move it toward your thumb. Follow with your middle, ring and smallest fingers one at a time. Repeat and switch hands.

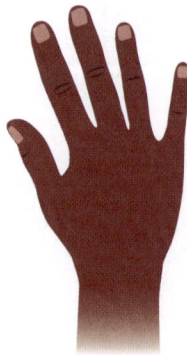

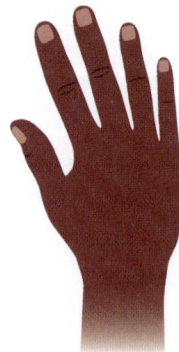

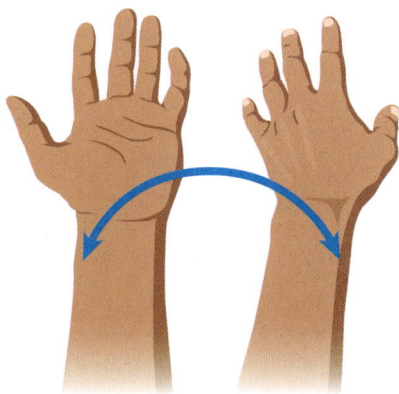

Forearm twist

Hold your forearm out with your palm up. Slowly rotate your forearm, turning your thumb up and over. Rotate back to the starting position. Relax and repeat. Switch arms.

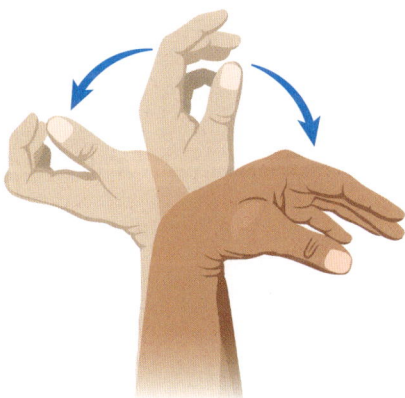

Wrist stretch

Hold your wrist out away from your body with your thumb pointing toward the ceiling. Bend your wrist so that your palm is facing you. Hold briefly. Then bend your wrist so your palm is facing away from you. Hold briefly. Repeat and switch wrists.

TAILORING YOUR PROGRAM

Your healthcare team can provide you with guidelines and recommendations for activity. These may be based on the type of arthritis you have, the severity of your symptoms and your health goals. Make sure you understand their recommendations and restrictions. (Ask questions until you do!) Then choose workouts that you enjoy and that are convenient for you.

You'll be more likely to stay motivated if you figure out what it takes to get you moving. What interests you? What's fun? The following options are good choices for exercising with arthritis. Combine them to create a well-rounded exercise plan that meets all your activity goals.

Group exercise programs

Some people enjoy participating with others in exercise programs and classes designed for people with arthritis. Group programs may be a good fit for you if you're feeling hesitant to take charge of your own activity plan or if you would feel safer getting started under the guidance of a trained instructor. You'll also like these programs if you find support in working out with people who have similar symptoms and challenges to yours. Groups can be a great source of motivation and new friendships.

On the other hand, maybe you'd prefer to swim in solitude. Consider your personality and social comfort level before signing up for a group class.

Many communities offer a range of classes and activities tailored for people with arthritis, including special walking events, regular walking programs, tai chi, aquatic classes and more. Group exercise programs vary — some meet once a week and others take place more often. Some programs focus on aerobic exercise, while others combine a mix of activities.

Figure out how group exercise fits your weekly exercise goals and plan other

FINDING A GROUP PROGRAM

The Arthritis Foundation has developed several exercise programs for people with arthritis, including walking, tai chi and warm-water aquatic exercise. These programs are offered in communities across the country. Programs are led by certified instructors and can be modified to meet your needs. Search online to find a Walk With Ease program or another Arthritis Foundation exercise program in your area. Community and fitness centers also may offer tai chi and other group programs.

Many kinds of exercise instruction are available online, through streaming services and on DVD. If there isn't an instructional class available in your community — or if it doesn't work with your schedule — you can find videos you like and exercise from the comfort of your own living room.

activities accordingly. Your physical therapist or another member of your healthcare team can provide information about options in your area.

Walking

If you can walk comfortably, then a walking program is your best bet for a starter aerobic exercise. It's an excellent activity for overall conditioning. It improves cardiovascular health and bone density. Walking also helps to nourish your muscles and joints. And it leads to improved mobility, strength and balance, all of which help keep stumbles from becoming falls.

Walking is inexpensive and usually convenient — it can be done almost anywhere and anytime. At first, walk only as far or as fast as you feel comfortable.

Plan a route that's close by and accessible. Being able to step out the door to start your walk is both convenient and motivating. Use stores, downtown areas or public spaces as destinations. Or see if a local shopping mall caters to walkers. Many large malls allow walkers in the early morning hours before retail stores open their doors. This may be a good option when it's too hot, too cold, rainy or icy outside.

Choose a walking route that's varied. Make it interesting, but don't involve too many stops, turns and busy intersections. You'll benefit most from a sustained, steady stride. Note where there are uneven sidewalks, inclines, loose gravel or dirt paths to help you avoid falls.

Make personal safety a priority. Walk in the daytime or in well-lit areas. Carry a cell phone or a whistle with you.

Tai chi

The Chinese martial art of tai chi was developed more than 1,000 years ago. Today, people continue to use this exercise to relax and strengthen muscles and joints and reduce tension.

Tai chi combines slow, deliberate circular movements and postures with deep, regular breathing that can increase circulation, relax the mind and body, and ease chronic pain. Studies show that this practice may be particularly helpful for osteoarthritis of the knee.

When learned correctly and practiced regularly, tai chi is an excellent source of balance and mobility exercises. But it will take a commitment of time and effort. You can use videos to learn tai chi or look for classes in your area. Local health clubs, recreation departments and martial arts centers may offer tai chi classes. Some are designed specifically for people with arthritis.

Water exercise

If pain and stiffness make it difficult for you to exercise, a warm-water exercise program may do wonders for you. These programs typically take place in pools heated to between 83 and 88 F. The buoyancy of the water reduces the weight that your joints, bones and muscles have to bear. And the soothing warmth relaxes your muscles, which may decrease muscle spasms and tightness. Combined, these factors decrease joint pain while building strength, range of motion and aerobic fitness — all in one class.

Many health clinics, gyms and local swimming pools offer aquatic exercise classes. You don't have to be a good swimmer to participate. Once you're comfortable exercising in the water, you can ease your way into land-based activities.

Sports and other activities

If you enjoy sports and are comfortable doing them, don't let arthritis slow you down. Discuss your interests with your healthcare team. You might enjoy swimming, biking, cross-country skiing, golfing or tennis. With good judgment and a little creativity, you can make many favorite activities work for you.

Just remember to modify the activities as needed. Ask your care team for assistance. If you golf, you might try playing nine holes of golf instead of 18. Use a golf cart instead of walking. Play in a scramble tournament on a team so you're not hitting every ball yourself. If you have hand or finger arthritis, try using molded golf grips on your clubs. They provide cushion and surface tack for an easier grip and help absorb the impact of hitting a golf ball.

Mixing different athletic activities into your workout, a practice known as cross-training, is a good way to keep exercise boredom at bay. Cross-training may also reduce your chances of injuring or overusing one specific muscle or joint.

STAYING MOTIVATED

When you have arthritis, regular exercise isn't about having bigger biceps or enduring more miles. It's an essential therapy for minimizing stiffness and pain, maintaining or improving your range of motion, and building muscle strength around affected joints. These are important accomplishments!

The key to exercise motivation is that it has to be personal. The reasons that help you stay active day after day and week after week should be your reasons and not someone else's. How do you discover your inner motivation? Start by asking yourself a simple question: "What can exercise do for me?"

You may need exercise to help relieve your symptoms, such as pain and fatigue — that's the most common motivation. Perhaps there are specific tasks that you want to continue doing, for example, being able to raise your arms above your shoulders in order to brush your hair or grasp buttons when putting on a shirt. Maybe you're interested in maintaining a high quality of life for as long as you can, for example, so you can continue living independently at home.

Maybe the idea of living with a chronic disease has scared you a little bit. Use that emotion to your advantage — fear is a great motivator. The point is that there are no wrong reasons for going out to exercise, as long as they are your reasons. The best motivation comes from within you, and without that internal drive, any long-term goal will be difficult to achieve.

Be sure to note any changes that may occur in your symptoms or in your physical capabilities while you're active. And celebrate success when you reach your goals — even the minor ones.

Of course, there will be days when you feel frustrated, discouraged or unenthusiastic. Here are tips for sticking with your activity goals:

Use realistic strategies

Set measurable activity goals at the beginning of each week, such as walking for 30 minutes on five days or attending your first water aerobics class.

Review your progress at the end of the week. Did you achieve your goals? If so, congratulate yourself and set new goals for the following week. If not, ask yourself if the goals you set were achievable. Then set more realistic goals for the next week.

Find an exercise buddy

Knowing that someone is expecting you to show up in the park or at the gym is a powerful incentive to get moving. Working out with a friend, co-worker or family member can bring a new level of motivation to your workouts.

Enlist your family's support

You'll need your family's help to make time to exercise and to provide support on the days when you're feeling sluggish. Ideally, you'll be able to do things together, too. Plan family outings that include swimming or walking.

Reward achievements

Reward yourself for small accomplishments. Treat yourself to a massage, an hour to yourself, a movie or a new book.

Enjoy the outdoors

If you love fresh air and nature, go outside and be active. Check out different parks for walking or biking.

Finally, always have a Plan B to fall back on. The normal ebb and flow of arthritis symptoms can put a kink in your best-laid exercise plans. If you scheduled a tennis lesson for Wednesday morning or a bike ride for Friday afternoon, you may feel defeated if symptoms flare during these times and you can't stick with your commitments.

Flare-ups can also get in the way as you try to increase your level of physical activity. Every time you take two steps forward, it may seem that your symptoms push you two steps back.

This is an undeniable challenge that you'll likely face. It's how you respond to the challenge that makes all the difference. For long-term success, you may need several strategies at the ready to solve problems as they arise.

To do that, it helps to plan ahead. Try to identify the barriers that are most likely to stop you from exercising: Your work schedule is unpredictable, you struggle with motivation, you don't like to exercise alone or you worry about injury.

Once you've identified the most common barriers, try to come up with specific solutions that may remove or change them. Maybe you can carve out an extra period of time for exercise each week, in case your regular schedule suddenly fills up. Or maybe you can keep an easy exercise video to follow at home during times when you're not feeling well.

Come up with your own solutions to potential roadblocks. The benefits of physical activity are worth it.

16

Eating a healthy diet

You might expect treatment for joint pain to involve your doctor's office, the pharmacy and perhaps physical therapy. But what about the grocery store? Or your daily lunch stop? The food choices you make can have a significant effect on your overall health and well-being, especially if you have arthritis.

To feel healthy, it's important to eat well. That doesn't mean you have to count calories or that you can never eat french fries or chocolate chip cookies. Rather, try to choose healthy foods most of the time. In fact, instead of focusing on limiting or avoiding foods, you may want to focus on adding healthy foods and habits to your routine.

Strive for a flavorful, balanced diet based on plant foods. It's your best bet for fighting inflammation, increasing your energy and controlling your weight — all of which can help to reduce your symptoms of arthritis.

DIET AND ARTHRITIS

A healthy diet can increase your energy, brighten your mood, improve your job performance, and lower your risk of heart disease, high blood pressure and diabetes. It's also beneficial for arthritis. A healthy, plant-based diet, emphasizing fruits, vegetables, whole grains, low-fat dairy products and lean proteins, can help:

- *Minimize arthritis symptoms and medication side effects.* Fruits, vegetables and foods made from whole grains contain beneficial vitamins, minerals, fiber and compounds called phytochemicals. These healthy compounds are associated with reducing inflammation, which can be a primary cause of pain and discomfort. Fruits and vegetables are also naturally low in calories and sodium and high in potassium. That makes them a good choice if you're coping with side effects of arthritis medications, such as fluid retention and weight gain.

- **Support bone strength.** You're at increased risk of developing osteoporosis if you have a type of inflammatory arthritis or connective tissue disease, such as rheumatoid arthritis or lupus, or if you take corticosteroid medications. Getting enough calcium and vitamin D in your diet through low-fat dairy products may help slow bone loss and reduce your risk of suffering a fracture.
- **Promote a healthy weight.** Most plant foods are relatively low in calories, so a plant-based diet can help with weight control. Maintaining a healthy weight is good for your overall health, but it's especially important when you have arthritis. That's because excess weight adds stress to your weight-bearing joints, especially your knees, which can aggravate pain, stiffness and inflammation.

You'll learn more about these three benefits as you read this chapter. And you'll learn how to use the Mayo Clinic Healthy Weight Pyramid to help you make smart food choices to help control your arthritis. You can find more information on the pyramid on pages 252-260, but the basic idea is simple: Use the shape of the pyramid to help you select healthy foods. Eat most of your food from the food groups at the base of the pyramid and less from the groups at the top.

It's best to see your healthcare professional before you begin any healthy weight plan.

REDUCING ARTHRITIS SYMPTOMS

For people with arthritis, the old saying "You are what you eat" tends to ring true. Many people with rheumatoid arthritis find that the food they eat plays a role in the severity of pain and other symptoms they experience.

Scientists and physicians have long suspected a connection between nutrition and arthritis, too. Early research dating back to the late 1920s looked for food allergies among people with arthritis. Today, research seems to indicate a direct link between diet and inflammation. Researchers have found different ways that some foods may offer protection against inflammation, while other foods may trigger or exacerbate the inflammation process.

A great deal of study is now focused on identifying particular foods that fall on either side of the inflammation equation. Researchers are still trying to understand exactly how foods may contribute to — or help — arthritis symptoms. Meanwhile, the following theories can help guide your eating choices.

Protection against inflammation

Research shows that some fats and certain nutrients or compounds found in foods may reduce the pain, inflammation and joint tenderness caused by rheumatoid arthritis.

Foods considered to be the most beneficial are part of an overall healthy diet, so there's no reason to wait for conclusive studies before eating more of these foods. To help reduce inflammation and pain, eat foods that contain these substances:

Omega-3 fats

Prepare more meals with cold-water fish, such as tuna, salmon, mackerel and herring, which are rich in omega-3 fatty acids. Walnuts, chia seeds, ground flaxseed and soy foods (tofu, edamame, and soy-based milk, yogurt or cheese) also are good sources of omega-3s. These inflammation-fighting unsaturated fats seem to modify the inflammatory process and may play a role in regulating pain. Although extra virgin olive oil doesn't contain omega-3s, it's been shown to have anti-inflammatory properties, too. (For more on omega-3s in fish oil supplements, see page 203.)

Antioxidants

Antioxidants are dietary substances that may help protect cells from damage. These substances appear to slow oxidation, a natural process associated with inflammatory arthritis that leads to cell and tissue damage. Common antioxidants include vitamins C and E, carotene, lycopene, and flavonoids.

In general, the most colorful vegetables and fruits have the highest levels of these substances. Think of spinach, kale, beets, blueberries and cherries. Studies have shown that blueberries, cherry juice and pomegranate juice — all rich in

flavonoids — can improve knee arthritis pain and decrease inflammation. Other foods that are rich in antioxidants include beans, nuts, green tea, red wine, dark chocolate, cinnamon, ginger root and turmeric powder. However, supplements containing antioxidants don't seem to have a similar effect.

Fiber

Dietary fiber — found mainly in fruits, vegetables, whole grains and legumes — includes the parts of plant foods that your body can't digest or absorb. Fiber passes relatively intact through your digestive system, and it's probably best known for its ability to prevent or relieve constipation. But diets high in fiber can provide other health benefits as well, such as reduced inflammation. The fiber feeds bacteria in your digestive tract, improving the diversity and balance of your gut bacteria. A healthier gut has been shown to help reduce inflammation in people with arthritis. In addition, eating high-fiber foods may help you reach or maintain a healthy weight and lower your risk of diabetes, heart disease and some types of cancer.

Special diets

In addition to studying specific nutrients, scientists have been investigating whether certain diets can reduce the severity of rheumatoid arthritis.

Some research suggests that following a vegetarian or vegan diet may be benefi-

TESTING YOUR SYMPTOMS

Arthritis symptoms vary from day to day, so it can be difficult to determine if particular foods are affecting how you feel. In general, red meats, processed sugary foods and fried foods tend to be associated with inflammation.

For a small number of people with arthritis, it's possible that sensitivities to certain foods — even foods considered healthy, such as dairy products or nightshade vegetables including potatoes and eggplant — may trigger or worsen symptoms.

If you believe that a particular food increases arthritis symptoms, you might try a test: Drop the item from your diet for a short time and then resume using it again. Note whether the change affects your symptoms. However, don't omit whole food groups or a large number of foods without first consulting a registered dietitian or your healthcare professional. Without proper guidance, you could become deficient in nutrients that are important to maintaining good health. This, in turn, could affect your arthritis symptoms. Be skeptical of any diet that eliminates an entire group of foods or stresses only a few foods while eliminating others.

cial. While research is ongoing, several studies have found that following a vegan diet for as little as three weeks is associated with lower levels of C-reactive protein, a marker of inflammation.

Researchers have also been exploring whether a gluten-free diet may help with arthritis. Some studies have found that after following a gluten-free vegan diet, people with rheumatoid arthritis had reduced symptoms or markers of inflammation. It's not clear if those effects are due to avoiding gluten, eating a vegan diet or other factors. Some people do notice improved joint symptoms after going gluten-free — including people with celiac disease. However, more study is still needed.

The Mediterranean diet is one of the most widely studied. Overall it's considered very healthy, and research has found many anti-inflammatory and disease-fighting benefits. This way of eating emphasizes vegetables, fruits, whole grains, nuts, fish, legumes and healthier types of oils such as olive oil. Meanwhile, it limits red meat and sugary or processed food. Studies suggest that the diet helps curb inflammation, which may relieve joint pain and stiffness. It has also been shown to protect against heart disease and other chronic diseases, including dementia and certain cancers. It may even help you live longer.

Research has also suggested that intermittent fasting may help with arthritis symptoms. Intermittent fasting means that you don't eat for a period of time each day or week. For losing weight, intermittent fasting seems to be about as effective as any other type of diet that reduces overall calories. In addition, some research suggests that intermittent fasting may be more beneficial than other diets for reducing inflammation and improving conditions associated with inflammation. Those include arthritis, along with Alzheimer's disease, asthma, multiple sclerosis and stroke. Still, intermittent fasting can have unpleasant side effects and isn't for everyone.

Work with your healthcare professional or a registered dietitian as you make the switch to a special diet or eliminate certain foods in order to ensure that you're getting all the nutrients you need.

THE MAYO CLINIC HEALTHY WEIGHT PYRAMID

The Mayo Clinic Healthy Weight Pyramid is built on the underlying principle of energy density — the amount of energy, measured in calories, in a given amount or volume of food. Foods that form the base of the pyramid, such as fruits and vegetables, are low in energy density. Most of them have few calories in a relatively large amount of food. In contrast, foods at the top of the pyramid are high in energy density. They have a lot of calories in a relatively small amount.

The pyramid helps you focus on foods that provide a lot of volume and nutrients without overloading on calories and unhealthy fats. As a result, you'll eat well and feel full while losing or maintaining weight. Plus, you reap the benefits of the nutrient-rich foods that make up the bulk of the pyramid.

Here's a closer look at the six food groups that make up the pyramid.

Vegetables and fruits

Vegetables and fruits share many attributes. They offer a wide array of flavors, textures and colors, as well as many disease-fighting nutrients.

Most vegetables and fruits are also low in energy density. They are high in water and fiber, which provide no calories. You can improve your diet simply by eating more vegetables and fruits in place of other foods.

Vegetables

Vegetables include a wide array of plant foods: roots and tubers, such as carrots and sweet potatoes; salad greens, such as lettuce and spinach; and broccoli, kale, cabbage and many more. Other plant foods, such as tomatoes, peppers and cucumbers, are included in this group, although they're botanically considered fruits because they contain the seeds of the plant.

Vegetables contain no cholesterol, and they are naturally low in fat, high in dietary fiber and generally low in calories. In addition, they're low in sodium and high in essential minerals such as potassium and magnesium. This makes them a good choice to help offset fluid retention or weight gain that may be caused by arthritis medications.

Another benefit of vegetables is that many of them are great sources of inflammation-fighting antioxidants. In general, the more colorful the vegetable is, the higher its antioxidant levels. Good examples include red bell peppers, beets, tomatoes, carrots, and dark green vegetables, including kale, spinach, broccoli and Brussels sprouts.

Fresh, frozen and canned vegetables are all good sources of nutrients. However, canned vegetables may be high in sodium because sodium is used as a preservative in the canning process. If you use canned vegetables, look for labels that indicate that no salt has been added, or rinse the vegetables before using them.

Fruits

Any food that contains seeds surrounded by an edible layer is generally considered a fruit. As with vegetables, you want to eat a variety of colorful ones. Strawberries, raspberries, blueberries, apples,

MAYO CLINIC HEALTHY WEIGHT PYRAMID

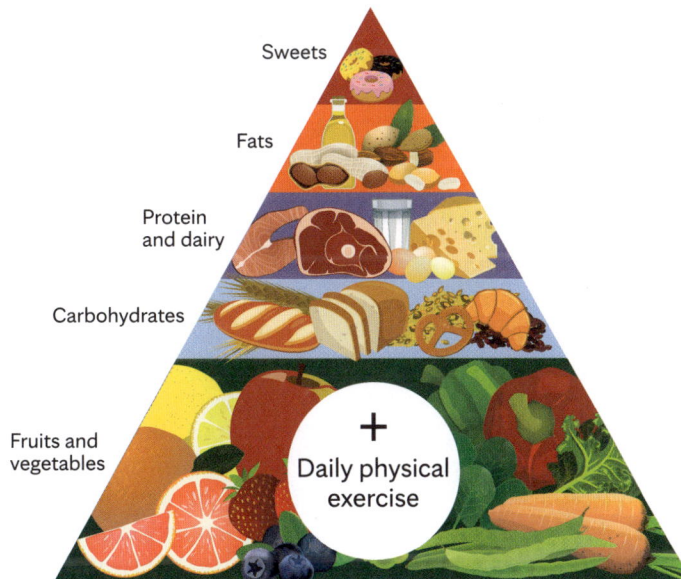

In many ways, the recommended diet of the Mayo Clinic Healthy Weight Pyramid is similar to the Mediterranean diet. Both are plant-based with an emphasis on fruits and vegetables, and both encourage whole grains over refined grains. Both include a moderate amount of fish and lean animal protein, such as poultry and dairy. And both diets encourage healthy fats such as olive oil over other forms, and limited but high-quality sweets.

oranges, peaches, plums, grapes, melons, mangos and papayas are all flavor-packed, nutritious powerhouses.

Like vegetables, fruits are great sources of fiber, vitamins, minerals and other phytochemicals. The most colorful fruits tend to have the most antioxidants. And since most fruits have a sweet or sweet-tart taste, they're good options as healthy snacks or dessert.

Fresh fruit is best, but frozen fruits with no added sugar and fruits canned in water or their own juices also are great choices. Because of processing, fruit juice and dried fruits, such as cherry juice, raisins or dehydrated bananas, can be a concentrated source of calories. They still provide some nutrients, but it's best to measure your portion.

Carbohydrates

Carbohydrates are your body's main energy source, and they are found in a wide range of foods. Most carbohydrate foods are plant-based. They include grain products, such as bread, cereals, rice and pasta. This food group also includes certain starchy vegetables, such as potatoes and corn.

Which kind of carbs should you eat? Think of all the carbohydrate-containing foods placed in a straight line. At one end are oats, brown rice and whole wheat flour. In the middle you'll find potatoes, white rice, white flour and pasta. And at the other end are highly processed products such as cookies, candies, french fries (or fried potatoes), chips, and soft drinks.

The foods in this lineup incorporate all three kinds of carbohydrates: fiber, starch and sugar. It's not hard to identify the healthiest and least healthy sections — less refined whole grains on one end, highly refined sugar on the other end.

The health benefits of many of the items in the middle aren't as clear. The nutrient value of foods such as rice, pasta, bread and potatoes vary and can shift depending on how they're processed and served.

Consider, for example, white and whole-grain breads. Both begin as nutrient-rich grains, typically wheat. With white bread, however, the grain's bran and germ are removed, taking away many natural vitamins and almost all the fiber. That's why it's best to choose whole-grain breads, because most of the vitamins and fiber are retained. The same goes for whole-grain pastas and cereals as well as brown rice. Similarly, the edible skins often removed from potatoes and sweet potatoes are full of nutrients and fiber.

When choosing carbohydrates, the key term to look for on labels is *whole*. Generally, the less refined a carbohydrate food, the better it is for you. Whole grains are particularly important if you have diabetes or you take corticosteroid medications, because they can help slow down the rise in blood sugar as you digest them. Better control of your blood sugar may also help reduce inflammation, which can help improve arthritis symptoms.

TIPS FOR USING THE PYRAMID

Although it may seem difficult at first to adapt to a new healthy-eating plan, it will become part of your routine with time and practice. Here are tips to make this new approach work for you:

- *Plan by the week.* You may find it more efficient and less stressful to plan menus for the next 3 to 7 days rather than figure out what you're going to eat one day at a time — or at the very minute you step into the kitchen to start preparing a meal.
- *Focus on the produce.* If you're a meat-and-potatoes eater, the pyramid's focus on fruits and vegetables may be a challenge. Try filling the biggest part of your plate with vegetables at dinnertime while moving the meat to the side. Snack on vegetables and fruits that require little preparation, such as baby carrots, cherry tomatoes, bananas and grapes. Or try making your regular soups, pastas and casseroles with less meat or no meat. Try adding extra vegetables, beans or other legumes instead.
- *Make pleasure a priority.* You may have to cut back on some of your favorite foods to lose weight and curb inflammation. But you don't have to sacrifice your enjoyment of eating. Be sure to include the flavors, colors and textures you enjoy at every meal. If you have a sweet tooth, try satisfying it with naturally sweet fruit. If you're a chocolate lover, opt for small bits of dark chocolate, which has more antioxidants than milk chocolate does.
- *Adapt menus to the season.* Use the freshest foods available for your meals — asparagus, peas and cherries in late spring, tomatoes, corn and peaches in the summer. Recently harvested produce is often available at local farmers markets. And produce is generally cheapest when it's in season.
- *Look for shortcuts.* As you adapt to a new way of eating, make it as simple as possible. Try buying pre-cut vegetables and fruits, bagged salads, and precooked meats such as a rotisserie chicken or canned tuna. You can also try using shredded low-fat cheeses and frozen vegetables and fruits to save on prep time and see what works for you.
- *Don't forget convenience.* You don't have to cook every meal from scratch. Keep convenience foods, such as a favorite frozen entrée or side dish, on hand for those days when there's little time to fix meals. Just be selective about what you choose. Read the nutrition labels carefully.
- *Be flexible.* Every food you eat doesn't have to be an excellent source of nutrition. It's OK to eat high-fat, high-calorie, inflammatory foods on occasion — sometimes it may be your only option. Your main goal is to choose foods that promote good health most of the time.

Protein and dairy

Protein is essential to human life. Your skin, bones, muscles and internal organs are made up of protein, and it's present in your blood, too. Protein is often associated with animal products, but it's also found in plants.

Choose proteins from animal products wisely. All meats, including chicken and fish, contain cholesterol. And many cuts of meat, as well as poultry products with the skin on, can be high in saturated fat, which can increase inflammation. Red meat has also been associated with inflammation. If you're used to eating a lot of red meat, try to eat it less frequently and only in small portions (about 3 ounces). Fill up on healthy foods such as vegetables, fruits and whole grains so that smaller portions of meat are enough.

You also get protein, as well as calcium, from dairy products. Low-fat dairy products have the same nutrients as whole-milk versions, but with less fat and fewer calories. Good choices include vitamin D-fortified low-fat milk and yogurt. Vitamin D works with calcium to protect your bones, which is especially important when you have arthritis.

Of course, if you have a milk allergy or you're lactose-intolerant, you'll want to get these nutrients from other sources, such as lower-lactose or lactose-free milk and plant-based milks. Eating dairy increases inflammation in people with milk allergies.

Research has been somewhat mixed on how dairy foods affect arthritis. Saturated fat in cheese and high-fat dairy products is thought to increase inflammation. But in a recent large review, researchers found that eating dairy

10 WAYS TO SPOT A BOGUS "ARTHRITIS DIET"

While some foods may have anti-inflammatory effects, there is no quick-fix diet for arthritis pain. Approach any product, diet pill, supplement or expensive diet plan with a healthy dose of skepticism. Steer clear of diets that promote:

1. Rapid weight loss
2. Permanent weight loss without an ongoing maintenance program
3. No need for exercise
4. Unlimited quantities of your favorite foods
5. Strict, rigid restrictions on entire food groups
6. Lists of "good" and "bad" foods
7. Lists of "right" and "wrong" food combinations
8. One-size-fits-all recommendations that ignore differences among individuals or groups
9. Claims that sound too good to be true
10. Simplistic conclusions drawn from a complex study or clinical trial

WHAT'S A SINGLE SERVING?

One serving is not always the same amount of food. Knowing what a serving is can help you align your eating habits with the Healthy Weight Pyramid or other dietary goals.

Vegetables	Visual cue	
1 cup cut-up vegetables	1 closed fist	
2 cups raw, leafy greens	2 closed fists	

Fruits	Visual cue	
1 small apple or medium orange	Tennis ball	
½ cup sliced fruit	Tennis ball	

Carbohydrates	Visual cue	
½ cup whole-grain pasta or cereal	Cupped handful	
½ small whole-grain bagel	Front of a fist	
1 slice whole-grain bread	DVD	

Protein and dairy	Visual cue	
2½ ounces chicken or 3 ounces of fish	Deck of cards	
1½ ounces lean beef	½ deck of cards	
1½-2 ounces of hard cheese	⅓ deck of cards	

Fats	Visual cue	
1 tablespoon peanut butter	1 thumb	
1 teaspoon butter or margarine	Tip of thumb	

products actually had an anti-inflammatory impact overall.

Legumes, which include beans, peas and lentils, also are good sources of protein.

Legumes are typically low in fat, contain no cholesterol, and are high in protein, fiber, folate, potassium, iron and magnesium. They're a great substitute for meat in soups and stews. And they may help reduce inflammation.

Finally, fish and shellfish are good sources of protein, and some also contain omega-3 fatty acids. Omega-3s can help lower triglycerides — fat particles in blood that can raise your risk of heart disease. Omega-3s may also improve the function of your immune system, help regulate your blood pressure, and reduce inflammation and arthritis pain. Research suggests that most people would benefit from eating at least two servings of fish a week.

Fats

Fats are essential to the life and function of your body's cells. Along with providing reserves of stored energy, fats help maintain cell structure. They also play a role in immune system functioning and the regulation of many body processes, including some processes associated with inflammation. In short, you need some fat in your diet.

The key is that you want the right quantity and quality. The fat group near the

A RISK OF BEING UNDERWEIGHT

Being overweight can worsen the symptoms of arthritis, but for people with rheumatoid arthritis there's also risk in being too thin. In a study conducted at Mayo Clinic, researchers found that people with rheumatoid arthritis who had a low body mass index (BMI) were three times more likely to die of cardiovascular disease than individuals without rheumatoid arthritis who had a normal weight. It's likely that people with the most severe forms of rheumatoid arthritis have an active and extensive inflammatory response, which can be associated with weight loss. For these individuals, the best course of action may be finding a healthcare team that will pay close attention to cardiovascular disease prevention and care.

If your BMI is normal or low (refer to the table on page 265), it's also important to be careful as you make healthy changes to your diet or eliminate foods that seem to trigger your symptoms. Sometimes these changes can result in unexpected weight loss. Talk to your healthcare professional or dietitian if you lose weight without trying.

top of the Mayo Clinic Healthy Weight Pyramid refers to fats that are typically added to foods during preparation, not the fat within foods in the other groups. These added fats include cooking oils, spreads and salad dressings. Some plant foods that are rich sources of fat also fit in this category, including avocados, olives, seeds and nuts.

There are several different kinds of fat in food. In terms of their healthfulness, not all fats are equal. Monounsaturated and polyunsaturated fats are the best choices. Look for products with little or no saturated fats, and avoid trans fats. Just remember that all fats are dense sources of energy — even the healthiest ones. Eat them in moderation.

Monounsaturated fats

These fats are found in olive oil, flaxseed oil, peanut oil and canola oil, as well as most nuts and avocados. This type of fat helps reduce low-density lipoprotein (LDL) cholesterol and helps clear arteries by maintaining high-density lipoprotein (HDL) cholesterol. In addition, extra virgin olive oil contains antioxidants, and canola and flaxseed oils and some nuts also contain omega-3 fatty acids — poly-unsaturated fats that may help reduce inflammation.

Polyunsaturated fats

These fats are found in plant-based oils such as safflower, corn, sunflower and soybean oils. Cold-water fish, such as

salmon, provide omega-3s — a heart-healthy form of this fat.

Saturated fats

Saturated fats are found in animal-based foods, such as meats, poultry, lard, egg yolks and whole-fat dairy foods.

They're also in coconut oil, palm oil and other tropical oils, which are used in coffee creamers, snack crackers, commercial baked goods and other processed foods. Saturated fat is the main dietary culprit in raising blood cholesterol and narrowing the heart's coronary arteries. These types of fats are also associated with inflammation.

Trans fats

Small amounts of trans fats occur naturally in dairy and meat products. The main dietary sources of trans fat, though, are processed foods made with partially hydrogenated oil. This type of fat has been used in stick margarine and vegetable shortening and in foods made with them, including many cookies, crackers and cakes, as well as candies, snack foods and deep-fried foods. Trans fat raises "bad" (LDL) cholesterol levels and lowers "good" (HDL) cholesterol levels, along with other harmful effects. Like saturated fats, trans fats seem to be associated with increased inflammation.

In 2015, the FDA determined that partially hydrogenated oil is no longer generally recognized as safe, and it has

GOUT AND DIET

Gout is a complex form of arthritis characterized by sudden, severe attacks of pain, redness and tenderness in your joints. It occurs when there's too much uric acid in your blood, a condition called hyperuricemia. Your body produces uric acid when it breaks down purines. Purines are substances made naturally in your body. They're also found in certain foods, such as organ meats, anchovies, herring, asparagus and mushrooms.

Normally, uric acid dissolves in your blood and passes through your kidneys into your urine. But sometimes your body produces too much uric acid. In other cases, the kidneys don't get rid of enough uric acid.

To prevent gout attacks and to reduce the risk of other chronic conditions associated with gout, such as heart disease, try the following tips:

- *Limit red meats.* Red meats such as beef, pork and lamb can increase the level of uric acid in your blood. Organ meats (liver, brain and kidney) are particularly high in purines. Because all meat, including poultry, contains purines, limit meat to a few ounces daily. To get protein in your diet, eat low-fat dairy products, nuts, beans and peas.
- *Eat fish and seafood in moderation.* Although fish and seafood are heart healthy, both have been linked to higher uric acid levels and gout. Eating moderate (4-ounce) portions of fish and seafood twice weekly may have benefits overall. You can also get the benefits of omega-3 fatty acids found in fish from plant foods such as ground flaxseed, chia seeds, soy foods and walnuts.
- *Cut back on fat.* High-fat meals contribute to obesity, which is linked to gout. Some evidence suggests they may trigger inflammation

been phased out of the production of foods. However, some foods that were manufactured outside the United States may still include trans fats.

Sweets

Foods in the sweets group include sugar-sweetened beverages, such as sodas, as well as candies, cakes, cookies, doughnuts and other desserts. And don't forget the table sugar you add to tea or coffee.

Sweets are typically a dense source of calories, mostly from sugar and fat. Yet they offer very little nutrition. In addition, sweets can cause spikes in blood sugar, which can lead to problems if you have

- *Reduce or avoid alcohol.* Alcohol interferes with the elimination of uric acid from your body. Beer and liquor have each been linked to an increased risk of gout attacks, even in moderate amounts. One recent study found that drinking wine also was associated with gout attacks, although previous research had not shown a link. To play it safe, limit or avoid all types of alcohol.
- *Prioritize whole foods.* Including more fruits, vegetables, whole grains and minimally processed foods aligns with the Mediterranean diet and the DASH diet — Dietary Approaches to Stop Hypertension.
- *Drink plenty of fluids, particularly water.* Fluids help remove uric acid from your body. Aim for 8 to 16 8-ounce glasses a day. There's also some evidence that drinking coffee in moderation is associated with decreased gout risk. But avoid sugary drinks high in calories.
- *Limit foods or beverages sweetened with high-fructose corn syrup.* Fructose, the type of sugar found in fruit and honey that is also used in high-fructose corn syrup, is known to increase uric acid. Avoid soft drinks and other beverages that include this common sweetener. It's smart to limit naturally sweet fruit juices, too.
- *Add cherries to the menu.* There is some evidence that eating cherries is associated with a reduced risk of gout attacks.
- *Get your vitamin C.* Vitamin C may help lower uric acid levels. Talk to your doctor about whether a 500-milligram vitamin C supplement fits into your diet and medication plan.
- *Lose weight if you're overweight.* Weight loss helps lessen the load on weight-bearing joints such as your knees and ankles, and it may also decrease uric acid levels. But avoid rapid-weight-loss diets, which could increase uric acid levels in your blood.

diabetes or if you manage high blood sugar levels as a side effect of taking corticosteroid medications.

You don't have to avoid sweets entirely, but be smart about your selections and portion sizes. The pyramid recommends limiting sweets to 75 calories a day. When possible, select healthier desserts, such as a small amount of dark chocolate.

FEED YOUR BONES

If your arthritis keeps you from getting regular exercise, you may be at an increased risk of osteoporosis — a condition that causes bones to become weak, brittle and susceptible to fractures. Weight-bearing exercise helps your body build and maintain bone. But if you aren't able to stay active, you may lose bone mass. Your risk of developing osteoporosis is also higher if you have a type of inflammatory arthritis or connective tissue disease such as rheumatoid arthritis or lupus, or if you take corticosteroid medications.

To reduce your risk, it's important to get enough calcium in your diet. This mineral is one of the building blocks of bone, and it may help slow bone loss. You also need adequate vitamin D to help keep your bones strong. You get some vitamin D from food. You also get this vitamin from sunlight — your body makes vitamin D when your skin is exposed to the sun's rays. Still, you may need a vitamin D supplement if you don't get enough calcium and vitamin D in food or you are not getting much direct sunlight outdoors.

How much calcium and vitamin D you need depends on your age and sex. (See the chart below.) The best way to get these nutrients is with a balanced diet. You probably know that dairy products are rich in calcium. You can also get a healthy dose of calcium from tofu, salmon, fortified cereal and dark leafy greens such as kale. What about vitamin D? Milk and yogurt are often fortified with it, to help with calcium absorption. Other good sources include fish such as sockeye salmon and canned tuna, fortified orange juice, and eggs.

If you think your diet frequently misses the mark, check with your healthcare team or a registered dietitian to see if you should take a calcium or vitamin D supplement. In some instances, your provider may also recommend medica-

RECOMMENDED DAILY INTAKE OF CALCIUM AND VITAMIN D FOR MEN AND WOMEN

Age (years)	Recommended calcium intake (mg/day)	Upper limit of calcium (mg/day)	Recommended vitamin D intake (IU/day)	Upper limit of vitamin D (IU per day)
19 to 50	1,000	2,500	600	4,000
51 to 70	1,000 (men) 1,200 (women)	2,000	600	4,000
71 and older	1,200	2,000	800	4,000

Source: Institute of Medicine, 2010

Some postmenopausal women need a higher amount of calcium or vitamin D, depending on osteoporosis risk.

tions to prevent osteoporosis, especially if you're taking steroid medications over the long term to treat your arthritis.

For most people, the best way to keep your bones strong — along with getting those essential nutrients — is through regular weight-bearing exercise and strength or resistance training. Even going for a walk can help. The greater the demands you place on your bones, the stronger and denser they become.

BENEFITS OF A HEALTHY WEIGHT

Research has shown that being overweight or obese increases your risk of osteoarthritis of the knee. Being overweight or obese also tends to worsen the signs and symptoms of arthritis. Excess weight adds stress to your weight-bearing joints, especially your knees, which has the effect of aggravating pain, stiffness and inflammation. Being obese can even cause pain in the neck and hands.

As a result, it's important to lose weight if you're overweight. And if you're at a healthy weight, it's critical to avoid weight gain.

Weight loss is especially important if you and your healthcare professional are considering joint surgery as a treatment option for arthritis, because excess weight can make surgery more difficult and more risky. In fact, some surgeons insist that their patients who are overweight lose weight before they undergo elective operations.

The good news is that if you have osteoarthritis or rheumatoid arthritis and you're carrying extra weight, shedding some of those excess pounds can reduce the stress on your back, hips, knees and feet — all places where you may develop arthritis pain. In fact, weight loss has been shown to improve symptoms and reduce the need for knee surgery no matter how much structural damage has occurred in the knee. A loss of 5% to 10% of your total body weight may:

- Decrease pain
- Provide a sense of control
- Increase mobility
- Increase your ability to exercise
- Increase your energy level
- Improve your balance

All these benefits in turn help decrease fatigue, prevent falls and improve your self-image.

And if you have pounds to lose, greater results may reap bigger rewards. A recent study found that people who lost 20% of their total body weight helped reduce pain and improve walking function significantly more than those who lost 5% to 10% of their body weight.

Weight-control basics

At first glance, the basic formula for weight control seems simple. If you burn more calories than you consume from food, you'll lose weight. If you take in more calories than you spend (through daily activity, exercise and basic body functions), you'll gain weight, which can worsen arthritis pain. However, it can be challenging to implement a practical, effective and sustainable weight-loss plan.

You may need to make changes to what you eat in order to control your weight, but it shouldn't be at the cost of good health, taste and practicality. The diet you choose should be simple, relatively inexpensive, enjoyable and satisfying so that you'll stick with it. Adding regular moderate physical activity also is important.

Even with arthritis, you have many physical activities to choose from that can help burn calories and increase muscle mass. You don't have to lift heavy weights to counteract muscle loss as you age. You can exercise your muscles with resistance bands or by using the weight of your own body, as in push-ups, lunges and standing squats. Normal daily activities such as cleaning, shopping and doing laundry help you burn calories, too.

The more active you are, the easier it is to maintain and even increase your muscle mass and maintain a healthy weight. (For more on exercise, see Chapter 15.) On days when you're not feeling well, try to stay active with lower-intensity activities.

Guide for weight loss

Before starting a weight-loss plan, it's important to work with your healthcare professional. However, you can use the Healthy Weight Pyramid as your guide to making smart eating choices. Following the pyramid ensures that you're getting a balanced diet — including foods that may help reduce inflammation but won't overload you with calories and unhealthy fat. It's a great plan for lifelong healthy eating.

Each food group in the pyramid comes with a recommended range of servings. How many servings you should eat depends on a variety of factors, including your weight, activity level and sex. If you're trying to lose weight, you'll want to aim for servings in the lower range for each food group rather than in the higher range. It's important, however, that you eat at least the minimum daily servings for each food group to maintain good health. Your doctor or dietitian can also help you find the right number of servings.

It's also important to remember that a serving is not the same thing as a portion. A serving is an exact amount of food defined by common measurements, such as cups, ounces and tablespoons. A portion is the amount of food put on your plate. And if you're used to restaurant-sized portions, one meal often contains several servings of each food.

You can use common visual cues to estimate servings. (For helpful examples, check out the table on page 257.)

Appetite control

Long-term use of some arthritis drugs may increase your appetite, making it more difficult to keep your weight under control. Eat slowly and stretch mealtimes to a minimum of 20 to 30 minutes to

WHAT'S YOUR BMI?

Body mass index (BMI) is a tool for determining your weight-to-height ratio. When looking at populations, BMI can be a reasonably accurate measure of health risk. It does not, however, take individual body composition into consideration. Whatever your BMI, you will benefit from a discussion about your weight and overall fitness with your healthcare professional.

To determine your BMI, find your height in the left column. Follow that row across to the weight nearest yours. Look at the top of that column for your approximate BMI.

	Normal		Overweight*					Obese				
BMI	19	24	25	26	27	28	29	30	35	40	45	50
Height						Weight in pounds						
4'10"	91	115	119	124	129	134	138	143	167	191	215	239
4'11"	94	119	124	128	133	138	143	148	173	198	222	247
5'0"	97	123	128	133	138	143	148	153	179	204	230	255
5'1"	100	127	132	137	143	148	153	158	185	211	238	264
5'2"	104	131	136	142	147	153	158	164	191	218	246	273
5'3"	107	135	141	146	152	158	163	169	197	225	254	282
5'4"	110	140	145	151	157	163	169	174	204	232	262	291
5'5"	114	144	150	156	162	168	174	180	210	240	270	300
5'6"	118	148	155	161	167	173	179	186	216	247	278	309
5'7"	121	153	159	166	172	178	185	191	223	255	287	319
5'8"	125	158	164	171	177	184	190	197	230	262	295	328
5'9"	128	162	169	176	182	189	196	203	236	270	304	338
5'10"	132	167	174	181	188	195	202	209	243	278	313	348
5'11"	136	172	179	186	183	200	208	215	250	286	322	358
6'0"	140	177	184	191	199	206	213	221	258	294	331	369
6'1"	144	182	189	197	204	212	219	227	265	302	340	378
6'2"	148	186	194	202	210	218	225	233	272	311	350	389
6'3"	152	192	200	208	216	224	232	240	279	319	359	399
6'4"	156	197	205	213	221	230	238	246	287	328	369	410

Source: National Institutes of Health, 1998

*People of Asian descent with a BMI of 23 or higher may have an increased risk of health problems.

allow your natural appetite-control mechanism to work.

Increasing the amount of high-fiber foods in your diet can help you feel full more quickly. To get more fiber, try whole-grain breads instead of white bread, fresh fruit instead of juice, and raw vegetables and fruits in place of salty snacks. These tips also may help you curb an overactive appetite:

- *Eat a healthy breakfast.* Make breakfast a high-fiber cereal, whole-grain bread and fresh fruit so you're less tempted to eat unhealthy snacks throughout the morning. Starting the day with a good breakfast can also set you up for eating a more balanced lunch.
- *Be sure you're hungry.* Are you eating because you're stressed or bored? On those occasions, try reading, being active or calling a friend in place of eating.
- *Eat slowly.* Savor the flavor and texture of individual foods to boost your satisfaction. Remember, it takes about 20 minutes for your brain to receive the signal that you're full. Make sure your meals last at least this long.
- *Ride out the urge.* Cravings generally pass within minutes, sometimes even seconds. If you're not actually hungry, busy yourself with an activity unrelated to food until the desire to eat passes.
- *Start small.* If you feel you always need to finish what's in front of you, start with half the amount of food on your plate that you normally eat. You may find that a smaller amount is still

enough. To make less food seem like more, serve your main course on a salad or dessert plate.

- *Enjoy a treat now and then.* Keep tempting treats out of the house so you don't overindulge. But allow for an occasional ice cream cone or small piece of apple pie when you're out.

Balance your diet: pair vegetables and/or fruits with lean protein and/or a small amount of healthy fat. Example: yogurt and fruit, veggies and hummus, apple and 1 tbsp peanut butter.

STRATEGIES FOR SUCCESS

Whether you're trying to lose weight or eat more healthfully to improve arthritic symptoms, the following strategies may help. Healthy eating isn't just about adding up calories and eating servings of salmon and kale. It's about organization, planning and practicality — at restaurants, in the grocery store and in your own kitchen.

Make a menu

You'll be more likely to stick with a healthy diet if you have a plan. With the right ingredients on hand, healthy meals come together from scratch almost as fast as they do with processed convenience foods.

Try planning your meals one week at a time. Consider your calendar as you plan. If you're invited to a friend's house for dinner on Saturday, cross that meal off your list. If you're volunteering on Wednesday evening and that will delay dinner, pencil in leftovers or an extra-quick meal that won't take much time and energy to prepare. Make sure your plan includes healthy options for breakfast, lunch and snacks, too. And don't forget to take your plan with you to the store.

Menu planning may take a little getting used to. But it's one of your best defenses against unplanned, unhealthy eating — such as grabbing chips or cookies when you need a break at work or arrive home hungry. Planning also helps you get a healthy meal on the table when your energy is low or you're in pain.

Plan for leftovers

Make a double batch of chili so it stretches over two dinners instead of one. Prepare two lasagnas and freeze one for later. Or roast a chicken and turn the leftover meat into a stir-fry later in the week. No matter how you do it, preparing for two meals at once is always a time-saver.

Prep and cook ahead

Make Tuesday night's stew during a free Sunday afternoon. Prep your vegetables for multiple meals in the morning so they're ready to use at dinnertime. If you are chopping veggies for a stir fry, chop more for toppings for a salad or soup for later in the week. Prepare a simple balsamic vinaigrette while you're talking on the phone. You may find many occasions when you can do small tasks in advance, making cooking less daunting later on.

Look for shortcuts

When you go to the grocery store, feel free to purchase pre-cut or frozen fruits and vegetables, meats sliced for stir-fry meals, and other items that save you time in the kitchen. They may cost a little more but can be worth it when you're not feeling well. Even prepared foods from the grocery store are generally less expensive than take-out or restaurant foods of similar nutritional value.

Keep a list of menu ideas

Make a file of recipes that require few ingredients and take 20 minutes or less to make. Refer to the list as you plan weekly menus, or pull it out when an unexpected event disrupts your day and you can't stick to your original meal plan.

Include family members

Ask family members what they'd like to eat that's different and healthy. They may be willing to assist you and experiment along with you.

Create a kitchen that really cooks

When you have arthritis, the time you have for meal preparation and the amount of effort you're able to manage can be major factors in deciding what foods you serve. Help yourself by making your kitchen efficient and easy to use.

Tools for organization

Arrange your kitchen so that the most common or important things you use are within easy reach.

Make use of energy-saving storage devices such as lazy Susans. You may also want to buy easy-to-open containers to keep food and equipment handy.

If you have the space, it may help to have a small cart with wheels for tasks that involve moving supplies from one place to another, to minimize the loads you have to carry.

For example, use the cart to gather ingredients from the refrigerator and pantry or while setting the table. Arrange one complete place setting at a time and work your way around the table. You can also use the cart to clear the table and carry items to the sink for cleanup.

Lightening your workload

Keep utensils nearby as you cook, to save steps and motions. Use a small electric food processor to chop and dice foods and grate cheese. Rinse dirty cooking utensils and equipment immediately so that cleanup will be easier later on.

Here are a few cooking-with-ease tips:
- Use utensils with thick handles that are easy to grip.
- Keep your knives sharpened for easy cutting.
- Slide heavy objects along the counter rather than lifting them.
- Serve hot items from the stove directly on the plates rather than lifting heavy pots and pans to serve in large serving dishes.
- Cook and serve in the same dish whenever possible.
- Use a slotted spoon to remove vegetables from water instead of lifting the pot and pouring the contents into a colander.
- Place a nonslip pad or wet cloth under a mixing bowl to help hold it stationary without gripping.

Tips for eating out

You can dine out and still stay true to your dietary goals. The following tips can help you stay on track when you're eating away from home:

Choose restaurants carefully

Look for places that offer lots of variety, where you can find a healthy meal that's appealing. Restaurants that prepare the food you order from start to finish are more likely to accommodate special requests. Many restaurants post menus and nutritional information on their websites, so you can look for healthy options and decide what to order beforehand.

Keep hunger under control

Don't skip meals on days you're eating out. If you're ravenous when you go into a restaurant, you're more prone to order too much food.

In fact, you may want to have a light snack of vegetables or fruit an hour or so before the meal to avoid overeating.

Look for plant-based options

Many restaurants have special listings for healthy eating. However, foods in the diet or light section may still be a heftier meal than you think. Look for items that contain small amounts of meat, poultry or fish, and lots of vegetables and low-fat carbohydrates — for example, a baked potato, brown rice or a slice of whole-grain bread.

Order wisely

If you can't find a healthy dinner item, order à la carte. Make a meal out of a broth-based (not creamy) soup or a salad and one appetizer. Choose something that's broiled, baked or steamed, not fried. Also consider sharing the meal with a companion or asking for a take-home box to arrive with your food so that you can immediately save half to take home for another time.

ADDING NUTRITION TO CONVENIENCE FOODS

It's OK to eat convenience foods, such as frozen entrées or side dishes, on busy days. Just be selective about what you choose. Look for items that are relatively low in fat, calories and sodium. Then, give them a nutritional boost:

Add spinach, fresh peppers, grated carrots, mushrooms and onions to prepared spaghetti sauce to increase fiber, nutrients and flavor.

Top frozen pizza with fresh tomatoes or thinly sliced peppers before heating. Or add a handful of arugula and a drizzle of olive oil or lemon juice after heating.

When preparing packaged whole-grain (brown) rice, toss in vegetables (peas, broccoli, corn) or fruit (raisins, apple, apricots).

Serve fruits and vegetables as side dishes when eating convenience foods, such as frozen microwave dinners.

Speak up

Ask your server to clarify any unfamiliar terms or explain how a dish is prepared. Request smaller portions and substitutions, such as fresh fruit for french fries. Ask whether items can be broiled instead of fried.

Cut out the condiments

Taste your food before instinctively adding salt, butter, sauces and dressing. Well-prepared food often needs only minimal enhancement. Ask for sauces or dressing on the side. Dab your fork in the sauce before using it to pick up your food. This allows you to enjoy the sauce but limits the amount.

FOOD AND DRUG INTERACTIONS

You may have heard that certain foods you eat can alter the effectiveness of some medications. On the flip side, some arthritis medications can interfere with how well your body uses certain nutrients. So, you may need higher amounts of certain vitamins or minerals to help make up for their reduced effectiveness.

Make sure you understand how your medication should be taken. Some of the drugs used to treat arthritis are most effective if you take them on an empty stomach. Others should be taken with food to prevent stomach irritation. Carefully follow the instructions from your healthcare team.

Two of the most common side effects of arthritis medications are heartburn and stomach upset, often described as a gnawing pain or empty feeling in the stomach. These symptoms might be caused by the food or the medication or a combination of both.

To help prevent the symptoms, sit upright for at least 15 to 30 minutes after eating meals or taking medications. Try to avoid eating for at least one hour before bedtime. Limit foods that tend to trigger reactions, such as alcohol, caffeine, cola, spicy foods, fried foods and black pepper.

Be sure to discuss your medications with your healthcare professional. Learn whether you need to avoid any foods because of medications, if you have any need to take supplements, and what is the most effective way to take the medication. In the end, it's important that your medications and your healthy-eating plan are working together. Both play important roles in helping you live well with arthritis.

17

Your mind and your health

Your mind is a collection of thoughts, feelings, beliefs and emotions — the infrastructure that processes and supports the continuous flow of information through your brain. It's a subtle yet powerful tool guiding your conduct in daily life. The health and vitality of your mind is extraordinarily important to maintaining your physical health and allowing you to live a balanced, satisfying life.

Thoughts and feelings you have about yourself and your place in life can powerfully influence your perception of and ability to cope with a condition like arthritis. How well you're able to manage your joint pain may be based on whether you're an optimist or pessimist, whether you feel confident or insecure about yourself, and whether or not you feel in control of your own life.

Put simply, positive or optimistic thoughts can have health-enhancing

benefits. Negative or pessimistic thoughts can intensify stress and pain. In general, optimists are convinced they can change and make things work out. They tend to react to adversity by taking action. Having a positive attitude may provide a buffer from stress, and it enables you to face life's difficulties with a greater sense of hope.

The mind-body connection works in various ways. For example, if you believe your life is under control, you tend to take better care of yourself — such as eating right, exercising and getting enough rest — than if you think nothing you do matters. Feelings of helplessness, meanwhile, may weaken your immune system by inhibiting the response of certain cells to invading bacteria, viruses and tumor cells. People with a pessimistic outlook also may isolate themselves from the proven, health-enhancing benefits of companionship, love and support from family and friends.

With arthritis, how well you manage the condition depends at least as much on your own actions as on the skill of your healthcare team.

If you believe you can manage arthritis — if you believe that you can handle pain and fatigue — you're more likely to use medical resources effectively than people with less faith in their coping skills. Between two people with the same level of physical impairment, the one with the better coping skills is likely to experience less pain and have less difficulty functioning.

Research has proven certain ways the powerful link between mind and body can affect your health. If you're convinced that you're doomed to live in pain with arthritis, you may be subjecting your body to extra stress and feelings of helplessness, making day-to-day activities more of a struggle.

But if you believe in yourself and in your abilities, you're already giving yourself a boost that will help you learn how to manage arthritis while living a full and satisfying life.

YOUR BODY AND STRESS

For years, scientists have closely studied the complex interactions of emotions, stress and disease, and the body's immune system and nervous system. It's the job of your immune system to maintain your health and facilitate healing by warding off invaders, such as bacteria and viruses, and abnormal cells.

Your nervous system provides communication links between organs that are part of your immune system, such as the spleen, lymph nodes and thymus. The nervous system also regulates hormones — body chemicals that control the immune response.

Stress can have a powerful impact on these functions. When you're under stress, your brain triggers the release of hormones as your body gears up to face the challenge. It's what you feel when you're scared or excited. Your heart beats faster, your breathing speeds up and your muscles tense.

These physiological reactions can be a positive thing, giving you an energy boost that's necessary to pass a test, give a speech or perform onstage. They can also "rev up" your immune system, preparing your body to heal injury or fight infection.

There's a downside to this process. Research shows that when stress is ongoing, or chronic, the continuous release of hormones begins to suppress your immune system, making you more susceptible to illness. If you're older or already have an illness, you become more prone to stress-related changes.

With a chronic condition such as arthritis, stress makes it harder to manage your symptoms. One of the most negative effects of stress is increased pain resulting from muscle tension and fatigue. The pain, in turn, reduces your stamina, causes feelings of helplessness, and intensifies anger, anxiety and frustration. As a result, you may become depressed and feel more and more helpless.

Stress is a part of life that can't be avoided. While you can control many stressful occurrences, you can't control all of them. Accidents or illness occur. Even positive events in your life, such as a job promotion or a wedding, may cause you stress.

For most of us, minor stressors are more common than major ones. Research indicates that these minor events can have a significant impact on how you feel day to day. Stress can also be generated from within — your reaction to an event is often what determines the amount of stress you experience. This reinforces the stress cycle of pain, reduced coping abilities and depression.

Heed the warning signs

The first step in breaking the stress cycle is learning to recognize when you're under stress. People experience stress differently in varying combinations of physical symptoms, emotional changes and behavioral changes.

Physical effects of stress may include:
- Headaches
- Chest pain
- Heart pounding
- High blood pressure
- Shortness of breath
- Muscle aches or pain
- Clenched jaw
- Teeth grinding
- Tight, dry throat
- Indigestion
- Constipation or diarrhea
- Stomach cramping or bloating
- Increased perspiration, often causing cold, sweaty hands
- Fatigue
- Insomnia
- Weight gain or loss
- Diminished sex drive
- Skin problems, such as hives

Emotional effects of stress may include:
- Anxiety
- Restlessness
- Worrying
- Irritability
- Depression
- Sadness
- Anger
- Mood swings
- Feelings of insecurity
- Lack of concentration
- Confusion
- Forgetfulness
- Resentment
- Assigning blame to others
- Guilt
- Pessimism

Behavioral effects of stress may include:
- Overeating
- Loss of appetite
- Poor anger management
- Increased use of alcohol and drugs
- Increased smoking
- Withdrawal or isolation
- Crying spells
- Changes in close relationships
- Job dissatisfaction
- Decreased productivity
- Burnout

If you experience any of these changes, try to determine if they are caused by something other than stress, possibly with the help of your healthcare professional or psychologist. If your symptoms appear to be stress-related, try to figure out what's triggering them. Obviously, situations such as divorce or a death in the family are major stressors. But what about the day-to-day occurrences that rev up your stress reactors?

Take note of the things that make your heart beat faster and your neck muscles tighter. Is it arguing with a co-worker, sitting in rush-hour traffic, juggling too many commitments or maybe all of these? Keeping a written log for a few weeks can give you a better handle on what sets your nerves on edge.

If you can identify your symptoms and what triggers them, you may be able to better control stress by avoiding the triggers, changing the circumstances, if possible, or altering your reaction.

FOCUS ON THE POSITIVE

OK, so you have arthritis. That's no reason to think of yourself as hopeless, alone or unhealthy.

Remember, you have choices. Taking care of yourself by eating well, exercising and getting enough rest can go a long way toward making you feel better and staying active. But what if you believe you're not in control of your situation? Chances are your thoughts are working against you.

DEPRESSION AND ARTHRITIS

Depression is more than just feeling down or blue. It's a biochemical imbalance of the brain, causing certain symptoms that, if extreme, can be life-threatening. When you have arthritis, it's not unusual for you to become depressed.

Depression can lead to many emotional and physical problems. Symptoms may include persistent sadness, irritability, anxiety, loss of interest or pleasure in life, neglect of personal care, changes in eating or sleeping habits, persistent fatigue, loss of energy, and feelings of worthlessness or guilt. Symptoms of depression tend to magnify the pain and discomfort of arthritis.

Please see a medical professional if you think you may be depressed. The condition usually requires long-term treatment involving medication and psychological counseling.

If you're reluctant to seek treatment for depression, consider this: It may help reduce pain. Research has found that for older adults with both arthritis and depression, taking antidepressant medications or attending therapy sessions reduced the symptoms of both conditions. The individuals also reported better joint function and overall health.

Self-talk is rapid-fire or automatic thoughts that pass through your brain constantly, although you may not be aware of it. If you pause for a moment and listen to what's going through your mind, you might be surprised by how negative your self-talk can be.

For example, you start a walking program and instead of focusing on the benefits the activity brings, you chide yourself for being out of shape. Or before you give a presentation, you tell yourself, "I'm lousy at speaking under pressure."

Negative self-talk may underlie some of the stress you're feeling. Cognitive behavioral therapy, a common type of talk therapy, may help you transform that self-talk from negative to positive. It can be an effective tool for anyone wishing to learn how to better manage stressful life situations such as arthritis.

To use cognitive behavioral therapy, you'll work with a counselor or psychotherapist who will help you become more aware of your inaccurate or negative way of thinking. Some interactive CBT apps also may be useful between sessions or on your own.

Therapy allows you to view challenging situations clearly and respond to them in a more effective manner. Therapy is generally focused on specific problems — for example, the struggles you may be having with mobility or your worries about the appearance of a deformed finger joint — using a goal-oriented approach. Sessions help you to:

- Identify the difficult situations
- Become aware of your thoughts, emotions and beliefs about these situations
- Identify the negative or inaccurate thoughts you have
- Challenge your negative or inaccurate thinking

Your therapist will encourage you to consider whether your view of a situation is based on facts or on your inaccurate perception of what's going on. This can be difficult if you have long-standing ways of thinking about your life and yourself. With practice, your ability to develop positive thinking and behavior will become a habit and won't take as much effort.

Instead of thinking, "I'll never be able to do anything I enjoy," you can tell yourself, "I'll take good care of myself so I can still do many things" or "I may have to slow down, but I don't have to give up." By changing your outlook, you'll find more constructive ways to cope with arthritis.

REDUCE STRESS

In addition to redirecting negative thoughts, there are other strategies for managing stress. You may talk about your problems with others, listen to soothing music or take a short evening walk. Even if you usually do pretty well in getting through life's crises as they arise, at times you may need a little extra help.

The following tips may help you better manage stress:

DIFFERENCES IN STRESS RESPONSE OVER TIME

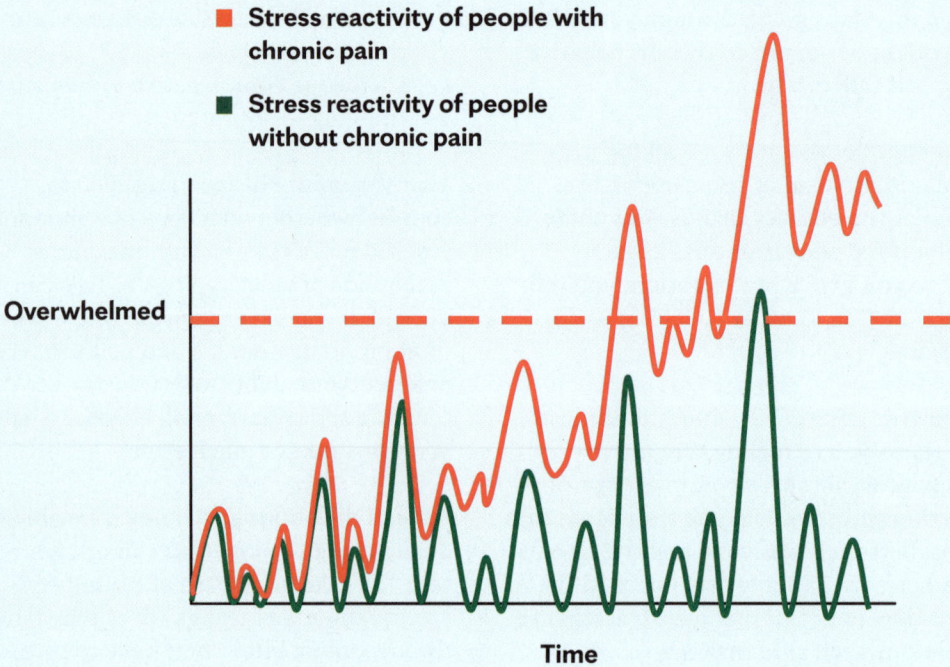

■ Stress reactivity of people with chronic pain

■ Stress reactivity of people without chronic pain

Overwhelmed

Time

The green line represents typical stress response fluctuations in people without chronic pain. The red line represents stress response fluctuations in people with chronic pain. Early on, stress responses are similar between the two groups. But over time, as the stress system of the chronic pain group is consistently activated by pain and the stress that pain causes, the system increases its response. The result is that people with chronic pain experience continually elevated stress responses both at baseline and peak levels.

- **Try to be more tolerant.** Learn to be more accepting of yourself and of situations over which you have no control. A starting point is the recognition that you'll always experience a certain amount of stress — and that is normal. Consider adopting a mantra to remind yourself of this and practice acceptance, such as "I focus on what I can control and let go of what I can't."
- **Plan your day.** Having a schedule of your daily activities and appointments may help you feel more in control of your life.
- **Get organized.** Declutter living and work spaces so that you don't have to spend time and energy searching for misplaced items. If organizing feels overwhelming, try setting a timer and working on one space for 15 minutes.
- **Manage your time.** Often stress is a result of too much to do and too little time. Setting priorities — and letting go of what doesn't realistically fit — may go a long way toward depressurizing your day.
- **Take occasional breaks.** Periodically during the day, take time to relax, stretch or walk. Set an alarm on your phone to remind you, or schedule breaks in your calendar.
- **Get adequate sleep, stay physically active and eat well.** A healthy body promotes good mental health. Sleep reinvigorates you. Physical activity burns off stress-related tension. And a balanced diet provides energy to handle daily stress. Make sure you're drinking enough water, too.
- **Discuss your concerns.** Talking with a family member or friend may help to relieve stress and cast events in a different light.
- **Get away.** Take a break from your normal routine. You might benefit from a change of scenery or a different pace of life. This could be as simple as visiting a new coffee shop or a new spot to walk.
- **Enjoy a good laugh.** It's healthy to spend time with people who make you laugh. Laughter is scientifically proven to help reduce and relieve tension.

If self-help measures don't reduce stress, seeking help from a counselor, psychiatrist, psychologist or clergyperson may be your next step. Seeking help is a sign of strength and self-awareness — and good judgment. Depending on your insurance coverage, you may even be able to talk with a therapist via video from your home.

LEARN TO RELAX

Relaxation helps reduce the muscle tension that can increase pain. If you need help relaxing, there are relaxation techniques you might try. Finding one that works for you helps decrease pain and increase your comfort level.

Relaxation techniques typically are most effective when you practice them regularly. You might initially follow some direction and then form a routine. Yoga, tai chi and other techniques that involve defined postures and repetitive movements can help you relax. Prayer and meditation, especially when kept simple, familiar and repetitive, also may help.

These quiet, reflective exercises can help you reverse the mental arousal from stress. Regular practice of relaxation techniques may also reduce stress by changing your thought patterns. It can be another powerful means of shifting thoughts from negative to positive.

The following are several relaxation techniques to try. If you're new to them, there are many apps, instructional products, streaming videos and classes that may help you. Pick a quiet time and place where you won't be disturbed. Practice regularly, preferably daily, for at least 15 to 20 minutes. And try to be patient — it may take several weeks to get the hang of it and start to see some benefit.

Meditation

This ancient practice has been called an altered state of consciousness and a unique state of relaxation. There are almost as many ways to meditate as there are people who meditate.

The basic premise of meditation is to sit quietly and focus on the rhythm of your breathing or on a simple word or phrase repeated over and over. When distracting thoughts arise — and they will — you simply notice them and let them go, always returning to your focus. With meditation, you enter a deeply restful state that reduces your body's stress response.

There are different types of meditation, including mindful meditation, relaxation response and transcendental meditation.

All forms work similarly. By meditating often, you can learn to relax your breathing, slow brain waves, and decrease muscle tension and your heart rate. Like other relaxation techniques, meditation can help lessen your response to the chemicals that your body produces when you're stressed, such as adrenaline. Too much adrenaline on a regular basis can be harmful.

Guided imagery

With this practice, also known as visualization, you enter a relaxed state brought on by meditation or self-hypnosis. In this state, you employ all your senses to imagine a setting that helps alleviate the physical symptoms of stress.

Studies of guided imagery suggest that when you imagine something, the same parts of your brain are stimulated as when you actually experience it. When you visualize a calming environment, your brain receives messages of relaxation that are passed on to your autonomic nervous and endocrine systems, which regulate key functions such as heart rate and blood pressure.

Progressive muscle relaxation

This relaxation technique works on the theory that to learn how to relax your muscles, you must first know how they feel when they're tensed. Therefore, progressive relaxation is a series of exercises that takes you through each of the major muscle groups from head to toe

— tensing and releasing tension as you go. Along the way, you focus on how the relaxed muscles feel compared with the tense muscles.

A similar technique to progressive muscle relaxation is called body scanning. You systematically focus on each muscle group, noting any tension and then letting it go without tensing the muscles. Instead of physically tensing and relaxing muscles, you focus on the sensations in each part of your body.

Self-hypnosis

Self-hypnosis is an induced state of relaxation that enhances your focus and helps make you more open to act on suggestions given to you — or that you give to yourself — in a hypnotic state. Self-hypnosis alters brain wave patterns in much the same way as other relaxation techniques. This stress-relieving result may be why it works to ease pain and stress and alter behavior.

Massage therapy

Massage therapy involves the manipulation of soft tissues of your body. There are several forms of massage, including the traditional kneading and rubbing of Swedish massage and the application of pressure at specific points of the body, which characterizes acupressure massage, also known as shiatsu.

Massage can lower your heart rate, increase blood circulation, relax mus-cles, improve range of motion and increase endorphins, which can help relieve pain. Massage can also be effective at relieving stress, depression and anxiety. It can decrease the perception of pain and has been shown to reduce arthritis pain.

The environment in which you receive massage is important. A warm, quiet area that is free from distracting noise or interruption can help relieve muscle tension. Low-volume sound or music also relaxes muscles. Your massage therapist may use a mineral oil to reduce friction, contributing to smooth, effective massage strokes.

Keep a journal

Writing down your thoughts and feelings can help you blow off steam, increase self-awareness, solve problems and put things in perspective. By writing regularly, you can also create a record of your symptoms, see patterns in their occurrence, gain a better understanding of your disease and find wording to better communicate about your condition. You may also be able to determine whether medications are affecting your mood or whether your arthritis flares when you're under stress.

Some research has even suggested that for people with chronic illnesses such as rheumatoid arthritis, writing about their stressful experiences may be linked to improved symptoms. One theory is that the emotional processing involved in the act of writing can help to reduce stress.

YOUR HEALTH-RELATED QUALITY OF LIFE

Recent research has explored how arthritis affects quality of life for adults —
including physical function, social roles and activities, sleep, fatigue, pain, anxiety and
depression.

Some factors that affect health-related quality of life (HRQOL) may be out of your
control. For example, you may not be able to change the type of arthritis you have or
other medical conditions you're managing. However, certain factors seem to help
improve the chance of a better HRQOL — while others contribute to the risk of poorer
HRQOL. Strong social connections and an emotional support network may especially
help you maintain a happier, healthier life with arthritis. So it's worth some extra effort
to stay connected through work, exercise, activities and staying in touch with friends.

Talk with your healthcare team about whether there are changes you could make in
the areas below that may tip the scale toward a better quality of life.

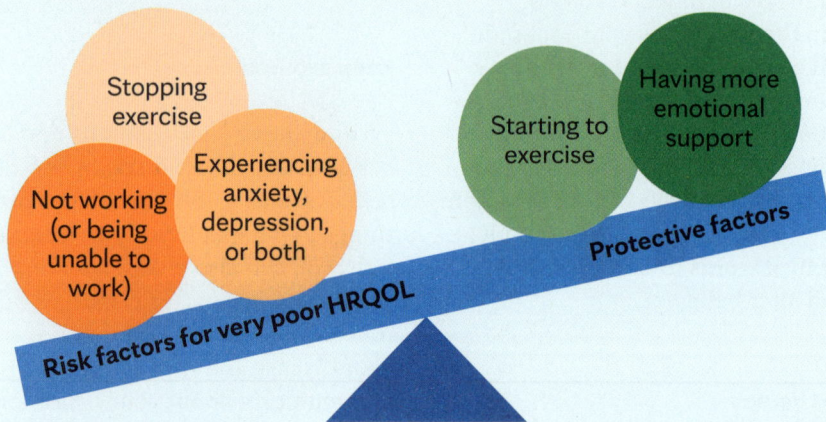

Stopping exercise

Not working (or being unable to work)

Experiencing anxiety, depression, or both

Starting to exercise

Having more emotional support

Protective factors

Risk factors for very poor HRQOL

SEEK SUPPORT

Having friends and loved ones to talk to
can help you feel less alone and overwhelmed and more able to cope. This may
be especially true when you're dealing
with the pain and fatigue of arthritis.
Having people who care about you also

makes you more likely to take better care
of yourself.

In addition, having support may help to
improve your physical functioning.
Receiving daily doses of friendliness and
understanding from others may improve
your psychological well-being. And

having social companionship — being asked to join in — appears to be beneficial both physically and psychologically. In short, staying connected and maintaining close relationships is good for your health.

Support groups may offer benefits similar to individual support. In fact, in a group of relative strangers, you might feel more comfortable expressing your deepest fears and daily concerns without worrying about scaring or burdening your loved ones. Depending on the nature of the group, you can deal with difficult problems, share experiences, learn how others cope with the same challenges and change your perspective.

You may get the most benefit from a support group if you're interested in learning about the experiences of others and if you're willing to share your thoughts and feelings. To find a group, talk to your healthcare team, your local Arthritis Foundation chapter or others you know who have arthritis.

If you're not comfortable in a group setting but feel a need to express and process your feelings about arthritis, you might consider individual counseling. A therapist can also help you learn meditation or self-hypnosis to practice on your own. Talk to your healthcare professional for a recommendation.

INTIMACY

Sexuality is a natural, healthy part of living and part of your identity. When the chronic pain of arthritis invades your life, the pleasures of sexuality often disappear. You may be concerned that sexual intercourse will cause physical pain, especially if you have arthritis in your back or hip. You may be worried that your partner finds you less attractive because of pain or swollen joints. Or you may have simply lost interest in sex as a result of the symptoms.

It doesn't have to be this way. You can have a healthy and satisfying sexual relationship while managing arthritis. The key is honest communication. It also helps to be creative and willing to change.

No matter what your health condition is, it's important not to lose sight of your sexuality. Here are strategies for enhancing your sex life and achieving greater satisfaction:

- *Communicate openly.* Talk with your partner about how you feel, what you want or need from the relationship, and how to be intimate in a way that's enjoyable for both of you. If you have unspoken fears regarding sexual contact, tell your partner about them. Talking openly together can ease your concerns and open the door for creative problem-solving.
- *Rekindle your romance.* Go on a date, plan a picnic, send flowers or just spend extra time together. Set the stage for sexual intimacy with dinner by candlelight or holding hands during an evening stroll.
- *Prepare your body.* Do gentle range-of-motion exercises for a few minutes before having sex. This may help prevent pain and stiffness. A warm

bath or shower with your partner also may help relax your muscles and prepare you for intimacy. Taking a pain medication or muscle relaxant before sex might be another option — but first, talk with your healthcare professional about which type of drug you can use and what dose is right for you.

- *Expand your definition of intimacy.* For many people with arthritis, it's the act of intercourse that causes the most problems. Consider alternatives that might be more comfortable and fulfilling, including cuddling, fondling, sensual massage, masturbation, oral sex or use of a vibrator.
- *Experiment to make intercourse more comfortable.* Instead of a conventional posture that may be painful, try a different position, for example, lying side by side, kneeling or sitting. Many good books are available that describe different ways to have intercourse.
- *Change your routine.* Many people have higher pain levels in the evening. If this is true for you, try being intimate in the morning — when you're refreshed from a good night's sleep and may have the most energy.

If you continue to have sexual problems, talk with your healthcare professional. Describe when and how your sexual desire or performance has been affected by arthritis. Pain and fatigue can reduce your libido, but many medications, including glucocorticoids and antidepressants, also can reduce your sex drive.

Your healthcare professional may be able to change your medication, change the dosage or recommend other strategies to enhance your sex life.

However, even if you suspect a medication may be affecting sexual performance, it's important that you don't stop taking it without first consulting your doctor.

In all partnerships, it takes effort to maintain what is good and to correct what isn't. Be willing to make that effort. A healthy sexual relationship can positively affect all aspects of your life, including your physical health, self-esteem and productivity.

Remind yourself that problems can also be opportunities. In your efforts to become more intimate again, you may discover something about your partner that you otherwise might have missed. The relationship you recover may be even better than the one you had before you developed arthritis.

SIMPLIFY YOUR LIFE

We live in an era of multitasking — doing (or trying to do) several things at once. Yet many people long for a simpler, slower-paced, more meaningful life. Arthritis may force you to slow down and focus on individual tasks. That may not mean quitting your job or hobbies, but you may need to allow more time for rest and self-care. As a result, you might pay more attention to the things in your life that give you satisfaction and pleasure.

The following suggestions can help simplify your life.

Reassess success

If you have a fast-paced, competitive lifestyle, you may find it exciting, but it may not always be the right choice for you. You may make more money and have a higher profile in your community than you'd have with a less demanding job or lifestyle. But as you manage your health and navigate different phases, remember to consider periodically whether lower-stress options are open to you.

Accept things you can't change

Maybe you can't do all the things you did before you had arthritis. If you have rheumatoid arthritis, the wax-and-wane nature of your disease might make it difficult to plan ahead, and you may be too tired to pursue every interest. Don't fight it. Decide what's important. Give top priority to those things you must do and those things you want to do. For the rest, delegate them, drop them or ask for help.

Take a breath

When you're stressed, your breathing is rapid and shallow. Relaxed breathing is slow and deep. By slowing your breathing, you can decrease the stress response and force your body into a relaxed state. Practicing relaxed breathing for at least 15 minutes a day may even help you

control conditions such as high blood pressure.

Here's one way to practice deep breathing: Inhale slowly to a count of four, then exhale slowly to a count of four. Do this whenever you're under pressure — when you're waiting in line or working on a deadline.

Learn to say no

You can't do everything, especially when you have arthritis. The next time someone asks for help, think twice before you say yes. Do you have the time? Are you already overcommitted? Is this a project you really want to work on? Are you feeling overwhelmed or worn out?

For some people, saying no may make them feel like failures for not living up to their own high standards. They try to do things as they would have before having arthritis, which leads to fatigue.

It's OK to say no. Cognitive behavioral therapy is an excellent way to learn how to accept your condition without feeling like you've somehow failed. Besides, you won't be very helpful to anyone if you're tired and running on empty.

Own less, clean less

Unless it's edible, just about everything you bring into your house takes time and energy to maintain. Perhaps you once enjoyed souvenirs or trinkets that now just serve as dust collectors.

Apply the "pleasure principle" to your possessions. Do they really make you happy? Consider getting rid of anything that doesn't significantly add to your life. If you haven't used it in a year, maybe you should put it in storage or give it away. And avoid buying things you don't need.

GET YOUR REST

Throughout this chapter, you've read about simple steps you can take to reduce stress and gain control over arthritis. Certainly, another key step is getting adequate rest. Modern society tends to push a busy lifestyle at the expense of rest. Achievement is often valued over health and quality of life. For some, it's a source of pride not to get much sleep or not to need much sleep.

When should you get rest? Whenever you're tired. Arthritis, particularly rheumatoid arthritis, makes you more prone to fatigue. This condition makes it imperative that you listen to your body and give it what it needs, especially when it comes to rest.

Know your limits. Your energy is a limited resource to be budgeted. Let's say you have $10 to spend each day, and you can choose how you want to spend it — but you may not use tomorrow's money today, or tomorrow will be a very bad day. Learning to budget your resources is an important part of having a chronic disease. If you need to rest in a

LEARNING TO HELP YOURSELF

The Chronic Disease Self-Management Program teaches people with chronic conditions, such as heart disease, lung disease and arthritis, how to take better care of themselves, tackle problems such as pain and fatigue, and use medications wisely. Two trained leaders facilitate the small-group workshops, which typically meet once a week for 2.5 hours over a six-week period. Often, one or both leaders are non-healthcare professionals and have some form of chronic disease.

These self-management workshops take place in communities across the nation. You can locate the nearest workshop by visiting the National Council on Aging (NCOA) website at www.ncoa.org/ncoa-map.

The Arthritis Foundation sponsors fitness programs designed to help you reduce pain and increase strength and flexibility. Certified instructors lead separate group classes for walking, tai chi, aquatics and low-impact exercise. You can locate a local program by visiting the Arthritis Foundation website.

comfortable chair or nap during the day to reserve your energy, allow yourself to do it.

Be sure to get a good night's sleep. According to the Centers for Disease Control and Prevention, around one-third of U.S. adults usually don't get the recommended amount of sleep. Chronic sleep deprivation impairs your attention, coordination and reaction time. It also increases your risks of obesity, high blood pressure, heart attacks, diabetes and depression.

Sleep as many hours as you need, not the number you think you can survive on. There are no prizes awarded for getting by on only four hours a night, and you could aggravate your arthritis by not sleeping enough.

Most adults need between seven and nine hours of sleep each night. You can tell if you're getting quality sleep if you can awaken in the morning without an alarm clock and feel refreshed, alert, and able to carry out daily activities without being tired or dozing off. One caveat: It's possible to sleep too much. If you're depressed, you might seek refuge in sleep.

Midday naps are fine as long as they don't affect your sleep at night. Try to avoid napping after 3 p.m. And keep naps relatively short — generally about 10 to 30 minutes. It may be that all you need to do is sit down and take a break from activity. Find a comfortable chair and rest without falling asleep. It's OK to be a little tired. And be sure to intersperse rest periods with periods of exercise and other activity.

STAY IN CONTROL

Self-efficacy is a term that describes your ability to take action and achieve goals. It's based on believing that you can have control over things that affect your life and that you have confidence to succeed in particular situations.

Research shows that self-efficacy is the best predictor of success in health outcomes, including how well you cope with arthritis. A strong sense of self-efficacy means that you can look at the challenges of living with arthritis as tasks you take control of. It means that you remain committed to achieving these goals and have the ability to bounce back from setbacks.

At this moment, you may be feeling overwhelmed by your symptoms or just don't have confidence that you can change things for the better. You can increase your self-efficacy in small steps. Developing a more positive outlook, learning a relaxation technique or including short rest breaks during periods of activity to prevent fatigue — these are all steps that can increase your self-efficacy.

Use the power of your thoughts, feelings, and beliefs about your illness and your life to help you manage arthritis.

18

Protecting your joints

You wouldn't intentionally overload one of your joints — particularly if you have arthritis. The joint may already be stiff and painful, and injury would limit it even more. But it's easy to overload or injure your joints through daily movements. The good news is that you can learn ways to protect your joints throughout your day.

The goal of this chapter is to help you preserve your joints and protect them from harm. Much of permanent joint damage is due to chronic inflammation, which you can take steps to reduce. Medications are an important part of this but are not your only tool.

Joint protection starts with your posture — the positions that you hold your body in when you're standing, sitting or lying down. Good posture means that whether you're stationary or in motion, you're putting the least amount of strain on your bones and supporting muscles, tendons

and ligaments. It means there's less wear on your joint surfaces.

If you have poor posture, that means your joints are not ideally aligned. For example, when you sit with your shoulders rolled into a slouch, your head, neck and back may be curved forward. The supporting muscles and ligaments need to work harder at keeping you upright and balanced. This effort causes extra wear on your joints, which may lead to arthritis and associated symptoms such as fatigue.

Good posture evenly distributes the weight of your body and maintains the natural curvature of your spine. Staying in one position for a while should feel almost effortless. (For examples of good standing and sitting posture, see the illustrations on page 298.)

If you're trying to improve your posture, it may feel a little stiff at the beginning. Don't worry! Keep practicing good posture, and it will soon start feeling natural.

BASICS OF JOINT PROTECTION

The following principles can help preserve your joints and protect them from damage.

Use proper body mechanics

Body mechanics are the actions you take so you can function in daily life. These movements include lifting, carrying, pushing, pulling, and getting out of a chair or bed, as well as using tools for jobs such as vacuuming, shoveling, raking, and writing. The mechanics for some of these actions are illustrated on pages 297-301.

Using good body mechanics follows the principles for good posture. Better movements allow you to work efficiently, conserve energy, maintain balance and reduce stress on your joints. Stressful body mechanics may cause muscle strain, which can lead to pain and increase the wear on your joints.

Whatever the task, use the largest joint possible to accomplish it. That means if you can use your elbows rather than fingers and wrists to perform a job, do so — or, if it turns out that you can use your

TRIM EXTRA POUNDS

If you weigh more than what is a healthy weight for you, you have plenty of company. Most adults in the United States fall into this category. Being seriously overweight has significant implications for your health and for your joints.

If you're overweight, you're more likely to develop osteoarthritis of the knee or hand. Extra pounds can speed the breakdown of cartilage in the joint. Other joints, including the back, hips, ankles and big toes, also can be damaged by extra weight. Being overweight increases the risk of developing rheumatoid arthritis, too.

Of course, many factors may contribute to the development of arthritis. One is heredity — the genes you inherit from your parents. A previous joint injury can make arthritis more likely as well. There's also the wear and tear on a joint over time. Being overweight can accelerate the process.

Losing even a few pounds can reduce your chances for knee pain and disability. Good nutrition and proper exercise are keys to weight control. (For more on exercise and nutrition, see Chapters 15 and 16.)

shoulders rather than elbows, adjust your mechanics accordingly.

The better way to lift and carry something cradled in your arms is by allowing your hips and knees to do most of the work, with the object tucked close to your body.

Avoid placing constant or excessive pressure on your joints. For example, break the habit of resting your chin on the knuckles of your hand. Use a briefcase with a shoulder strap or wheels to avoid carrying heavy objects with your hands.

Avoid remaining in the same position for long periods of time. For example, if you're driving a car or seated at a desk, take frequent breaks to move around and flex your joints.

To preserve the joints in your fingers and hands, avoid tasks that require tight grasping, pinching or gripping. Assistive devices can help you do these tasks with less strain on the joints. These devices are described later in the chapter.

Get active

Reducing arthritis pain doesn't mean avoiding activity. In fact, regular exercise is one of the most effective ways to protect your joints, extending their life and usefulness.

Exercise can strengthen the muscles surrounding your arthritic joints, providing much-needed support. It increases

joint flexibility and range of motion. And it reduces fatigue, boosts energy levels and helps you lose weight, thereby reducing the load on your joints.

The following tips can help you get more active. If you're not accustomed to physical activity, check with your health-care team first. They can advise you on the best way to get started.

You may also be referred to an occupational therapist or physical therapist for guidance. They can help you learn the best ways to exercise with your particular joint pain.

Warm up and cool down

Before any exercise, warm up joints and muscles with a heating pad or hot pack, with massage, or by gently walking in place for a few minutes. A warm bath or shower also may help.

Hot packs, applied for 20 minutes, should feel warm and soothing but not uncomfortably hot to the touch. Because heat may increase swelling and pain, don't apply it to an already warm, swollen joint. After exercise, it may help to apply cold to the arthritic joints for 10 to 15 minutes.

Start slowly

To maintain mobility without damaging your joints, it's important to move each joint through its full pain-free range of motion — all the directions it can comfortably move in. Your pain-free range may vary from day to day or throughout the day.

Gently stretch the muscles around your affected joints at least once a day, perhaps in the morning when you get up. You may also want to stretch before you exercise and at the end of your exercise routine. If you have time and energy for only limited stretching, save it for after activity.

Always warm up for a few minutes before stretching, and take care not to overdo it, especially if you have rheumatoid arthritis. Gentle stretching loosens your muscles and increases a stiff joint's range of motion. Sudden jerking or bouncing may be harmful to your joints, so aim for slow, fluid motions.

Step it up gradually

Start exercising at a comfortable level. That might be no more than a walk to the end of your driveway and back. If that's all you can do at the moment, start with that. Once you're reasonably comfortable, increase the distance you walk a little at a time.

Try exercising at different times of the day. Find a time when you feel the least pain and stiffness.

Know your limits

The kind of exercise you do and how hard you do it will depend on what type of arthritis you have and how strong your symptoms are from day to day.

If you have rheumatoid arthritis, consider the amount of wear and tear the activity may have on affected joints. Non-weight-bearing activities, such as swimming or riding a stationary bike, are probably best. A low-impact activity such as walking also may be a good option. If the affected joint is not painful and a particular activity is not causing pain during or after the exercise, it's probably OK to proceed. If the activity causes pain, stop and consider an alternative exercise. For example, if riding an upright stationary bike seems to aggravate hip pain, try using a recumbent stationary bike.

If you have osteoarthritis of the hip or knee and the bones and cartilage of the affected joint aren't too worn down, then a low-impact activity such as walking might be what you need. However, if the bones and cartilage of the joint are significantly worn down, walking may cause even more damage. Non-weight-bearing activity may be a better choice.

Setting up a personal exercise program to suit your needs is discussed in more detail in Chapter 15.

Organize and prioritize

Planning your daily schedule is a good way to reduce strain on your joints. Start by prioritizing tasks. Get the important jobs done before you get tired or over-work yourself. Recognize which tasks require the most effort — you may need assistance for those.

You can also tailor your workspace to your needs. Adjust the height of a desk and chair to levels where you can sit comfortably and aren't required to stretch or strain. Keep frequently used tools and supplies within arm's length to minimize straining to reach them.

If you're on your feet a lot, make sure you're wearing shoes that fit well and provide firm support. Use long-handled versions of tools, such as a dustpan or garden trowel, for tasks that would usually involve bending and stooping. Move bags, boxes and heavy equipment on wheeled carts or baskets whenever possible.

Respect pain

Learn to tell the difference between the general discomfort you feel from arthritis and the pain that comes from overusing a joint, such as from exercising too much or too hard.

Adjust your level of activity or work method to avoid excessive pain. You're more likely to damage a joint when it's painful and swollen. Don't overwork tender, injured or badly inflamed joints. Pain is considered excessive if it alters your breathing pattern — you'll find that you're holding your breath or breathing more rapidly than normal. Excessive pain also doesn't subside when you stop an activity.

If pain increases, lasts more than an hour or two after the activity, or comes on more quickly day after day, chances are you're doing too much activity or moving in a way you shouldn't be.

Get your rest

This concept may seem confusing: On the one hand, you're told to be active. On the other hand, you're supposed to take frequent rest breaks.

In fact, it's a delicate balance to keep. At certain times you'll need rest to restore

BE KIND TO YOUR JOINTS

An important rule of joint protection is simply avoiding situations that aggravate your condition — increasing inflammation and wear on your joints. But how do you put that advice into practice? Try these tips:

- When writing, use good posture and lighting. Relax your hand often and stretch your neck often. Use a pen with a wider barrel or a special grip. Nylon tip or rolling ball pens require less pressure than pencils and ballpoint pens.
- Install lever-type handles instead of knobs on the doors in your home.
- When you're moving lawn supplies or groceries and doing other household tasks, use a utility cart to transport heavy items and to avoid extra trips.
- When traveling, use luggage with built-in wheels.
- During an activity, sit — with good posture — instead of standing when possible.

your energy. At other times you'll need exercise to maintain strength and stay reasonably flexible.

There are two forms of rest: joint rest and whole-body rest. It's important for you to give your body both.

Joint rest

Using a joint affected by arthritis helps keep it strong and flexible. Even so, the joint can easily become fatigued, swollen or painful after heavy exertion. When the muscles around a joint feel tired, that's usually a signal to sit down and rest.

If a joint is injured or badly inflamed, it will need recovery time. For example, you may need to wear a splint to keep the joint stationary. As the inflammation dies down, the splint can be removed and you can gradually start moving the joint.

Whole-body rest

If you have arthritis, especially rheumatoid arthritis, a well-rested body is an important goal to reach every day. Rheumatoid arthritis makes you especially vulnerable to fatigue. Joint pain can cause you to lose sleep or prevent you from sleeping well. The pain may cause you to change positions frequently to take weight off the affected joints.

Fatigue associated with arthritis is a deep-down exhaustion. It can make virtually everything you do seem like too great an effort, leaving you feeling almost helpless. When you're exhausted, you may not feel like doing much. But if you don't engage in enough physical activity, your muscles will only get weaker, and you'll find it even more difficult to get started with physical activity.

Alternatively, you may tend to keep going until a job is done, regardless of discomfort — whether walking to the corner or finishing the laundry. That strategy may not be the best, either. When you exercise too strenuously without breaks, you can strain muscles and joints and risk injury.

The key is to get rest before you become too tired. Pace yourself. Don't try to push through periods of feeling extra tired. If you experience a surge of joint inflammation (flare), you'll need to schedule more time to rest your joints.

Try dividing any exercise or work activity into short segments with frequent breaks. Plan 10 minutes of rest for every hour during periods of physical exertion. On the surface, that approach may sound disruptive, but it can help you get more done without pushing your joints to their limit.

From time to time during each day, find a comfortable position and relax for a while. An easy chair, couch, bed or reclined seat in your parked car are all potential options. You don't need to sleep, but you do need to give your body a break.

When it's bedtime, go to bed. Avoid the temptations of watching TV or reading. A good night's sleep gives your joints the rest they need. It can also help restore your energy and enable you to deal more effectively with pain.

If you have rheumatoid arthritis, set a goal of eight or nine hours of sleep each night. If you have trouble sleeping, talk to your healthcare professional about it promptly. When sleep disturbances are treated, fatigue usually improves.

ASSISTIVE DEVICES FOR DAILY TASKS

Putting the basic principles of joint protection into practice can help you extend the life of your joints. But even if you're doing your best to reduce wear and tear, it's still the case that proper activity, body mechanics and rest may not be enough. That's when you may look for help from assistive devices — tools and technology that have been adapted to help you perform daily tasks.

For example, your painful knee may need a brace to support it — that's a form of assistive device. Or you may opt for using a cane to help you walk. If your hands are affected by arthritis, special grips may be added to a toothbrush handle or a pen that allow you to hold them securely.

How do you know what kind of assistive device to look for or how to use it? That's typically the result of an in-depth evaluation by your healthcare team, which may include your physician, physical therapist, occupational therapist and other specialists. They will evaluate your condition in relation to how well you're able to function in daily life and match a

specific device to your needs. You may want to keep a list of activities that you find difficult, as a reminder when you discuss the issue with your healthcare team.

Your healthcare team also provides specialized training in the care and use of a device. And they provide follow-up, evaluating how successfully the device is helping you and making adjustments as your condition changes.

People sometimes avoid assistive devices, refusing to believe they need any help, or they think the use of special tools is a form of weakness. Some people worry that using an assistive device such as a cane will make them look old or lead to a loss of function.

In reality, assistive devices allow you to be more independent. In that way, they play an important role in helping you manage your arthritis. Think about it like this: Few people think twice about getting into a car to drive across town. But the car is an assistive device. It makes it easier for you to get from one place to another quickly and comfortably.

Assistive devices are simply a means to an end. They make it easier and safer for you to perform many everyday activities, such as opening a stubborn jar or taking a shower, without making your condition worse.

Medical supply stores and catalogs and many pharmacies offer a wide variety of assistive devices that are practical and affordable. Sometimes a little creativity is all you need. For example, you can use plastic foam tubing — the kind used to insulate plumbing — to make sleeves that fit on all kinds of handheld tools and utensils, making them easier to grasp. The foam insulation also reduces vibration.

Here are tips for selecting and using some of the many assistive devices available.

Handheld aids

If you have arthritis in your hands, avoid making a tight fist or tightly pinching an object. Most pencils and pens, for example, have thin handles that force you to grasp them tightly. This position puts painful stress on the joints of your fingers, thumb and wrist. Keeping your fingers and thumb unclenched is less physically stressful. So, look for grips or clips you can use with writing tools to give you a wider grip.

Grooming and personal hygiene

If you have limited range of motion, you may opt for long-handled brushes and combs. Bathing aids such as long-handled sponges and brushes can help you reach all parts of your body with less effort and pain. Use an electric toothbrush or one with a specially designed handle. Try mirrors with foam rubber handles for an easier grasp. Bath benches, grab bars and toilet seat risers provide greater ease, safety and independence with personal hygiene.

Getting dressed

If you have trouble reaching all the way to your feet, look for a shoehorn with an extension handle or a stocking aid that allows you to pull on your socks without bending forward.

Use special tools that help you grip buttons and zippers securely. Attach elasticized fabric fasteners in place of buttons on cuffs, or sew on the buttons with elasticized thread that stretches as you slip your hand through the sleeve.

Select pants or skirts with a stretch waist if a limited range of motion makes dressing a challenge. You might use clip-on neckties for convenience. If you prefer a regular necktie, leave the knot tied and slip the tie over your head.

In the kitchen

Organize your work area. Make sure the items you use often are within easy reach.

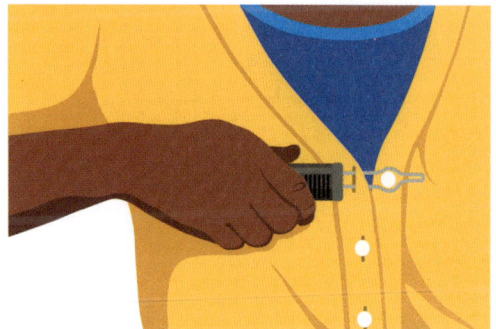

A buttonhook can help you grasp and fasten buttons on your clothes if pinching buttons is difficult for your fingers.

Store frequently used cookware and utensils in cabinets at hip-to-shoulder height. Seldom-used items may be stored in less easily accessible spots.

A single-lever faucet can make the numerous tasks you perform at the sink less taxing on your finger joints.

Operating an electric can opener puts less stress on your joints than a manual opener. In addition, use an electric jar opener or an opener that can be mounted under a cabinet or countertop.

If you have a hard time opening a refrigerator door with your hand, try looping a strap through the door handle. Pass your arm through the strap to pull the door open.

An electric knife can ease routine slicing and trimming tasks. You may also work on a cutting board with tiny raised

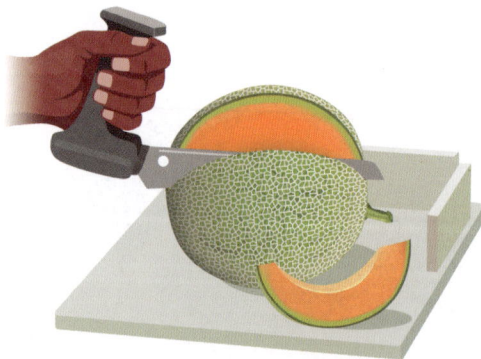

An L-shaped knife allows your hand and wrist to stay in a more neutral position, avoiding the pinch grip that you use with traditional knives.

spikes that hold food firmly in place as you cut it. If you use a nonelectric knife, buy one that's L-shaped with a wide-diameter vertical handle. Grasp the handle like a dagger and cut with a sawing motion without applying much pressure.

In the grocery store, it may help to select foods that don't require slicing and dicing. For example, cut-up fruit and vegetables in the produce section may cost more but will save you time and effort.

Doing housework

For cleaning, use a long-handled mop, dustpan and broom. Work with long, smooth strokes. Use a rocking motion while working with long-handled tools. Shift body weight onto the front foot when making a forward stroke, and then shift weight to the rear foot when making a backward stroke.

Fill a bucket only half full to help avoid heavy lifting. Wash windows with a firm sponge that allows you to hold it with an open hand. Kneel close to the side of the bathtub, maintaining a balanced posture, and use a long-handled brush to scrub the other side. Store cleaning supplies on each floor and within easy reach so that you don't need to transport them everywhere.

Do laundry on a regular basis to avoid having heavy loads accumulate. Place a table at a comfortable height near the washer for sorting and folding clothes. If you have a front-loading washer or dryer, place it on blocks for easier access. Protect your back by avoiding unnecessary bending or stooping whenever you can.

In the shop

For some tasks, there's no alternative to using a manual tool, which may require gripping, pushing or lifting. But often there's a power alternative that puts less stress on your joints than a manual tool does. For example, a power nail driver or screwdriver may be easier on your joints. Where appropriate, look for lighter versions of tools or handle extensions that can improve the leverage for turning a tool.

ASSISTIVE DEVICES FOR MOBILITY

Devices such as braces, canes and walkers help you move around safely and maintain your balance, both inside and outside. They can offer you a more independent lifestyle and allow you to accomplish many tasks that you might otherwise require assistance with. At the same time, these devices provide extra support, stability and protection for painful joints.

Using a brace

If you have osteoarthritis in a knee, wearing a brace can provide pain relief. It may also help correct a slight misalignment of the joint that could be contributing to your condition. Pain symptoms often improve in many cases of mild to moderate osteoarthritis.

The brace wraps around the joint, helping to relieve pressure on the affected parts and reduce pain and swelling. Any brace, especially a knee brace, should fit properly. It's important to work with your healthcare team to get a good fit. Depending on the type of brace, it may offer a long-term solution to the problem of pain.

Using a cane

When properly adjusted to your height and grip, a cane greatly improves your balance and mobility. A poorly fitted cane, by contrast, throws you off balance, makes you less stable on your feet and increases your arthritis symptoms.

It's a common mistake to choose a cane that's too long. This pushes one side of your body up, putting extra strain on your shoulders and arm muscles. On the other hand, a cane that's too short causes you to lean forward, putting extra pressure on your wrist.

Select the right style

When buying a cane, don't base your decision on looks alone. A distinctive cane may add fashionable flair, but there are more important factors to consider. For example, a lightweight cane is easier to lift than a heavy one. A physical therapist can recommend a cane to best meet your needs and can teach you to walk with it so that it feels natural.

Consider length

To determine the proper length of a cane, stand up straight with your shoes on. Hold your arms at your sides. The length should equal the distance from the crease in your wrist to the floor. When you hold your cane while standing, your elbow should bend at a comfortable angle, about 20 to 30 degrees.

If you walk in different shoes that have heels of varying heights, make sure you have an adjustable cane. Nonadjustable canes can only be cut one time to fit.

Get a good grip

Choosing a grip is generally a matter of personal preference. A good grip relieves unnecessary stress on your joints, while numbness or pain in your hand or fingers may signal a poor fit.

A handle with a large diameter is generally easier to hold for extended periods. Make sure your fingers and thumb don't overlap when you grip the handle. If you have trouble grasping with your fingers, ask your doctor or physical therapist for advice.

The traditional candy-cane-style grip may not be the best choice because it doesn't center your weight over the staff. Instead, consider one with a swan-neck grip or with a grip that straddles the pole part of the cane.

Check the tip

The end of your cane should have a supple rubber tip that grips the floor. The tip provides traction and safety while you use the cane. Check the tip regularly — maybe once a month. Replace the tip before it wears down and becomes smooth.

Elbow bent about 20 degrees

Cane lines up with wrist crease when arm is straight down

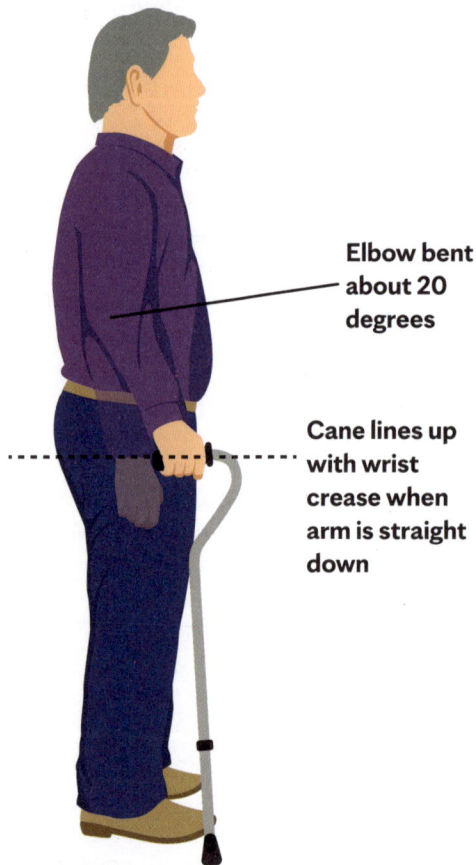

Fitting a cane
It's important that a cane fits properly. With the cane in your hand, the bend in your elbow should be at a 20-to-30-degree angle.

Learn proper technique

Hold your cane with the hand opposite your weaker leg. Stand tall and look ahead, not down at the floor. Pick up and move your cane in unison with the weaker leg. Keep the cane in place as you move the stronger leg forward.

Put as much weight on your cane as necessary to make walking comfortable, stable and smooth. Don't place the cane

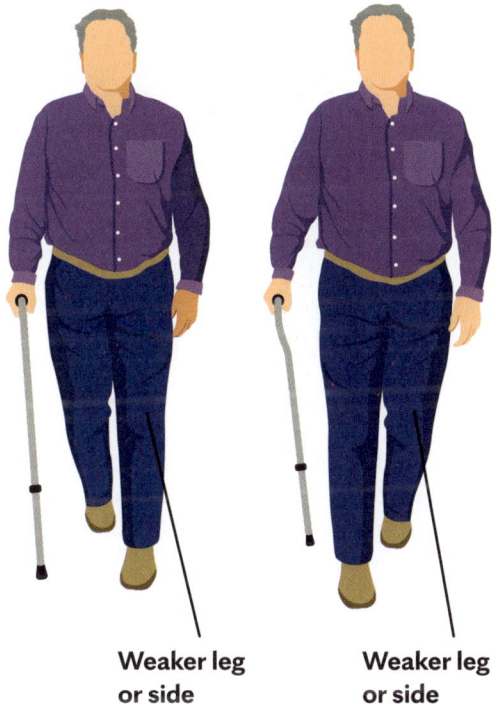

**Weaker leg   Weaker leg
or side   or side**

Walking with a cane
If you use a cane to assist one of your legs, grip the cane in the hand opposite the affected leg. Move the cane in unison with your affected leg.

too far ahead of you. Be careful when walking on uneven ground or on ice or other wet, slippery surfaces.

When going up stairs, remember "up with the strong" and lead with your stronger leg. Then pick up and move the cane at the same time you move your weaker leg up to the step.

When going down stairs, it's "down with the weak." Pick up and move the cane at the same time you move your weaker leg down the step. Then bring your stronger leg down to the step. When using stairs in either direction, use your free hand to hold the handrail, if there is one.

If you're receiving Medicare, the program will share the cost of a cane. But your healthcare professional has to write a prescription for the cane, indicating that it is "needed for walking." Most other health insurance plans also provide coverage if a cane is prescribed.

Once you've found a cane that fits and you've used it for a while, decide if the assistive device is a help or a hindrance. If you've fully recovered from joint replacement surgery, you can retire your cane — and relearn to walk without it.

MOVING IN THE RIGHT WAYS

The following pages demonstrate how to tailor your everyday movements to protect your joints. Follow these tips to ease arthritis pain and avoid further joint damage.

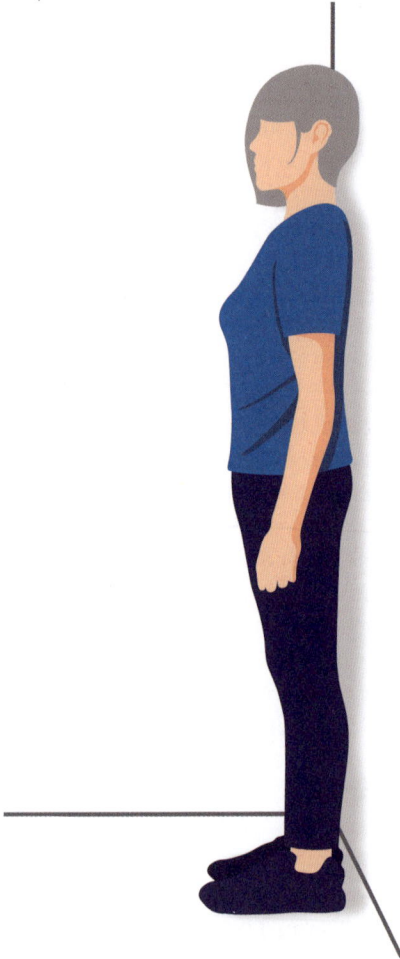

For good standing posture:

- Hold your chest high, keeping your shoulders back and relaxed.
- Gently pull your belly button toward your spine. Hold the position while breathing normally and looking straight ahead.
- Keep your feet parallel, with your weight evenly balanced on both feet.
- Keep your knees straight — not bent or in a locked position.

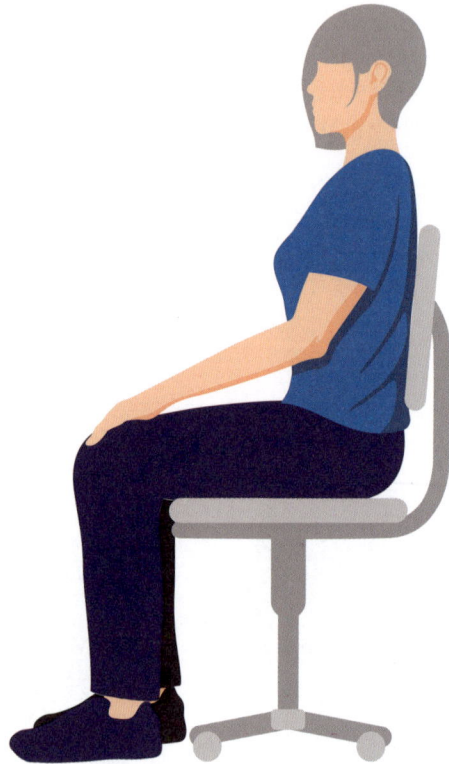

For good sitting posture:

- Rest both feet flat on the floor, keeping your knees level with your hips.
- Sit with your back pressed firmly against the chair. If necessary, support your lower back with a small cushion or rolled towel.
- Keep your upper back and neck comfortably straight, tucking your chin in slightly.
- Keep your shoulders relaxed — not elevated, rounded or pulled backward.

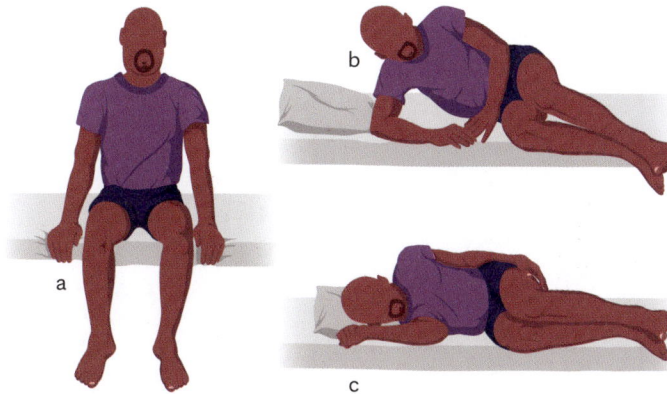

To properly lie down in bed:

- Start by sitting on the bed so that your head will hit the pillow when you lie down.
- Using your arms for support, slowly lower yourself onto the bed while bringing your legs up to a side-lying position.
- When sitting up from lying down, first bend your knees and then roll to your side. Slide your feet over the edge of the bed as you use your arms to push your body up to a sitting position.

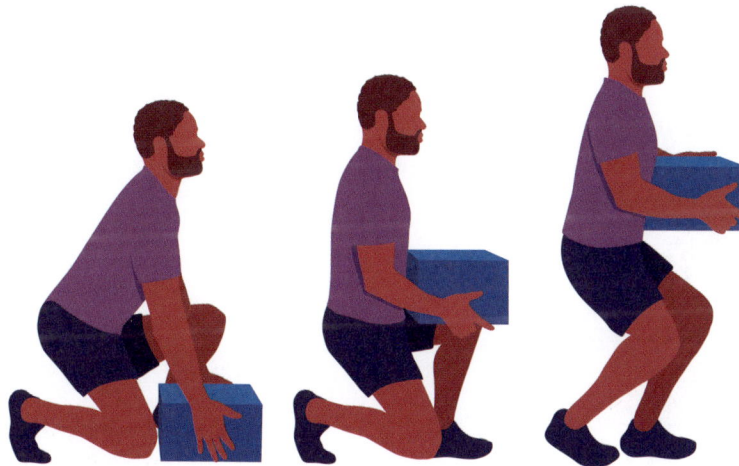

To properly lift objects:

- Keep your back straight and your feet apart, as in the standing position.
- Lower your body to get close to the object. Bend from your hips and knees. Do not bend at the waist.
- Hold the object by putting your hands around it, keeping it close to your body.
- Keeping your knees bent and your back straight, lift the object using your arm and leg muscles. Do not use your back muscles.
- If the object is too heavy, ask for help.

Protecting your joints   299

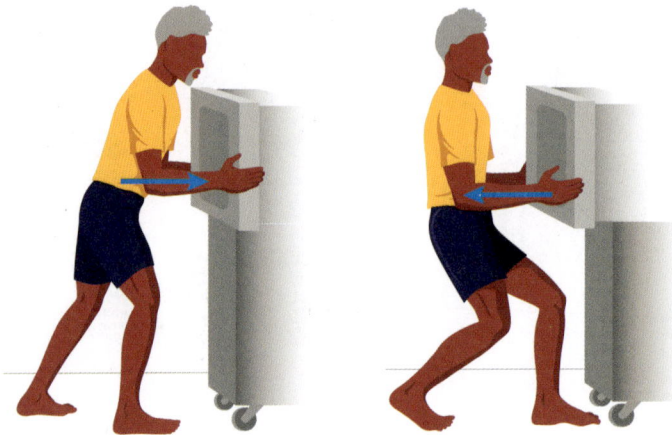

To properly push and pull objects:

- Keep your feet apart, as in the standing position.
- Keep your back straight.
- Lower your body to get close to the object. Bend from your hips and knees. Do not bend at the waist.
- Use the weight of your body to help move the object.
- If the object you're moving is too heavy, ask for help.

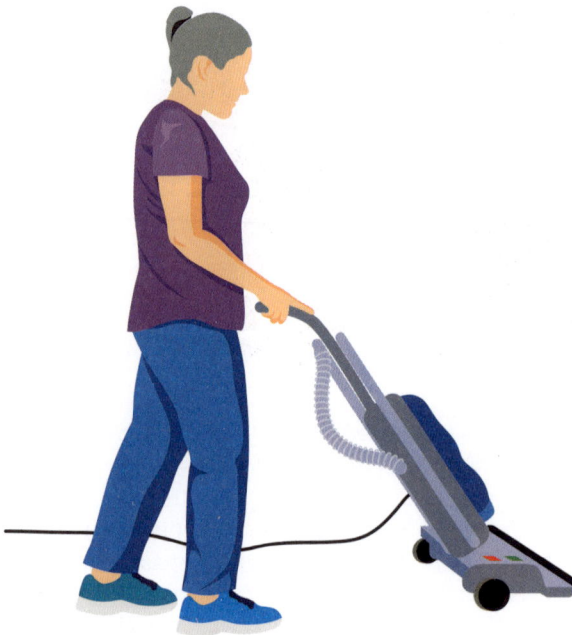

To properly use long-handled tools:

- Maintain a balanced posture with your back straight.
- Use a rocking motion, shifting your body weight from your front foot to your rear foot.
- Move your arms and legs rather than your back.
- Use long smooth strokes rather than short, choppy motions.

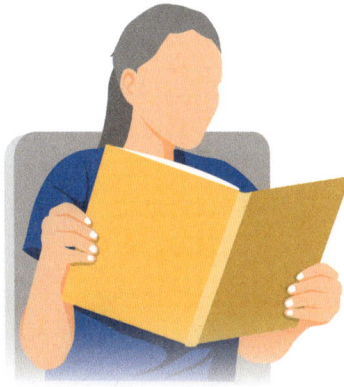

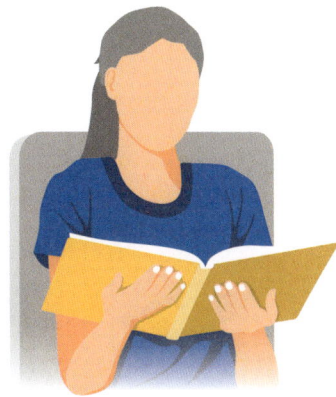

Holding a book

There are better and worse ways to hold a book, when considering your joints. A pinching grip (left) can strain your finger joints and cause pain. Instead, rest the book comfortably on your palms to ease pain (right).

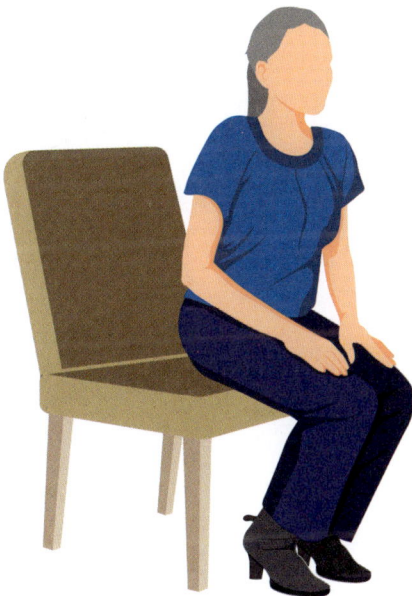

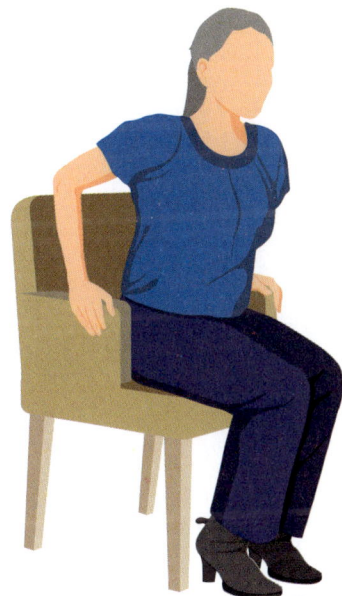

Getting up from a chair

When rising from a seated to a standing position, slide forward in the chair, but don't move your feet forward. Keeping your feet slightly apart, use your legs to stand up. If possible, push up on the arms of the chair with your palms as you rise.

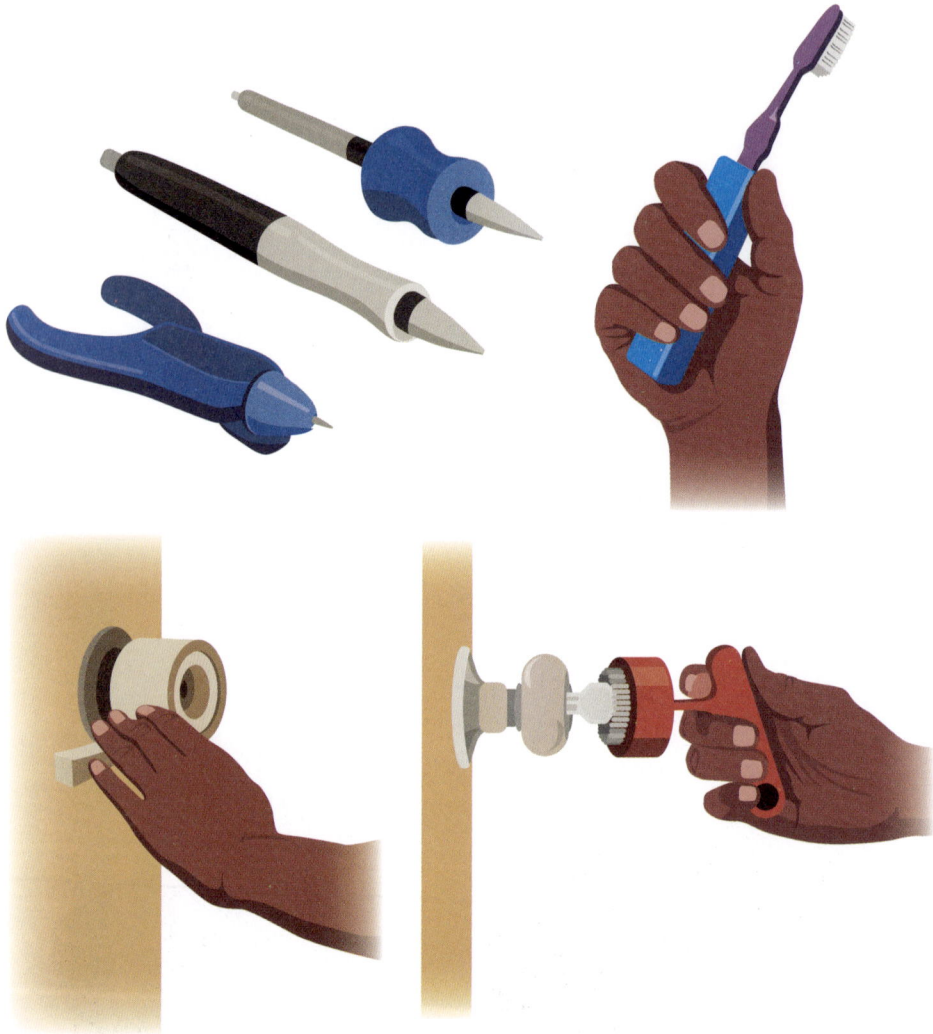

Devices that support and protect your joints

Handheld devices can help you perform many simple tasks. Large-barrel implements such as pens (upper left), toothbrushes (upper right) and eating utensils can reduce the stress on your finger and thumb joints. Squeezing a doorknob can be hard on finger joints. A lever attachment (lower left) makes it easier to open the door. A special turning tool (lower right) features a collection of collapsible metal pins that mold around objects such as oven knobs and keys.

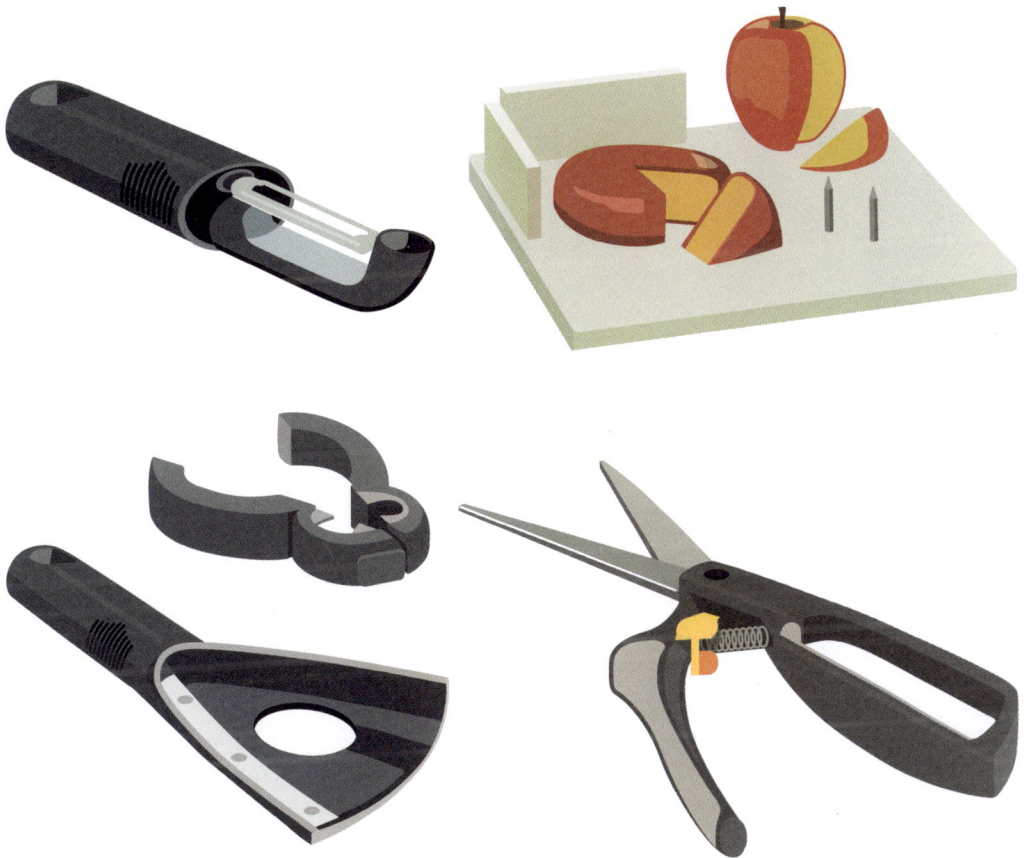

Helpful kitchen tools

Kitchen tools, such as vegetable peelers, can be purchased with wider handles (upper left). A cutting board equipped with nail pegs and a raised ledge (upper right) helps secure food during meal preparation, reducing the amount of force you need to hold food while chopping. When faced with a stubborn jar lid or bottle cap, different types of opening devices can reduce the amount of stress placed on your hand joints (lower left). Spring-loaded scissors (lower right) open automatically, reducing joint strain in your fingers and thumb.

19

Traveling with arthritis

Travel can be stressful even when you're healthy. But if you have arthritis, the thought of carrying luggage, changing planes or walking long distances can be enough to give you second thoughts about taking a trip.

However, having arthritis doesn't mean that you're stuck in one place. In fact, today it's easier to travel with a disability than ever before. Thanks to laws such as the Americans with Disabilities Act (ADA) and the Air Carrier Access Act, the travel industry, including airlines, hotels and cruise ships, has made travel more accommodating for people with special needs.

In addition, both new and established companies have recognized the growing market for travel clients with mildly to severely limited abilities. Special tours, vacation packages and activities are available for people with arthritis.

PLANNING A TRIP

Where in the world do you want to go? Maybe you dream of visiting the Louvre in Paris or hiking part of the Appalachian Trail. Maybe your employer just needs you to solve a problem in Cleveland.

The key to any successful trip starts with planning. With the right preparations, the world is yours to explore.

Naturally, you must be honest about your capabilities. Rock climbing may not be the best choice for you, but a mountain-top helicopter excursion might be an alternative. Whitewater rafting could be extremely painful with a neck condition, but a week in a riverside cabin might let you appreciate the water without discomfort.

Choose a vacation that has flexibility. Consider how you'll spend the day if your companions take on more strenuous activities or extensive sightseeing. Remember, frequent rest periods may be the most important ingredient of a satisfying trip.

Doing research before your trip is important. Read travel guides and websites, including those geared toward people with disabilities. Librarians at your public library may be able to point you toward helpful information. Search for tour companies that offer vacations that appeal to you. You might even request information directly from locations you want to visit.

In addition, talking with people who have taken similar trips will help you know what you can expect when you arrive.

Disability and disease-specific support groups, both in person and online, can help with details of planning. And make sure to get the advice of your healthcare team when planning a trip. They may have good insight into how much you can handle and how you can accomplish your travel goals.

Calling in the pros

Many people rely on travel agents and tour operators. Agents are professionals who can save you time and money, and they often do not charge for their services. Instead, they may receive commissions from the airlines and hotels they book with. Tour operators generally combine several travel components, such as airline tickets, hotels and ground transportation, into one package that is

SHOULD YOU BUY TRAVEL INSURANCE?

Without some form of travel insurance, hotels and airlines may refund your money if you become ill and can't make the trip or need to go home early. But it's probably best to purchase trip cancellation insurance if you think there's a chance you'll be unable to travel. Such policies are generally available from your travel agent, tour operator, booking website or AAA club. You may also want to search an independent website that lets you compare travel insurance options before buying. Your credit card may already provide some insurance for trips you book with it.

If you need to make a refund request, be sure to send a doctor's statement with the request. Be aware that trip cancellation insurance may not pay if you cancel because of a preexisting condition, so check the coverage before buying.

Review your medical insurance coverage before you travel. Policies sometimes include the costs of a medical illness while you're away from home, including travel back home if you become seriously ill, but many plans don't include this coverage. Again, some policies exclude preexisting conditions, so be certain to read the fine print.

usually less expensive than what you would pay if you put them together yourself. The fees of tour operators are usually included in these expenses.

To select a travel agent, start by asking friends and relatives for referrals. You can also call agencies and ask about their experience in arranging trips for travelers with physical limitations.

Choose an agent with whom you're comfortable discussing your needs, and make sure they are willing to spend the time required to arrange for those needs. Treat your agent as a travel partner who wants to continue working with you after the basic decisions about your destination have been made.

CHOOSING WHERE TO STAY

Where you sleep at night can make or break your trip, so keep your physical needs in mind when choosing lodging. You may be able to book an "accessible" room on a hotel's website, but it's smart to communicate directly with the hotel to make sure that it will suit your needs. Be sure to specify what you require well in advance of your travel date. Always get written confirmation of any guaranteed arrangements.

There are many questions you might ask about your lodging. For example, find out how close you'll be to other destinations, such as the convention center, restaurant or beach. Ask what floor you'll be on, where the elevators are located in relation to your room, whether the bathrooms have handrails, if there is a bathtub or a shower stall, whether the doors and faucets have levers instead of hard-to-grasp knobs, and whether the hotel has a shuttle that can be used by someone with physical limitations.

You might also ask if the hotel has porters to help carry your luggage and how you can arrange taxi or rideshare services. You may want to inquire about handicapped parking, fire exits and access ramps. If you'll be there awhile, you may want to check on the availability of laundry and other services at the hotel.

In many cases, hotels offer a range of special amenities and services, such as tours in accessible vans, heating pads for those unexpected flare-ups or in-house spas with whirlpools. It pays to ask as many questions as possible before you book.

Keep in mind that you're not limited to the major hotel chains. Many bed-and-breakfasts, inns and privately owned vacation rentals can host guests with disabilities. And on some travel websites or apps, you can even filter your search results for lodging with accessible features. That way, you'll only see options that work for you. To be safe, you may still want to contact the company or host to ask specific questions.

WHAT TO TAKE

Packing light is good advice for all travelers, but especially for people with arthritis. Try to plan carefully so that you'll have enough clothing, plus the important items that make your arthritis more manageable, without packing extra things you won't need.

Don't forget to bring any aids you use daily, such as a raised toilet seat, long-handled reacher, special pillow or heating pad. If you have electrical appliances and are traveling to a foreign country, you may need to pack a plug or voltage adapter.

To minimize strain on your joints, use lightweight luggage that's easy to trans-port. Check to see if porters and taxis or rideshares will be available at your destination, and ask the porters and drivers to carry your luggage whenever possible. At the airport, check your bags at the curb. Be sure to carry small bills for tipping the people who assist you.

Check weather forecasts for your destination to decide what type of clothing is most appropriate. Dressing in layers allows you to adapt easily to weather changes. You may be most comfortable wearing loose or stretchy clothing so you can move around easily, whether traveling or enjoying your destination.

PACKING YOUR BAGS

- Pack as few items as possible. Lay out the essentials in front of you. Choose articles of clothing that are easy to layer or combine with other items. Remove any duplicates or extras unless absolutely required.
- Travel with lightweight luggage that has sturdy wheels, telescoping handles and cross-body straps. Attach identification tags to all luggage.
- Airlines often allow one carry-on bag and one personal item, such as a purse, small backpack, personal computer or briefcase, onboard with you. Size matters — the smaller your baggage, the easier it will be to hoist into an overhead bin and the less likely it is to be checked at the gate. Also, make sure you're familiar with the baggage policies of the airline you're flying. Many charge fees for carry-on bags as well as checked luggage.
- In carry-on luggage, liquids, gels and aerosols are permitted in 3.4-ounce containers, placed in a quart-size, clear plastic, zip-close bag. One bag is allowed per traveler.
- Prescription medications and medical supplies will not count against your carry-on allowance, but if they exceed 3.4 ounces or cannot fit into a zip-close bag, you'll need to declare them to a security officer.
- Check with your airline or travel agent regarding the checked baggage policy, including the number of pieces you may bring and size and weight limitations.

Sunscreen, sunglasses, a hat (either for sun protection or warmth) and comfortable shoes also are essential.

When packing medications, you may not be able to "pack light." It's smart to take a supply that's more than enough for your trip and carry medications in original containers. Keep them in your carry-on luggage, in case you're separated from the bags you've checked — although some travelers pack a duplicate supply in their luggage. If you need medications to be kept cool, most attendants will gladly store them in a refrigerator for you, although you may prefer carrying them separately in a vacuum flask or insulated container.

Along with your medications, bring copies of your prescriptions, contact information for your healthcare professional, a summary of your medical history and a complete list of all the drugs you're currently taking. It's a good idea to leave copies of this information at home with a friend or relative, too, in case your healthcare professional is unavailable. If you have other medical problems in addition to arthritis, you might consider wearing a medical alert bracelet or necklace.

TRANSPORTATION

You'll want to take certain steps in planning, depending on the form of transportation you use. The good news is that over the years travel companies have become more accommodating to people with disabilities, including arthritis.

Traveling by air

Thanks to a U.S. law called the Air Carrier Access Act, regulations make it illegal to discriminate against disabled air travelers. These regulations clearly state the responsibilities of travelers, carriers, airport operators and contractors. For people with arthritis, the rules mean more time for boarding, accessible terminal parking and accessible restrooms, among other things.

Still, you must do your part. When you make airline reservations, state your special needs, such as seating or storage capacity for oversized arthritis aids. Allow extra time to get through the airport, request an airport wheelchair or other terminal transport if you need it, and check your luggage through to your final destination.

At all airports in the United States with scheduled airline service, passengers must go through a pre-boarding screening process for security. The Transportation Security Administration (TSA) has suggestions for people with disabilities and medical conditions to help make the screening process go smoothly. Those suggestions include:

- If you need assistance moving through the airport, contact your airline. The airline can provide someone to assist you through the terminal and screening line.
- If you require a companion or assistant to accompany you through the security checkpoint and to the boarding gate, request a gate pass for your companion from the airline. Do

TRAVELING WITH ARTHRITIS MEDICATIONS

Many types of medicine are easy to travel with. For example, pills or gelcaps are small and generally aren't affected by a range of temperatures as you travel through different environments. However, some medications used to treat arthritis must be kept cool to remain safe and effective. If you're planning to travel with medications, it's smart to be clear on whether you'll need insulated containers, refrigeration while traveling or other special considerations. Refer to the table below. If you have any questions, make sure to talk with your healthcare team before your trip.

STORAGE RECOMMENDATIONS FOR REFRIGERATED MEDICATIONS

Medication	Refrigeration required	Room temperature stability
Abatacept	Yes	6 hours
Adalimumab	Yes	14 days; may vary by product
Anakinra	Yes	12 hours
Bimekizumab	Yes	30 days
Canakinumab	Yes	60 minutes
Certolizumab pegol	Yes	7 days
Etanercept	Yes	30 days
Golimumab	Yes	30 days
Guselkumab	Yes	4 hours
Ixekizumab	Yes	5 days
Rilonacept	Yes	3 hours once reconstituted
Risankizumab	Yes	24 hours
Sarilumab	Yes	14 days
Secukinumab	Yes	4 days
Tildrakizumab	Yes	30 days
Tocilizumab	Yes	2 weeks
Ustekinumab	Yes	30 days

this before reaching the security checkpoint.

- The limit of one carry-on and one personal item does not apply to the medical supplies, equipment, mobility aids or assistive devices that you may require.
- Pack your medications and medical documentation in a separate bag to help speed the inspection process. Make sure that the medication container is not too densely filled and that it's clearly labeled.
- You may present any medical documentation about your condition to the screener. But such material is not required, and having it won't exempt you from the screening process.
- Tell the screener about any special equipment or devices that you're using or about any devices located in or on your body.
- Make sure that all your carry-on items, equipment, mobility aids and assistive devices have identification tags attached.
- Items such as wheelchairs, scooters, crutches, canes, walkers, prosthetic devices, braces and orthopedic shoes are permitted through the security checkpoint.
- If your prosthetic device requires tools for removal, the TSA recommends bringing them along in case you need to remove the prosthesis for any reason.
- If you have a medical device either inside or outside your body, check with your healthcare professional to learn if it's safe to pass through a metal detector or to be hand-wanded.

If your healthcare professional says it's unsafe, request a pat-down inspection from the screener.

- If a personal search is required, you may request a private area for screening. You may request a private area at any time during the screening process.
- Ask the screener for assistance if you need help as you proceed through the screening, including walking through the metal detector.
- Certain times of the day are less congested at airports, making the process easier to negotiate. A travel agent or airline representative may be able to suggest less crowded flights.
- If you will need to change planes, find out whether you'll have to change terminals and whether a shuttle between terminals is accessible to you. If not, ask for suggestions on how to reach your destination.

Traveling by train

Trains generally provide a good transportation option for people with disabilities. Throughout Europe and Asia, rail travel is relatively easy and accessible, with many trains accommodating disabled travelers on international routes. In the United States, Amtrak offers special assistance for disabled passengers and their travel companions.

When making Amtrak reservations online or on the phone, you can request an accessible seat or room and space to store a mobility device. Have written documentation of your disability ready at the ticket counter and when boarding the train. This may include a letter from your healthcare professional or a membership card from a disability organization.

Most train stations have personnel to provide baggage assistance and to help get passengers from the station entrance onto the train. Amtrak suggests that you make any requests for assistance when you make your reservations.

Amtrak can supply you with a wheelchair. If you have your own wheelchair, it must not exceed 30 inches wide and 48 inches long and should have a minimum ground clearance of 2 inches. It must weigh no more than 600 pounds occupied.

Traveling by bus

Many bus lines can provide assistance with boarding and getting off vehicles. The driver may also be able to help with stowing and retrieving your luggage and mobility devices. Most coach bus aisles are not wide enough for wheelchairs. If you use a wheelchair or have trouble using stairs, make the arrangements for assistance with customer service. Try to make your request at least 48 hours before your departure.

Bus travel is often slower, so you may want to schedule trips for the middle of the week, when fewer people travel. Keep medications and bottled water with you. For a long ride, take a pillow and snacks, too.

Traveling by car

When you travel by car, you'll enjoy more freedom than with other forms of transportation. You can stop whenever you want, you'll have more room to stretch out, and you can take along anything that fits in your vehicle.

There are ways to make the trip even more enjoyable. Be sure to stop frequently, getting out to stretch and move around. Keep medications, snacks, maps, an emergency kit and first-aid supplies in the car.

For safety, make sure your cell phone is charged before starting out, or carry a charger that can plug into the car. Make hotel reservations in advance, or stop early enough to find a place to stay. Don't let yourself get tired before finding lodging for the night.

If you rent a car, ask for amenities that will make driving more comfortable, such as hand controls, a transfer board if you use a wheelchair, swivel seats, a padded or built-up steering wheel, or a spinner knob on the steering wheel that allows easier turning. To get a car with special features, you may need to reserve your vehicle two to three business days in advance.

Traveling by ship

You may find travel aboard a cruise ship particularly relaxing. A number of design changes have been made to U.S. ships in recent years, such as the widening of passageways, doorways and elevators and the addition of accessible staterooms for wheelchair-using travelers. Special meals and exercise plans may be available, too.

Keep in mind that while the ADA requirements generally apply to all ships operating in U.S. waters, cruise lines operating in other countries may not have the same accessibility requirements. So before booking, make sure you check to see that the cruise ship will have the accommodations you need.

Before booking a particular cruise, ask your travel agent or a cruise line representative about the ship's design and accessibility. You may want to consider which onboard amenities you'll use most — such as restaurants, meeting rooms, pools or sun decks — and try to book a room nearby. It's difficult to arrange having all of them close by.

When choosing a cruise, also consider where it stops. Cobblestone streets or ancient stone stairways may make it difficult to enjoy a destination if you have arthritis. Find out how passengers embark and disembark at each destination, too. At some ports of call, a ship may anchor at sea and shuttle passengers to shore on smaller boats. If you anticipate difficulty with embarking or disembarking the ship, you may want to choose a cruise that has fewer stops or plan to stay aboard soaking up the ship's ambience while your companions go ashore.

Choices abound these days in cruises geared for the leisurely traveler, and

many shore excursions now accommodate those with an unhurried pace. Most ships employ healthcare professionals, but their pharmacies are usually limited. You'll want to take along more than enough medication to get you through the trip.

TRAVELING ABROAD

Whether you're touring Australia or Italy, Venezuela or Singapore, arthritis should not prevent you from having an enjoyable, stimulating adventure.

You may need to see a healthcare professional before you travel, depending on your general health and on your destination. If you're visiting a developing country, you should plan to consult your healthcare professional or a travel medicine clinic. This consultation should take place at least 4 to 8 weeks before the journey to ensure that any necessary medications can be prescribed and that vaccinations have time to take effect.

Services at travel medicine clinics vary widely. Some offer vaccinations and general information. Others offer comprehensive overviews of the health hazards along your itinerary, with detailed advice on how to stay well. The clinics are typically affiliated with medical centers or universities. Check the directory at the International Society of Travel Medicine website: www.istm.org.

In addition, the International Association for Medical Assistance to Travelers offers a free information packet detailing its services. These include free climate and sanitation information and advice on international disease and immunization requirements. You can learn more about this organization at www.iamat.org.

Although healthcare has improved in many world destinations, be sure to carry ample medications on overseas trips and pace yourself so that you won't need a healthcare professional to attend to a routine flare-up.

No matter where you're headed, take all reasonable precautions to keep yourself safe and healthy. Then relax and have fun. You can travel — and travel well — with arthritis!

20

On the job

Having arthritis is no reason to put a career on hold or start planning an early retirement. Focusing on what you can do instead of what you can't do may help you discover an inner strength you never thought you had and come up with creative solutions to the demands you face at work.

Your success in the workplace depends greatly on having a positive attitude, the confidence to work toward your goals, and the will to get on with life and not dwell on every obstacle that appears in your path.

One of the initial challenges you may face on the job will be deciding whether or not to inform your boss and co-workers about having arthritis. This is a personal choice, and deciding either way may carry potential downsides. In some cases, this knowledge may raise questions in your employer's mind about whether you're physically able to do the job. Some

supervisors consider arthritis to be just aches and pains, and they may wonder whether you're using the disease as an excuse for special treatment. And in some situations, unspoken discrimination shows up as denied opportunities, such as promotions you deserve but don't get.

For reasons such as these, many experts recommend that you say nothing about the disease if you can answer no to both of the following questions:
*   Is your arthritis obvious?
*   Do you need special accommodations or resources to do your job?

If you answer yes to either question, it may be best to inform your employer and co-workers that you have arthritis. Otherwise, they may come to believe that you're not doing your share of the work — and they may resent you for it.

Choosing not to disclose your arthritis may also have consequences for you. If you decide to say nothing, you may be more prone to ignore your body's warning signs and push yourself beyond your limits to maintain your secret. This will only make matters worse by increasing the pain and fatigue so common to arthritis.

If you decide that you need to tell your boss about your condition, schedule a meeting with care. Pick a time when distractions and job pressures for both of you are lower than usual. There is no required information that needs to be shared, but to advocate for yourself effectively, you may want to include:
- General information about your disability
- Why you are disclosing it
- How it affects your ability to perform key tasks for your job
- The types of accommodations that you have had in the past or one that you anticipate you might need

For example, if you have rheumatoid arthritis, you might disclose how long you have lived with this diagnosis, what it is, and explain that when pain flares up or fatigue sets in, these are signs that your affected joints need rest and repair.

At this meeting, have suggestions prepared for changes that will help you do your job better. If you need more rest breaks while at work, for example, you could note how that will help your productivity the rest of the time. Discuss your work responsibilities with your doctor or occupational therapist, too. They may have ideas to help you perform particular tasks more easily, perhaps with

the aid of assistive devices — even some as simple as putting armrests on your chair. They can also recommend exercises to increase your dexterity and range of motion for repeated movements you'll do during the workday.

KNOW YOUR RIGHTS

The Americans with Disabilities Act was passed by Congress in 1990. It's the most extensive bill of rights for people with disabilities that has ever been signed into law.

This law bans discrimination against people with disabilities and requires companies of 15 or more employees to make reasonable changes to help individuals do their jobs. In fact, a wise employer who values your experience will be willing to provide the tools necessary for you to do your job well.

Reasonable accommodations might include the following:
- Providing or modifying equipment to help you do certain tasks, such as a wheeled cart to carry supplies, a headset instead of a handheld phone or a chair with good back support. The cost of some assistive devices may qualify your employer for tax benefits.
- Installing a ramp if you have difficulty with stairs. Note that the employer can't make you pay for special equipment or accommodations like this. An exception would be if the changes place undue hardship on the employer, in which case you may be

asked to share some of the cost. But what constitutes undue hardship is judged on a case-by-case basis.

- Adapting workplace furniture to suit your needs, such as adjusting the height of your desk, allowing a stool for long periods of standing or providing a chair that ensures proper positioning.
- Allowing break periods for rest.
- Changing work responsibilities, eliminating tasks you have difficulty performing that aren't essential to your job.

If you believe that your employer is treating you unfairly and is unwilling to make reasonable changes to help you do your job, you can file a formal complaint with the Equal Employment Opportunity Commission (EEOC).

You can order free publications about the Americans with Disabilities Act and antidiscrimination legislation at the EEOC website: www.eeoc.gov. The state where you live (or work) also may have laws protecting you from discrimination. If you have questions about your legal rights, talk with a lawyer who specializes in employment law.

PROTECT YOUR JOINTS

Finding ways to reduce activities that irritate, inflame or damage your joints can help keep you off disability and in the workforce. Here are some ideas:

- Arrange your work area to reduce the need for lifting, walking or other movements that may be painful.

- Find the most comfortable positions, sitting or standing, for doing work. For tips on working at a computer, see page 318.
- If you perform repetitive motions, such as typing or assembly work, rest the affected joints every 20 to 30 minutes by stopping the activity and stretching your muscles. In fact, even if you don't perform repetitive motions, try to take a short break every half hour or hour to change positions, stretch and relax.
- If a task is always painful, search for other ways to do it. Occupational therapists specialize in solving such problems. Or ask a co-worker for help in exchange for your assistance with something else.
- Use special tools or assistive devices that reduce the strain on your joints: electric staplers, dictation services, chair leg extensions (to make it easier to get up), and enlarged grips for pencils and pens.
- Don't be afraid to ask for help if you need it.

Exercise

Maintaining muscle strength around your joints helps keep the joints stable and functional. Your doctor and physical therapist can design an exercise program that allows you to strengthen the joints that you use most often in your job. Some of the exercises can be simple and inconspicuous enough that you can do them during your lunch break or in momentary rest breaks. For example, if you work a lot with your hands, take a few seconds to bend your fingers, wrists and elbows as far as you can, then stretch them back out.

Relax

Job stress can aggravate arthritis pain, which in turn intensifies job stress. You can break the cycle by learning relaxation techniques.

Here are a few ideas:
- Let your mind wander to recall a happy memory.
- Look out a window and enjoy the scene.
- Listen to a recording of relaxing sounds, such as gentle rain.
- Take a short walk or sit outside.
- Lie down or sit quietly for a few minutes.

Conserve energy

You can help avoid the fatigue caused by arthritis by pacing yourself. Do the most important projects of the day during your time of peak energy. For example, if you know that you're a morning person, spend the morning doing the work that requires the most energy. Vary your schedule by alternating the more difficult tasks with easier ones. If possible, take a rest break of about 10 minutes every few hours.

COMMUTE WISELY

For some people with arthritis, the trip to work itself can be painful and exhausting.

These ideas may help make getting to work easier:
- Share rides with a co-worker. Pay for the service, or take turns driving.
- Use public transportation. It's usually slower but less exhausting than driving in heavy traffic. The Americans with Disabilities Act requires that accessible public transit vehicles be available to individuals with disabilities.
- If you need to drive, install equipment that minimizes the discomfort: a backrest, special mirrors, steering wheel modifications. Some automakers give you a rebate if you install this equipment in a new car. They may also provide a list of local companies that do the installation.
- If you have trouble walking, talk to your employer about possibilities for parking near the building entrance.
- You may be able to get a disabled parking permit from your state transportation department. You'll need to present a letter from your healthcare professional to get it. The permit allows you to use parking spaces reserved for people with disabilities.
- If you have difficulty climbing stairs, you may ask for a ramp leading into the building. You may also request a workspace closer to the entrance.
- If you can manage stairs with handrails, make sure rails are installed on the stairs close to your work area. If not, request them. The addition can be beneficial to the general public and enhance public safety as well.

GET COMFORTABLE WITH YOUR COMPUTER

Working at a keyboard for many hours can worsen the pain and fatigue of arthritis. If you work for most of the day at a computer, consider these tips for having better posture and position:

- As you sit in your chair, lean back slightly so that your lower back is firmly supported by the backrest. Keep your feet flat on the floor, with your knees bent at about 90 degrees. If you don't have firm back support, request a chair that allows you to adjust the backrest to different heights and angles.
- Move close to the keyboard so you aren't reaching for it. The keyboard should be 3 to 6 inches from your lap. Both the keyboard and the monitor should be directly in front of you. The top of the screen should be at eye level.
- A padded bar between the keyboard and your lap can provide wrist support. While you're typing, your wrists should be straight, with your forearms parallel to the floor. Chairs with armrests offer support for the forearms, and wrist braces can help keep your wrists comfortably aligned. If your wrists are usually bent as you type, you can develop carpal tunnel syndrome, which produces pain or numbness in your hands.
- Learning the proper technique for typing may be much easier on the joints than the hunt-and-peck method, which tends to put more pressure on individual joints.

- If typing is too difficult, use a mouse as much as possible. Voice-activated software is another option now available on many computers and smart devices.
- Take short breaks from the computer to stretch your legs, arms and fingers. Don't forget to give your eyes a break by focusing on an object at a distance.

KEEP AN OPEN MIND

Despite all that you and your employer do to accommodate for your arthritis, the nature of your job or the progression of your condition may require you to cut back on the number of hours you work or to find another line of work.

If your job requires heavy physical labor, such as construction, your healthcare professional may refer you to an occupational therapist or to a vocational rehabilitation agency. These specialists can help you build strength and determine how much weight you can safely lift.

If the physical restrictions are such that there's no work you can satisfactorily do at your company, a vocational rehabilitation agency can help you find other employment. Sometimes employees in these circumstances transition to a related profession or industry. A former construction worker, for example, may join a company that sells equipment to the construction industry.

JOB INTERVIEW TIPS

Although employers aren't allowed to ask if you have a disability, they may ask if you're able to perform specific job functions. A sample interview question might be: "Do you have any physical limitations that would hinder your performance of the job you're applying for?" Such questions can put you in an awkward situation if you think you'll need some kind of assistance in doing the work.

Some career counselors advise that you shouldn't disclose that you have arthritis. They suggest that doing so could eliminate you as a candidate with no chance to discuss the matter. In this line of reasoning, you should respond to the question with a no, under the presumption that the employer will provide the legally required reasonable accommodations if that becomes necessary. Another possible response, if you're not sure how arthritis will affect your job performance, is to answer "*will discuss*" on an application.

If your arthritis will be obvious at the interview, consider hinting about it during the interview setup (most likely in a phone conversation). But do so only after you make the interview appointment, and only if the person you're talking to is the one who will be interviewing you. Possible hint: "I sometimes have trouble with stairs. Do you have an elevator?" Hints like this may help reduce surprise, making it easier for the interviewer to concentrate on your needs.

Perhaps the most popular interview question is, "Tell me about yourself." As friendly as it may seem, this open-ended question is more than a pleasant ice-breaker to conversation.

The law prohibits employers from basing their hiring decisions on age, sex, race, religion, health or nonfelony arrests. They aren't supposed to ask, "How's your health?" But by describing yourself in response to their open question, you may reveal more than you intend. If you're prepared ahead of time, you can answer the question honestly and at the same time avoid revealing your condition — unless you want to do so.

During the interview, summarize the assets you would bring to the job, such as your education, certification or previous employment experience. Relate your personal strengths to the kinds of tasks you may be required to do. For example, highlight the fact that you're organized and thorough or good under pressure or an excellent team player. You could add that your experience, your desire to excel and your eagerness to accept new challenges have led you to apply for the job.

If your condition will be obvious at the interview, you may want to refer to it briefly. But don't shift the focus to your limitations. Remain focused on your strengths. Talk about the adjustments you've made that allow you to stay productive at work. For example, you can say something like: "I understand that you're legally prohibited from asking about my arthritis, except for questions about how I would perform specific tasks required for the job. I'll be happy to answer any questions because I'm certain I can do the work."

If your arthritis isn't obvious at the interview but will require job accommodations, you face a tough dilemma that has no easy solution. Should you say nothing until you receive a job offer? If so, you can be certain that you won't be ruled out of employment because of a disability. At the same time, the employer might feel misled. And this could generate hard feelings and a shaky start to your new job.

An alternate approach would be to tell the employer about your arthritis, especially if you're aware of aspects of the job in which you'll need some accommodation soon. If you decide this is the best solution for you, mention that the accommodations are usually inexpensive. You can also include a reminder of your qualities and experience that make you a particularly strong candidate for that role.

When you have a positive outlook and make thoughtful preparations, you have every right to be hopeful about your future in the workplace.

21

Your immune system and arthritis

Living with arthritis comes with challenges. As you've seen in previous chapters, there are many ways to overcome these challenges and make life easier.

Finding a healthcare team you trust is key. This team — including your primary physician or care provider, a rheumatologist, and other specialists — can guide you through treatments. They can also suggest exercises and lifestyle changes to help relieve arthritis pain and help you get back to your normal activities.

Along with relieving joint pain, the main goal of your healthcare team is keeping you healthy overall. For example, they'll work with you to keep your bones strong to prevent osteoporosis and lower your risk of fracture. Exercise, diet, and calcium and vitamin D supplements can all improve bone strength. Medications may help, too.

Another important way your healthcare team can help you stay healthy is by working with you to prevent infections. Arthritis — as well as the medications used to treat it — can weaken your immune system. That leaves your body at increased risk for an invading illness.

If your body can't fight back normally, a disease that typically isn't serious can take a larger toll on your health. It becomes especially important to prevent the spread of germs. In certain cases, your healthcare professional may prescribe an antibiotic to lower your risk for some infections.

The following sections discuss ways to boost your immune system while you're living with arthritis. By taking preventive measures such as these, you can give yourself the best chance of staying healthy and strong so you can live a fulfilling, productive and enjoyable life.

GET VACCINATED

For people of any age, the most effective way to prevent infectious diseases is to stay up-to-date on vaccinations. This is especially important for people with arthritis who are on medications that suppress or weaken the immune system. If you are taking a biologic medication or daily prednisone, you may be considered immunosuppressed.

The Centers for Disease Control and Prevention recommends certain schedules of vaccinations for children as well as adults. You can find these schedules and more information at www.cdc.gov /vaccines.

It's important to talk with your healthcare professional about your vaccination history and how arthritis affects your risk of disease. You may need to consult a specialist if a vaccine is in question.

Types of vaccines

For people who are immunosuppressed, vaccines are typically safe unless they contain live vaccine material. Live-attenuated vaccines use a weakened, or attenuated, form of a live virus. In healthy people, this prompts the immune system to develop antibodies against that virus, but it doesn't typically make them sick. However, if your immune system isn't healthy to begin with, it may not be able to fight off even the weakened virus from a live vaccine. You should avoid being around others for at least a week if they have received a

LIVE VACCINES

Live-attenuated vaccines include a weakened version of a live germ. If you have a weakened immune system because of arthritis medications or other health conditions, you'll likely need to avoid these vaccines. Because of the risk of infection, anyone who lives with an immunocompromised person should also avoid these vaccines.

Live vaccines include:
- Chickenpox (varicella)
- Nasal spray flu vaccine (not the flu shot)
- Measles, mumps and rubella (MMR)
- Oral polio (not the polio shot), not used in the United States
- Oral typhoid (not the typhoid shot)
- Yellow fever
- Zostavax for shingles (not Shingrix, a newer shingles vaccine)

The rotavirus vaccine can be administered to infants ages 2 months to 7 months who live with someone who is immunocompromised. However, for at least four weeks after an infant receives the rotavirus vaccine, no immunocompromised person should handle the infant's diapers.

If you have any questions about vaccinations or exposure to certain diseases, talk with your healthcare professional.

live vaccine. New types of vaccines were developed for COVID-19, including mRNA (Pfizer and Moderna), viral vector (Janssen and AstraZeneca) and protein subunit (Novavax) vaccines. All these are safe for immunosuppressed people to receive, but viral vector vaccines are no longer being used for COVID-19 due to concerns about an increased risk of clotting side effects seen with the Janssen vaccine and decline in demand for the AstraZeneca vaccine.

Common live vaccines include those for measles, mumps and rubella (MMR), chickenpox (varicella), and the nasally inhaled flu vaccine. Other live vaccines are given in special circumstances, usually for travel. See the sidebar on page 322 for more detailed information about live vaccines and other common examples.

Many vaccines are inactivated, meaning they use a dead version of the disease-causing germ. Others use just a part of the germ or a product of it. There's no risk of transmitting the disease with these types of vaccines. But they can still train your immune system to recognize certain invaders and quickly build up antibodies to defend against them. Vaccines that are generally safe for most people, including those with weakened immune systems, include the following:

- Diphtheria
- Flu (shot only)
- Hepatitis A
- Hepatitis B
- Human papillomavirus (HPV)
- Meningococcal disease
- Pneumococcal disease

- Polio
- Rabies
- Respiratory syncytial virus (RSV)
- Shingles (Shingrix, not Zostavax)
- Tetanus
- Whooping cough (pertussis)

Ideally, vaccines should be given before immune-suppressing medications are prescribed. If possible, they should be given 2 to 3 weeks before starting medications that weaken the immune system, so they have time to become fully effective. Alternatively, they may be given three months after immunosuppressing drugs are stopped. If you're breastfeeding, you can still receive vaccines.

Since 2019, the novel coronavirus disease (COVID-19) has been a leading cause of illness throughout the world. Unfortunately, COVID-19 will likely be a problem for years to come, similar to the flu. However, there are multiple ways to protect yourself from this infection. The first and most important step is vaccination. In those who become ill with COVID-19, oral antiviral therapies like nirmatrelvir and ritonavir (Paxlovid) may be helpful to stop severe disease and keep you out of the hospital. Those at highest risk for severe disease may benefit from intravenous (IV) antiviral medication if they become sick, or monoclonal antibodies for preventing infection. Therapies to prevent and treat COVID-19 are rapidly changing, so it is best to talk with your healthcare team about what options are best for you.

KEEP YOUR IMMUNE SYSTEM HEALTHY

Another key to staying healthy is caring for your immune system itself. As you age, your immune system ages, too. Your body's capacity to respond to infections slowly weakens over time. That leaves older adults more susceptible to inflammation, potentially increasing the risk for autoimmune diseases and other illnesses. Thus, improving and maintaining the health of your immune system is one of the most important steps you can take to live a long, healthy life.

Healthy living and behavioral choices are the cornerstones of immune health. To create the strongest foundation for your body's defense system, optimize your diet, exercise, sleep, and mental and spiritual health.

Just as making healthy choices in these areas can bolster your immune system, less healthy lifestyle factors can stress your body and hinder its ability to fight off attacks. Previous chapters have discussed many of these factors in more detail. To keep your defense system strong, make

any of the following lifestyle changes that aren't already part of your routine.

Stop smoking

If you smoke, quitting now is one of the most powerful ways you can help your body fight illness. Smoking is the single greatest negative influence on immune health.

Limit alcohol consumption and avoid substance misuse

While some alcohol such as red wine is thought to be beneficial in moderation, you should avoid excess alcohol and all illicit or recreational drugs. These can compromise your health in general.

Manage your weight

If you're carrying extra pounds, like many adults, losing some weight can improve your health. There is abundant data to suggest that being significantly overweight contributes to increased inflammation and a compromised immune system. Keep an eye on your weight as you get older, too. The body's natural metabolism tends to slow down with age, making it easier to gain weight.

Watch what you eat

Foods that have anti-inflammatory effects, such as in the Mediterranean diet, may help maintain your immune system.

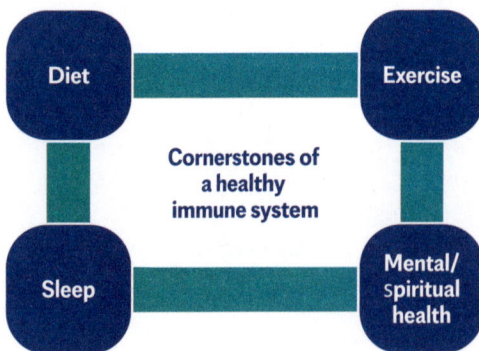

Diet — Exercise
Cornerstones of a healthy immune system
Sleep — Mental/spiritual health

On the other hand, processed foods and diets high in sugar, alcohol and red meat have all been shown to negatively affect immune cells and processes. So, eating for immunity may be as simple as a healthy, plant-based diet. Eat more fruits and vegetables, nourishing fats such as monounsaturated fats, a variety of whole grains, and lean protein. In addition, staying well hydrated can help your body flush out toxins, curbing inflammation.

Consider supplements with caution

Echinacea, elderberry, ginseng and garlic oil are discussed in the popular media as supplements that may improve immune health. However, there is no high-quality evidence to suggest that these prevent infections. While many think that supplements are safe because they are natural, some can be dangerous, especially if used at high doses or in combination with arthritis medications. Remember that these supplements, unlike prescription medicine, are not subject to government requirements for quality control and evidence for effectiveness before being sold.

Exercise

You already know that being active is important for your health. Exercise is one of the best medicines for life, and it's perhaps even more vital for people with arthritis. In fact, research shows that exercise benefits the immune system, boosting its function to fight disease. Frequent activity may even change how the immune system ages. Find a fun way to incorporate exercise into your daily routine. If you've avoided exercise because high-impact activity hurts your joints, try tai chi, dancing, yoga, gardening or walking.

Get better sleep

Missing out on sleep can make you more likely to get sick after being exposed to a virus. During sleep, your immune system releases cytokines, which help the body fight infection or inflammation. Sleep deprivation may decrease production of cytokines. In addition, infection-fighting antibodies and cells are reduced during periods when you don't get enough sleep. To stay healthy, make sleep a strict part of your to-do list. Schedule a "pre-sleep buffer" before bed to prepare for a good night's sleep — cut out nighttime caffeine, put down your phone, turn off the TV or tablet, and create a dreamy sleep environment.

Manage stress

Daily life is often stressful and busy, but it pays to manage your stress effectively, as studies show that stress contributes to health decline. You can take steps to lessen the toll stress takes on your body by trying mind-body interventions such as listening to music, spending time on your hobbies, meditating, doing yoga and getting out into nature. You might also benefit from counseling, focusing on time management and exercise. (For more on stress relief, see Chapter 17.)

Avoid harmful environmental exposures

To keep your immune system healthy, avoid carcinogens — substances that cause cancer. This includes avoiding excessive sun exposure, limiting your exposure to smoke and staying safe from harmful chemicals that may be around your work or home.

STAY UP AND RUNNING

Maintaining a healthy immune system is important for everyone. But especially for people with arthritis and on medications that suppress the immune system, helping this complex system stay strong and functional is key. Avoiding sickness helps you feel well enough to engage with family and friends, thrive at work, and keep up the activities you enjoy.

Researchers are continually making discoveries that give us a deeper understanding of how immune cells and processes work, but there's no question that the steps in this chapter can help boost your immunity. As you take steps to gain control of your joint pain, keeping your whole body healthy overall is vital to your progress.

BIOLOGIC MEDICATIONS AND INFECTIONS

The body's immune system is a well-regulated system. When bacteria, viruses and other invaders are discovered, white blood cells produce certain cytokines. These cytokines, including TNF, IL-1, IL-6, IL-12 and IL-23, mobilize the cells to engage and destroy the invaders. This temporarily causes inflammation. Usually, after the infection is cleared up, your body stops making these excess cytokines. If you have rheumatoid arthritis, that production doesn't decrease. As proinflammatory cytokines build up, more white blood cells collect in an area, causing inflammation, pain and tissue damage. Cytokine inhibitor medications block the action of the specific cytokine they target, reducing inflammation.

Because of how they work, biologics also limit your ability to fight infections. In general, this risk isn't greater than that of some nonbiologic medications. Most people who develop a serious infection while taking a biologic are also taking other medications that suppress the immune system, such as methotrexate or a corticosteroid. The risk also increases if you take a combination of cytokine inhibitors.

Due to an overactive immune system, people with rheumatoid arthritis have an increased risk of some cancers, such as lymphoma. It's not yet clear whether cytokine inhibitors can affect the risk of certain cancers. More high-quality evidence is needed.

Additional resources

WHERE TO GET MORE HELP

You can find a lot of health information on the internet and social media. Some of it is very good advice, but some of it is downright bad. Don't believe everything that you find. The online environment has a way of making all health information appear of equal quality. The key is making sure to get information from trusted sources. Carefully read reports and check if the information comes from respected publications, organizations or medical professionals. If something you find seems questionable or conflicts with conventional wisdom, you have the right to be skeptical.

Also beware of fraudulent medical products or information promising an arthritis cure. At worst, the products may actually be dangerous. Even vitamins can be harmful if they're taken in large doses. Watch out for glowing testimonials or medical treatments described as secret,

miracle, foreign, breakthrough or overnight.

Listed here are resources and organizations that you can depend on for quality information on arthritis and guidance on living an active life with joint pain. Your medical care team may be able to point you to others.

At the time of this writing, all sources cited in this book were publicly available. However, the availability of online health information can change over time, so if a link is no longer accessible, consider checking the organization's website or searching for updated sources.

American College of Rheumatology
www.rheumatology.org

The website of this organization for healthcare professionals in rheumatology contains information on causes, symptoms and treatments for many forms of arthritis.

Americans with Disabilities Act (ADA)
800-514-0301 (toll-free)
www.ada.gov

This website and toll-free number can help you find official information on the ADA, receive technical assistance or file a complaint.

Arthritis Foundation
www.arthritis.org

The Arthritis Foundation is an excellent resource for knowledge and support. This national organization provides self-help materials and can lead you to local support groups, classes and medical care providers who are experienced in working with people who have arthritis. The Arthritis Foundation's magazine, *Arthritis Today,* features current news and advice for easing symptoms.

Choose PT
www.choosept.com

This website from the American Physical Therapy Association offers information on how physical therapy may help you recover from many conditions, including arthritis.

Equal Employment Opportunity Commission (EEOC)
www1.eeoc.gov/eeoc/publications /index.cfm

Find fact sheets about discrimination, information on your legal rights in the workplace, guidance on the ADA for employers and more on the EEOC's website.

Job Accommodation Network
800-526-7234 (toll-free)
https://askjan.org

Provided by the Office of Disability Employment Policy, this resource offers free guidance on workplace accommodations and disability employment issues.

Healthy Aging - Mayo Clinic Press
https://mcpress.mayoclinic.org/healthy -aging/

Find expertise on hot topics, practical tips for every day and reliable insights to help you care for your physical and mental health at any age.

Mayo Clinic
www.MayoClinic.org

Visit Mayo Clinic's website for additional information on many health conditions, medications and other treatments.

National Institute of Arthritis and Musculoskeletal and Skin Diseases
www.niams.nih.gov

This organization, also known as NIAMS, is part of the National Institutes of Health. Its website offers more information on many forms of arthritis and related conditions, including who's at risk, what a diagnosis may involve and types of treatment.

National Institute on Aging
www.nia.nih.gov

The National Institute on Aging provides information and resources to help people age 50 and older incorporate exercise and physical activity into their daily lives.

National Rehabilitation Information Center (NARIC)
https://naric.com

This database is the library of the National Institute on Disability, Independent Living, and Rehabilitation Research (NIDILRR). Visit the website to search for articles and guides on independent living, technology and more from research projects funded by NIDILRR.

Office of Disability Employment Policy (ODEP)
www.dol.gov/odep

This federal agency of the Department of Labor works to improve employment opportunities for people with disabilities. Its website provides information on relevant laws and many other resources.

Your local library

Your public library may offer helpful books related to arthritis, as well as online access to information from around the world. Ask a librarian about the best way to search for the information you need — for example, the latest update on clinical trials or product reviews before you purchase equipment.

Index

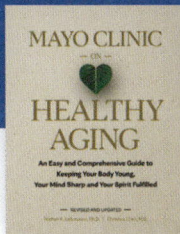

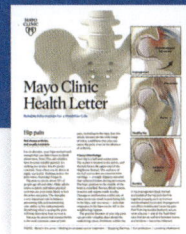

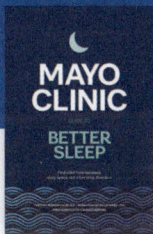

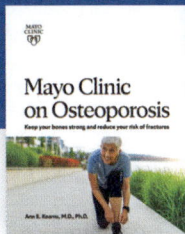

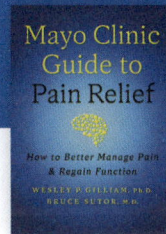

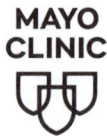

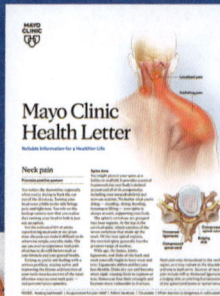

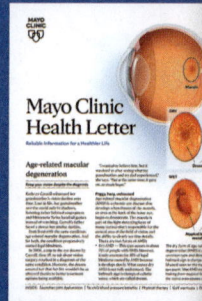

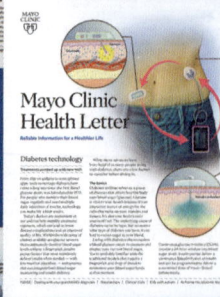

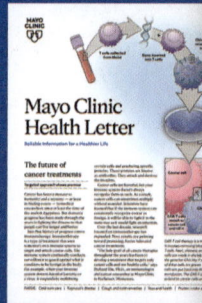

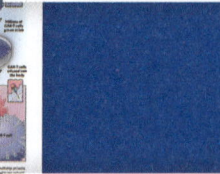

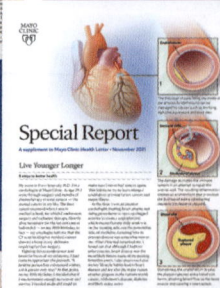

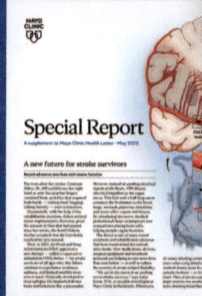